Advances in Neurosurgery 21

R. Lorenz, M. Klinger, M. Brock (Eds.)

Intracerebral Hemorrhage

Hydrocephalus malresorptivus

Peripheral Nerves

With 120 Figures

Springer-Verlag
Berlin Heidelberg New York London Paris
Tokyo Hong Kong Barcelona Budapest

Proceedings of the 43th Annual Meeting
of the Deutsche Gesellschaft für Neurochirurgie
Frankfurt/Main, May 10-13, 1992

Dr. Dr. h.c. Rüdiger Lorenz
Neurochirurgische Universitätsklinik
Schleusenweg 2-16, W-6000 Frankfurt/M., FRG

Prof. Dr. Margareta Klinger
Neurochirurgische Klinik der Universitätsklinik Erlangen-Nürnberg
Schwabachanlage 6, (Kopfklinikum), W-8520 Erlangen, FRG

Prof. Dr. Dr. h.c. Mario Brock
Neurochirurgische Klinik und Poliklinik
Universitätsklinikum Steglitz, Freie Universität Berlin
Hindenburgdamm 30, W-1000 Berlin 45, FRG

ISBN 3-540-56304-0 Springer-Verlag Berlin Heidelberg New York
ISBN 0-387-56304-0 Springer-Verlag New York Berlin Heidelberg

Typesetting: M. Masson-Scheurer, Kirkel

25/3130 - 5 4 3 2 1 0 – Printed on acid-free paper

Contents

Hydrocephalus malresorptivus

List of Contributors

You will find the addresses at the beginning of the respective contribution

Introduction

R. Lorenz[1]

This, the 21st volume of *Advances in Neurosurgery*, contains a selection of papers presented at the 43rd annual congress of the Deutsche Gesellschaft für Neurochirurgie (German Society of Neurosurgery), held in Frankfurt am Main, Germany, from 10 to 13 May 1992.

This annual meeting had five scientific themes. The opening cycle of lectures concerned structural questions and problems in and around neurosurgery, and articles will be published in the *Zentralblatt für Neurochirurgie,* no. 4 (1992). The neuroscientific themes – spontaneous intracerebral hematomas, hydrocephalus malresorptivus, problems of neurosurgical intensive care, and peripheral nerves – are represented in this book. It contains 60 contributions selected from a total of 107 papers, 50 posters, and 12 morning seminars given at the congress.

Neurosurgery started in Frankfurt am Main in 1934. The young doctor Traugott Riechert, some decades later to become well known because of his work on functional stereotactic neurosurgery, finished his medical studies in 1931, became a doctor of medicine in 1932, and worked for 2 years in an ophthalmology center, before coming to Frankfurt as an assistant at the neurological clinic in order to establish neurosurgery at the medical faculty of the Johann Wolfgang Goethe University of Frankfurt, nowadays (since 1967) in the state of Hesse. His chief was the neurologist Prof. Dr. Karl Kleist. With the support of Kleist Traugott Riechert started training with the neurosurgeon Wilhelm Tönnis on 1st September 1936 in Würzburg and later with the radiologist W. Löhr in Magdeburg. On 1st October 1936 he started "Operative Neurology" in the building of the Neurological Clinic and served additionally as a (neuro-)radiologist. From 1st September 1939 onwards the "neurosurgical department" was housed in the clinic of surgery. By this time, Riechert could report on 212 brain operations, 32 operations on the spinal cord, 1070 encephalographies, and 223 carotid angiographies.

In 1980, Traugott Riechert was awarded an honorary degree in medicine for his fundamental work in neurosurgery by the Medical Faculty of the Johann Wolfgang Goethe University of Frankfurt am Main.

After the turmoil of World War II, the Department of Neurosurgery did not have a chairman until 1951. At this time two departments were established, one in the clinic for surgery, headed by Bertold Hübner, and one headed by Hugo Ruf as part of the neurological clinic. Hübner, was a pupil of Gerhard Okonek in Göt-

[1] Neurochirurgische Universitätsklinik, Schleusenweg 2–16, W-6000 Frankfurt, FRG.

Advances in Neurosurgery, Vol. 21
R. Lorenz, M. Klinger, M. Brock (Eds.)

tingen, was hired by the surgeon R. Geissendörfer, and Ruf, a pupil of Riechert in Freiburg, brought in by the neurologist Jürg Zutt.

In 1965, Hugo Ruf got a completely new, extensive clinic for neurosurgery with 135 beds and many facilities for basic research and special neurosurgical – stereotactic and functional – work. It was the largest clinic in Europe, situated in the neighbourhood of the neurological clinic and the orthopedic institute in Niederrad, and near to the other clinics of the medical faculty to the west.

In 1968–1970 the universities all over West Germany were changed and restructured. The department of neurosurgery at the clinic of surgery was closed. Bertold Hübner went to head the department of neurosurgery-neurotraumatology in the Berufsgenossenschaftliche Unfallklinik Frankfurt (Employee's Liability Insurance Association Clinic for Traumatology) at the request of Contzen, the successor to the well-known spine-specialist Herbert Junghanns. The neurosurgical clinic took over the department for neurology, headed by P. A. Fischer, the number of beds being reduced to 70 and the research facilities shared. So three departments were formed: the Department of Neurology (P. A. Fischer), the Department of Neurosurgery (H. Ruf), and the Department of Neuroradiology (H. Hacker). As a subdivision of the Department of (General) Neurosurgery, a Department of Functional Neurosurgery was founded, headed by G. Thomalske. After G. Thomalske's retirement in 1990, stereotactic neurosurgery became reintegrated into General Neurosurgery because of the reduced role of functional neurosurgery in favor of drug treatment of most functional illnesses.

Since the retirement of H. Ruf in 1979, the Department of Neurosurgery has been chaired by R. Lorenz, a pupil of H. W. Pia in Giessen.

We were all pleased and honored to host the 43rd Annual Meeting of the Deutsche Gesellschaft für Neurochirurgie and to welcome so many neurosurgeons and guests. Especially, we were delighted to receive a large delegation from the Polish Society of Neurosurgery, including its president Prof. J. Bidzinsky from Warsaw and the president elect Prof. J. Wronski of Wroclaw. They have taken an important step in promoting the friendship between the Polish and the German Societies of Neurosurgery as a continuation of efforts on both sides. As special thanks they were accepted by the German Society of Neurosurgery as corresponding members.

On behalf of the organizers, the board of the Deutsche Gesellschaft für Neurochirurgie and the program committee, I would like to thank all who contributed to the success of the 43rd annual meeting, especially the speakers and lecturers. Prof. Margareta Klinger has had the arduous task of selecting the papers to be published here according to the votes of the chairmen of the individual sessions and the program committee. She has done it, as ever, in an excellent and successful way. Most of all, she is to be thanked for the timely appearance of this book.

Intracerebral Hemorrhage

Spontaneous Intracerebral Hematomas: Clinical Appraisal of Surgical and Conservative Treatment

B. L. Imielinski[1] and W. Kloc[1]

Introduction

Spontaneous intracerebral hematomas (ICH) present a major problem with a high mortality rate and a significant functional impairment in survivors. The pathogenesis of hemorrhage is heterogeneous and complex, but whether hypertensive or of other origin, it constitutes a devastating cause of neurological damage [5, 6]. Surgical treatment of spontaneous ICH is still a matter of controversy. Since the report of Cushing [2] in 1903 on a surgically treated case of hypertensive ICH, many other reports have been published [1–5, 7, 8, 13].

Clinical Materials and Methods

Over a period of 7 years (1984–1990) 145 patients with spontaneous ICH were treated in the Department of Neurosurgery at the Medical School of Gdańsk. Bleedings caused by trauma, neoplasms, and blood dyscrasias were excluded. Angiography was restricted to patients with lobar localization suggestive of aneurysms and was performed in 67 patients (46.2%): in 48 hypertensives and in 19 patients with undetermined etiology. Of the total number of 145, hypertensive etiology was established in 109 patients (75.2%), while in 36 (24.8%) the cause of bleeding remained undetermined. There was a distinct prevalence of males and only a slight preponderance of the left-side localization (Table 1).

The mean age was 51 years (55 for hypertensives and 38 for unclassified patients) with the peak within the fifth to seventh decades of life. Arterial hypertension proved to be a frequent finding within the limits of the same decades. The youngest hypertensive patient was a female of 24 and the oldest one – also a female – was 78 years of age. The majority of patients (75.8%) were submitted to surgery (Table 2), and in 40.9% of them (45/110) the localization of hematoma was lobar. Complete evacuation was never attempted, tough parts of the clot were left behind. Among the patients treated conservatively, half the hematomas (18/35) were located in the basal ganglia. The total mortality (Table 3) reached 40.9% and was higher in patients who were operated on (49.1%) than in those treated

[1] Department of Neurosurgery, Medical School Gdańsk, ul. Dębinki 7, 80–211 Gdańsk, Poland.

Advances in Neurosurgery, Vol. 21
R. Lorenz, M. Klinger, M. Brock (Eds.)

Table 1. Analysis of etiology, sex, and localization

Etiology	Sex				Localization										Total	
	Males		Females		L		R		Lobar		Basal ganglia		Posterior fossa			
	(n)	(%)	(n)	(%)	(n)	(%)	(n)	(%)	(n)	(%)	(n)	(%)	(n)	(%)	(n)	(%)
Hypertensive	63		46		59		50		38	34.9	65	59.6	6	5.5	109	75.2
Unknown	31		5		20		16		23	63.9	10	27.8	3	8.3	36	24.8
Total	94	64.8	51	35.2	79	54	66	45	61	42.1	75	51.7	9	6.2	145	100

Table 2. Relation of alertness on admission to mortality

Glasgow Coma Score	Surgery		Conservative treatment		Total		Mortality				Total	
							Surgery		Conservative treatment			
	(*n*)	(%)	(*n*)	(%)	(*n*)	(%)	(*n*)	(%)	(*n*)	(%)	(*n*)	(%)
4–9	61		8		69		43	70	2	25	45	65
10–15	49		27		79		11	22	2	7	13	17
Total	110	75.8	35	24.2	145	100	54	49.1	4	11.4	58	40

medically (11.4%), and in hypertensive patients (53/109, 48.6%) when compared with unclassified patients (5/36, 13.9%).

The consciousness level appears to be an important factor in determining risks: patients with a lower level had a worse prognosis than alert ones.

Another important agent proved to be age: below 60 years of age mortality was 37/110 (33.6%), while above this limit it was 21/35 (60%). For the hypertensive group it reached 32/76 (42.1%) and 21/33 (63.6%), respectively.

Computed tomographic (CT) scan, being the safest, fastest, and most accurate diagnostic method, also provided important data to calculate the volume of the hematoma. This was done by the use of "the best-fit method" [9].

Table 3. Analysis of mortality depending on mass effect and mode of treatment

	Mortality					
	Surgery		Conservative treatment		Total	
	(*n*)	(%)	(*n*)	(%)	(*n*)	(%)
Volume of hematoma						
< 50 cm^3	15/48	31.3	2/27	7.4	17/75	22.7
> 50 cm^3	39/62	63.4	2/8	25	41/70	58.6
Medial shift						
No shift	10/32	31.2	0/19	0	10/51	19.6
Up to 10 mm	29/53	54.75	4/15	26.6	33/68	48.5
Over 10 mm	15/25	60	0/1	0	15/26	57.6
Basal cistern obliteration						
No obliteration	7/26	26.9	0/23	0	7/49	14.2
Slight obliteration	17/39	43.5	2/9	22.2	19/48	39.5
Complete obliteration	30/45	66.6	2/3	66.6	32/48	66.6
Total mortality	54/110	49.1	4/35	11.4	58/145	40.9

Table 4. Results of treatment in Glasgow outcome scale (GOS)

GOS	Surgery (*n*)	(%)	Conservative treatment (*n*)	(%)	Total (*n*)	(%)
I	21	19.1	18	51.4	39	26.9
II	27	24.5	12	34.3	39	26.9
III	7	6.4	1	2.9	8	5.5
IV	1	0.9	0	0	1	0.7
V	54	49.1	4	11.4	58	40

In the group of patients with hematoma below 50 ml in volume, mortality was lower than that in patients whose hematoma had a volume above this value. Mass effects were manifested by ventricular collapse and deformity as well as by a midline deviation, which was regarded as a more ominous symptom in proportion to the degree of the shift. Certain prognostic meaning could also be seen in obliteration of the basal cisterns, depending on its intensity. These parameters indicate an increased intracranial pressure (ICP) and consequently an unfavorable prognosis.

The relation of timing of surgery to mortality revealed that among the patients operated within 24 h, mortality reached 64.7% (22/34), in the group operated between the 2nd and 3rd days – 45.5% (15/33), for the group operated between the 4th and 7th days – 46.2% (12/26), and after 8 days – 29.4% (5/17).

Discussion and Conclusions

The distribution of patients according to age, sex, and lateralization does not differ much from that indicated by data from the literature [2, 7, 10–12, 14, 15]. The attributable risk of hypertension for ICH indicates a high proportion of hypertensive patients in this series and in the literature [5, 10, 12–14]. Hypertension accounts for about 50%–75% of ICH and is known as the most common risk factor. In the cases where hypertension is not the likely cause and in the lobar localization angiography is necessary to exclude vascular malformation or a tumor [12].

Advancing age not only correlated positively with an increasing incidence of hemorrhage [5], but it also influenced the results of treatment, including mortality [1, 7]. The consciousness level in ICH varied extremely but was important in determining risk [3, 11, 14]. It was the best guide to prognosis. The mass effect must be defined as an active process which incorporates the failure of a compensatory mechanism to maintain functional and organic equilibrium [3, 4]. The dislocation of the ventricular system and medial shift bear a significant relationship to the outcome [3]. Certain prognostic value can also be found in the obliteration of the basal cisterns. These CT parameters should influence the decision towards surgery [3].

To sum up, the survival rate and the quality of survival are higher when the patients are preoperatively alert or somnolent, under 60 years of age [1, 7], and the hematoma is of a volume below 50 ml [1, 3, 4, 9, 10]. When the patients develop signs of increasing neurological deficit in spite of medical therapy, surgical removal of the clot is indicated [4, 7, 12]. Cerebellar hemorrhage causing a life-threatening syndrome requires prompt surgical treatment, even in a deep coma [8, 10, 15]. Opinions regarding timing of operation are not uniform. Some authors advocate delaying operation by 48–72 h after the ictus [2, 14]. Mortality in groups of patients who have been operated on nevertheless remains high, and many survivors are disabled even after prompt surgical evacuation [6, 7, 10, 12]. It seems that the optimal time for operation should be chosen depending on the clinical condition.

Evaluation of surgical versus conservative treatment is widely debated in the literature [14], and most neurosurgeons agree that the operation should be carried out, at least in selected cases [3, 6–8, 14]. However, it would be a difficult task to elaborate uniform criteria or standard rules to indicate whether conservative or surgical treatment is preferable. The patients who benefit most from surgical removal are those with subcortical hematoma [10, 12], especially of hypertensive etiology [2, 7, 12, 14]. On the other hand, at least part of this subgroup can be treated medically [15] and will make a good recovery without surgery [14]. If the patient is developing an increasing neurological deficit, surgical removal is indicated [14]. But in a thalamocapsular type of hematoma, in which increased ICP is absent, no significant differences in outcome between medical and surgical treatment were noted [7, 11, 12]. One should also take into account the damage done by surgery, depending on the localization and accessibility of the hematoma [3].

The comparison of late results in surgically and conservatively treated groups does not reveal clear differences [7]: or, as in this series, morbidity and mortality are higher in the former group. One should not forget, however, that patients in the surgical group were generally in a worse condition and had a larger hematoma than those treated conservatively. Because of that, any attempt to compare will be not free from bias, taking into consideration the specific selection of patients referred for surgery [3, 16].

It seems that formulation of clear-cut indications for surgery is not possible. Our opinion is consistent with the views of Benaim [2] and partly with those of Ronsohoff et al. [14]. Surgery should be considered in the case of:

1. Progressive neurological deficit
2. Functional impairment persisting longer than 1 week
3. Development of intracranial hypertension.

Surgery is not indicated in the case of:

1. Absence or regression of neurological deficit
2. Deep coma
3. Vegetative disorders

On the basis of CT scan information, surgery should be considered when the hematoma is characterized by:

1. Large volume
2. Superficial localization
3. Increasing size
4. Mass effects

On the contrary, surgery is not indicated in the case of:

1. Small volume
2. Absence of mass effect
3. Deep localization

Keeping in mind the two fundamental aims of saving life and preservering function, the surgeon must make a correct decision on whom and when to operate.

References

1. Auer LM, Deinsberger W, Niederkorn K, Geli G, Kleinert R, Schneider G, Holzer P, Bone G, Mokry M, Koerner E, Kleinert G, Hanusch S (1989) Endoscopic surgery versus medical treatment for spontaneous intracerebral hematoma: a randomized study. J Neurosurg 70:530–535
2. Benaim J (1983) Hypertensive intracerebral hemorrhage in South America. Progress in surgical treatment. In: Mizukami M, Kogure K, Kanaya H, Yamori Y (eds) Hypertensive intracerebral hemorrhage. Raven, New York, pp 123–145
3. Bolander HG, Kourtopoulos H, Liliequis B, Wittboldt S (1983) Treatment of spontaneous intracerebral hemorrhage. A retrospective analysis of 74 consecutive cases with special reference to computer tomographic data. Acta Neurochir Wien 67:19–28
4. Broderick JP, Brott TG, Tomsick T, Barsen W, Spilker J (1990) Ultra-early evaluation of intracerebral hemorrhage. J Neurosurg 72:195–199
5. Brott T, Thalinger K, Hertzberg V (1986) Hypertension as a risk factor for spontaneous intracerebral hemorrhage. Stroke 17:1078–1083
6. Bullock R, Brock-Utne J, van Dellen J, Blake G (1988) Intracerebral hemorrhage in a primate model: effect on regional cerebral blood flow. Surg Neurol 29:101–107
7. Fujitsu K, Muramoto M, Ikeda Y, Inada Y, Kim I, Kuwabara T (1990) Indications for surgical treatment of putaminal hemorrhage: comparative study based on serial CT and time-course analysis. J Neurosurg 73:518–525
8. Kanaya H, Saiki I, Ohuci T, Kamata K, Endo H, Mizukami M, Kagawa M, Kaneko M, Ito Z (1983) Hypertensive intracerebral hemorrhage in Japan: update on surgical treatment. In: Mizukami M, Kogure K, Yamori Y (eds) Hypertensive intracerebral hemorrhage. Raven, New York, pp 147–163
9. Kloc W, Wasilewski W, Imielinski BL (1992) A trial of evaluation of the ICH treatment results according to their volume calculated on the ground of "the best fit method" (in Polish). Neurol Neurochir Pol Suppl 1:283–288
10. Luessenhop AJ (1983) Hypertensive intracerebral hemorrhage (HIH) in the United States: update on surgical treatment. In: Mizukami M, Kogure K, Kanaya H, Yamori Y (eds) Hypertensive intracerebral hemorrhage. Raven, New York, pp 123–131
11. Ojemann RG (1983) Spontaneous brain hemorrhage: what treatment should we recommend? Stroke 14:467
12. Ojemann RG, Heros RC (1983) Spontaneous brain hemorrhage. Stroke 14:468–474
13. Omae T, Ueda K, Ogata J, Yamaguchi T (1989) Parenchymatous hemorrhage: etiology, pathology and clinical aspects. In: Vinken PJ, Bruyn GW, Klawans HL, Toole JF (eds) Vascular disease. Elsevier, (Handbook of clinical neurology, part 2) Amsterdam, pp 287–331

14. Ronsohoff J, Derby B, Kricheff I (1971) Spontaneous intracerebral hemorrhage. Clin Neurosurg 18:247–266
15. Yoshida Y, Shinkai H, Ooneda G (1983) Morphogenesis of microaneurysms and plasmatic arterionecrosis in hypertensive cerebral hemorrhage. In: Mizukami M, Kogure K, Kanaya H, Yamori Y (eds) Hypertensive intracerebral hemorrhage. Raven, New York, pp 181–190
16. Zierski J (1980) Hematoma in hemispheric lobes. In: Pia HW, Langmaid C, Zierski J (eds) Spontaneous intracerebral hematomas. Springer, Berlin Heidelberg New York, pp 135–140

Prognostic Factors and Surgical Indications in Spontaneous Lobar and Putaminal Hematomas

A. Krone[1], M. Glaser[1], D. Pfeuffer-Hess[1], U. Bogdahn[2], I. Haubitz[3], and E. Hofmann[4]

Introduction

Since McKissock et al. published their historical study in 1961 [9] which showed no benefit from surgical treatment, the role of surgery in the treatment of spontaneous intracerebral hematomas has remained a matter of debate. After the introduction of computed tomography (CT) still no generally recognized criteria for a surgical indication are available despite several recent studies [1, 4, 5, 7, 10]. Facing the ethical problems of a prospective randomized trial the following questions were investigated by a retrospective clinical study: What is the impact of clinical and radiological factors on patients' outcome? Are there subgroups defined by these prognostic parameters which are significantly different after conservative or surgical treatment?

Patients and Methods

The files, questionnaires to the general practitioner, and CT data on all 152 patients with lobar and putaminal hematomas who were admitted to the Departments of Neurology and Neurosurgery, University of Würzburg, between January 1982 and July 1990 were analyzed retrospectively. The follow-up time was 1 year. The hematoma volume was calculated as the sum of the clot volume in each CT slice by multiplying the surface area of the hematoma by the thickness of the slice. The surface area was determined by planimetry of the hyperdense hematoma area (Evaluskop; Siemens, Erlangen, FRG). In all surgical cases conventional craniotomy and transcortical evacuation was performed. Hematomas due to vascular malformations, trauma, tumors, and plasmatic coagulation disorders were excluded. The activity of daily living (ADL) classification [6] was used to grade the outcome.

---

[1] Neurochirurgische Klinik und Poliklinik, Universität Würzburg, Josef-Schneider-Straße 11, W-8700 Würzburg, FRG.
[2] Neurologische Klinik und Poliklinik Universität Würzburg, Josef-Schneider-Straße 11, W-8700 Würzburg, FRG.
[3] Rechenzentrum, Universität Würzburg, Am Hubland, W-8700 Würzburg, FRG.
[4] Abteilung für Neuroradiologie, Universität Würzburg, Josef-Schneider-Straße 11, W-8700 Würzburg, FRG.

Advances in Neurosurgery, Vol. 21
R. Lorenz, M. Klinger, M. Brock (Eds.)

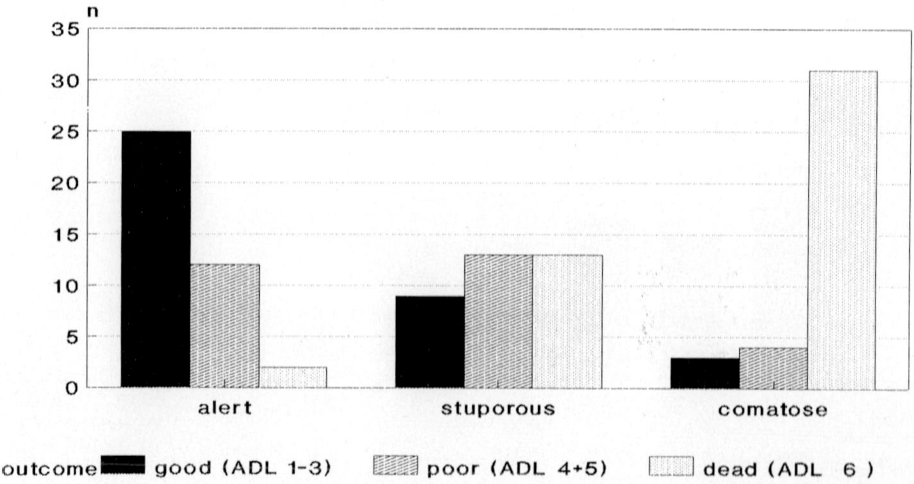

Fig. 1. Prognostic value of the level of consciousness in 112 conservatively treated patients with lobar and putaminal hematomas

Results

The mortality rate was 35% for lobar and 45% for putaminal hematomas. In lobar hematomas surgery was performed twice as frequently as in putaminal hemorrhage (37% versus 18%). The level of consciousness proved to be the statistically most significant prognostic factor regarding survival ($p < 0.01$, chi-square test) among clinical parameters. After conservative treatment over 90% of the patients survived if they were alert on admission whereas almost all comatose patients died (Fig. 1).

In stuporous patients the prognosis was uncertain. Among CT parameters the hematoma volume proved to be of highest prognostic significance, followed by intraventricular hemorrhage. A linear correlation between hematoma volume and outcome was found (Fig. 2). To determine the critical hematoma volume the discriminant analysis of Dirschedl was applied. Here a volume of 44 ml was calculated as representing the value which most significantly discriminated between survival and mortality rate by using the chi-square test. When the untreated patients were excluded ($n = 24$) and the data split according to a hematoma size of 44 ml, no benefit from surgery was seen in hematoma volumes of 44 ml or smaller. Patients with hematomas larger than 44 ml survived significantly more frequently ($p < 0.05$, chi-square test) after surgical treatment (Fig. 3). There were more patients with poor results in the surgical group because of the increased number of survivors. The relative number of good results related to all surviving patients was about the same as in the conservative group. Only stuporous and comatose patients with larger hematomas seemed to profit from surgery (Fig. 4). Patients with impaired consciousness and a hematoma size of greater than 44 ml survived in less than 20%, and not a single good outcome was found in this group. Comparable

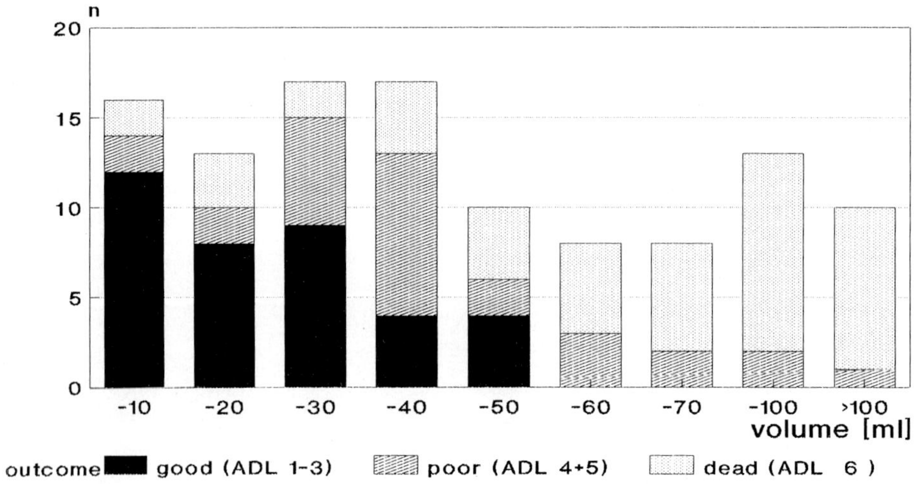

Fig. 2. Correlation of hematoma volume and outcome in the same group as in Fig. 1

surgical patients had a survival rate of over 50%. However, good clinical results (ADL 1–3, independent life) were as rare as 13% within this group.

When the conservative and surgical treatment groups were compared for patients' characteristics, they were found to be well balanced for mean age (55.6 versus 56.4 years), sex (86% versus 82% men), hypertension (64% versus 61%), mean hematoma volume (70.5 versus 69.7 ml), and midline shift over 5 mm (86% versus 79%). There was a tendency to better clinical performance on admission in the

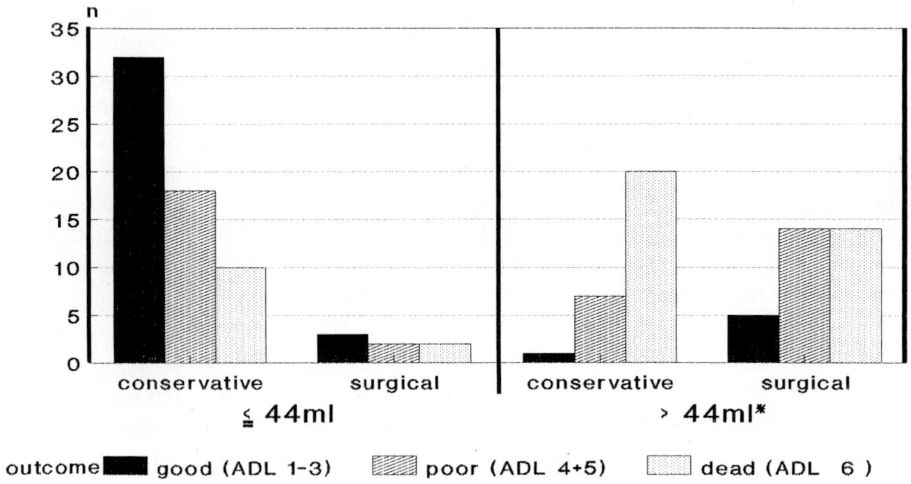

Fig. 3. Treatment results in 128 patients with lobar and putaminal hematomas. *Asterisk*, the survival rate is significantly higher in the surgical group with hematoma volumes over 44 ml ($p < 0.05$, chi-square test)

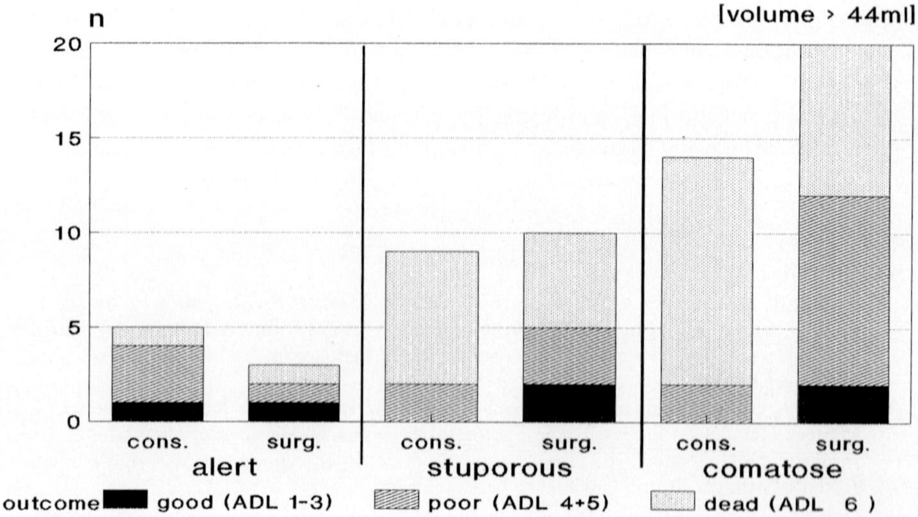

Fig. 4. Treatment results related to the level of consciousness in patients with hematoma volumes over 44 ml

conservative group: 18% versus 9% alert, 50% versus 61% comatose patients. Significant differences ($p < 0.05$) were found for the 1-year survival rate (29% versus 58%) and for the ratio of lobar (32% versus 64%) and putaminal (68% versus 36%) hematoma location. Therefore the results for lobar and putaminal hematomas were evaluated separately in addition.

A critical volume of 50 ml was calculated for lobar and one of 36 ml for putaminal hematomas. Above the critical volume the survival rate for patients with lobar hematomas was significantly higher for surgically than for conservatively treated patients (74% versus 33%; $p < 0.05\%$, Cox test). The small number of operated putaminal hematomas ($n = 15$) did not allow any conclusions regarding surgical indications in this group.

Discussion

Although evacuation of spontaneous intracerebral hematomas is common practice in neurosurgical institutions, uncertainty still exists concerning the criteria for surgical indications. While studies based only on clinical factors showed no benefit from surgery [8, 9], additional CT parameters seem to allow better definition of subgroups who may profit from hematoma evacuation [2–7, 10]. However, most studies suggesting surgery for certain subgroups are criticized for various reasons: lack of control group [7], exceptionally high mortality rate in the conservative group suggesting selection bias [1], and ignorance of hematoma location [10].

The present study confirms that generally available clinical (level of consciousness) and radiological (hematoma location and volume) parameters are statistically powerful prognostic parameters. There was statistical evidence that for subgroups with hematoma volumes above a critical size and impaired consciousness surgery significantly improves the survival rate. Functional results in these patients were mostly poor, but the few good results were found only after surgery. One small prospective [5] and the large cooperative study in Japan [6] support these results.

References

1. Auer LM, Deinsberger W, Niederkorn K, Gell G, Kleinert R, Schneider G, Holzer P, Bone G, Mokry M, Körner E, Kleinert G, Hanusch S (1989) Endoscopic surgery versus medical treatment for spontaneous intracerebral hematoma: a randomized study. J Neurosurg 70:530–535
2. Bogdahn U, Wortmann B, Boenighaus K, Haubitz I, Martin R, Kuhn W, Ratzka M, Mertens HG (1989) Prognostische Faktoren bei spontanen supratentoriellen Blutungen. In: Bogdahn U, Mertens HG (eds) Prognostik in der Intensivtherapie des Zentralnervensystems. Springer, Berlin Heidelberg New York, pp 112–123
3. Helweg-Larsen S, Sommer W, Strange P, Lester J, Boysen G (1984) Prognosis for patients treated conservatively for spontaneous intracerebral hematomas. Stroke 15:1045–1048
4. Hungerbühler JP, Regli F, Van Melle G, Bogousslavsky J (1983) Spontaneous intracerebral haemorrhages (SICHs). Clinical and CT features; immediate evaluation of prognosis. Arch Suis Neurol Neurochir Psychiatr 132:13–27
5. Juvela S, Heiskanen O, Poranen A, Valtonen S, Kuurne T, Kaste M, Troupp H (1989) The treatment of spontaneous intracerebral hemorrhage. A prospective randomized trial of surgical and conservative treatment. J Neurosurg 70:755–758
6. Kanaya H (1990) Results of conservative and surgical treatment in hypertensive intracerebral hemorrhage-cooperative study in Japan. Jpn J Stroke 12:509–524
7. Kaneko M, Tanaka K, Shimada T, Sato K, Uemura K (1983) Long-term evaluation of ultra-early operation for hypertensive intracerebral hemorrhage in 100 cases. J Neurosurg 58:838–842
8. Kanno T, Sano H, Shinomiya Y, Katada K, Nagata J, Hoshino M, Mitsuyama F (1984) Role of surgery in hypertensive intracerebral hematoma. A comparative study of 305 non-surgical and 154 surgical cases. J Neurosurg 61:1091–1099
9. McKissock W, Richardson A, Taylor J (1961) Primary intracerebral hemorrhage. A controlled trial of surgical and conservative treatment in 180 unselected cases. Lancet II: 221–226
10. Volpin L, Cervellini P, Colombo F, Zanusso M, Benedetti A (1984) Spontaneous intracerebral hematomas: a new proposal about the usefulness and limits of surgical treatment. Neurosurgery 15:663–666

Assessment of Prognosis and Indication for Surgery on the Basis of Cluster Analysis in Intracerebral Hematomas

H. G. Höllerhage[1], M. Zumkeller[1], M. Pröschel[1], and H. Dietz[1]

Introduction

Although the surgical evacuation of intracerebral hematomas is rather common, there is still considerable controversy regarding the indications for this treatment [2, 4, 5, 7]. The clinical trial of McKissock et al. [3] more than 30 years ago suggested that conservative treatment is preferable in most cases. Their conclusion was mainly due to the rather poor surgical outcomes of that time and not attributable to particularly successful medical therapy. In the meantime, the diagnosis has been facilitated by the availability of the computed tomographic (CT) scan. This has led to the improvement of the operative treatment owing to the better assessment of size and location of the lesion by CT imaging. Less invasive techniques, such as small craniectomies combined with stereotaxic or ultrasonic retrieval necessitating only minimal cortical incisions, have been developed. It can be assumed that this progress has made the results of this early clinical trial obsolete. However, more recent randomized trials are not available. Therefore we performed a retrospective study to answer the question of when to operate and when to treat conservatively. Like all retrospective trials, our study has the inevitable deficiency that no randomization was performed. To compensate for this, we performed a cluster analysis. This statistical procedure allows for objective grouping of the patients on the basis of clinical data. Thus it is possible to compare the results of conservative and surgical treatment within homogeneous groups of patients.

Clinical Material and Methods

The records of 125 successive patients were reviewed. Of these, 70 had a traumatic and 55 a spontaneous intracerebral hemorrhage. We entered the relevant clinical data, such as age, clinical grade on admission, location, and size of the lesion, presence of a midline shift, pupil reaction, type of treatment, and final outcome, into a database for further statistical analysis.

[1] Neurochirurgische Klinik, Medizinische Hochschule Hannover,
Konstanty-Gutschow-Straße 8, W-3000 Hannover 61, FRG.

Advances in Neurosurgery, Vol. 21
R. Lorenz, M. Klinger, M. Brock (Eds.)

Statistical Procedures

A statistical package developed at the University of Linz (Austria) (ALMO Statistik-System, Prof. Dr. Kurt Holm, University of Linz, Austria) was used. This includes a software implementation of a generalized linear model [1] as well as the procedure of cluster analysis. Using the generalized linear model we performed a stepwise multiple regression with the final outcome as target variable (criterion) and the other clinical data as predictors. This allows for the identification of relevant clinical data which significantly influence the outcome. In a further step of our study the cluster analysis was performed. By this procedure the patients are grouped into clusters on the basis of their similarity. There are many algorithms to calculate similarity and no incontestable standard has been established. We used the implemented standard procedure of the above-mentioned package without changing the algorithm by special options. This warrants the highest possible objectivity of the analysis. All clinical data except the outcome and the type of treatment formed the basis of clustering. The program allows the user to decide into how many clusters the original group should be divided. However, the resulting size of each cluster depends on the degree of similarity within the cluster, so that the program cannot be forced to generate, for example, six subgroups of the same size. We subsequently divided the original groups of spontaneous and traumatic intracerebral hematomas unless the number of patients in the smallest cluster fell short of six. Within all clusters, a comparison of the results of surgical and conservative treatment was performed by calculating the biserial tau coefficient.

Results

Tables 1 and 2 specify the relevant prognostic factors of spontaneous intracerebral and traumatic hematomas. The effect parameter is a quantification of the strength of the influence of the respective factor in the multivariate model. Interestingly both for spontaneous and traumatic intracerebral bleedings, the surgical treatment has a significant beneficial effect.

Tables 3 and 4 show the results of the cluster analysis. The group of spontaneous intracerebral hematomas could be divided into four subgroups, the group of traumatic intracerebral hematomas into three subgroups. Further subdivision of the original groups led to clusters of fewer than six patients. The tables show the number of patients and the assessment of the value of surgery within each of the groups. In the group of spontaneous intracerebral hematomas, a subgroup of 24 hematomas could be identified in which surgery had a highly significant beneficial effect. Interestingly, although the location was only one of the seven variables upon which the clustering was based, this subgroup represents all lobar hematomas. Further analysis of this cluster revealed an average patient age of 44 years, an average lesion size of 27 ml, an average Glasgow Coma Score (GCS) of 10 and an average midline shift of 3 mm. Within the group of traumatic hematomas, the assessment of the value of surgery by calculating the biserial tau

Table 1. Factors influencing the prognosis of spontaneous intracerebral hematomas identified by a stepwise multivariate regression analysis with the outcome as target variable (quantified as GCS)

Factor	Effect	
GCS below 8	– 0.51	*
Volume above 17 ml	– 0.35	*
Midline shift	– 0.32	
Pathological pupils	– 0.38	
Surgery	+ 0.39	*

Multiple correlation coefficient $r = 0.73$.
The values are the effects of the analysis of variance with dichotomous prognostic factors. Adverse effects have a *negative sign*, favorable effects a *positive sign*. Significant factors are marked by *asterisks*.

coefficient revealed no significant result in any cluster. There was a tendency in favor of operation except for one cluster. Further analysis of this cluster showed that it contained deep-seated bleedings of the pons and the midbrain. Surgery was done in these cases only when a younger patient was in extremis but proved to be unsuccessful.

Discussion

As a more recent controlled study of the value of surgery is not available and not even underway, retrospective studies have to do. The main deficiency of such studies is that they do not control for patient selection and are therefore inherently biased. We tried to overcome this by using a multivariate approach which correlates not only surgery versus conservative treatment, but takes variables which

Table 2. Factors influencing the outcome of traumatic intracerebral hematomas

Factor	Effect	
Age above 50	– 0.93	*
GCS below 8	– 0.34	*
Shift	– 0.3	
Pathological pupils	– 0.35	*
Surgery	+ 0.57	*

Multiple correlation coefficient $r = 0.66$.
The interpretation of values and signs is analogous to Table 1.

Table 3. Number of patients within each cluster after division of spontaneous bleedings into four clusters

Patients (n)		Surgery	Significance
1.	12	+	(*)
2.	8	+	(*)
3.	24	+	**
4.	11	+	(*)

The sign in the column "Surgery" indicates whether the effect of surgery was favorable (+) or adverse (–). * $p < 0.05$; ** $p < 0.01$; trend.

usually influence the selection into one or the other treatment group into account. The second step was a cluster analysis which divides the patients into more or less homogeneous subgroups according to their clinical and radiological data on admission. The multivariate analysis shows a significant beneficial effect of surgery for both spontaneous and traumatic hematomas. In a similar analysis by Portenoy et al. [6], these authors could not establish surgery as an independent prognostic factor. However, they do not give the exact number and the exact level of significance so that evaluation of their results is difficult. The cluster analysis shows a tendency in favor of surgery in nearly all subgroups except for deep-seated traumatic pontine and mesencephalic hematomas. We could show that the group of lobar hematomas presents a rather homogeneous entity in which surgery has a highly significant beneficial effect.

We conclude from our results that, as long as controlled trials are not available, surgery should be done in doubtful cases to be on the safe side. Such cases may be, for example, large hematomas of the basal ganglia, whereas in lobar hematomas we could prove a clear indication for surgery. This result is so clear that challenging it by a randomized trial may be ethically problematic. Probably only one clear contraindication for surgery exists: that is deep-seated traumatic pontine and mesencephalic hematomas. The well-established opinion that desolate cases are no candidates for surgery is not affected by this study.

Table 4. Number of patients within each cluster after division of traumatic bleedings into three clusters

Patients (n)		Surgery	Significance
1.	6	–	(*)
2.	13	+	(*)
3.	51	+	(*)

The numbers and signs are analogous to Table 3.

References

1. Holm K (1979) Das allgemeine lineare Modell. In: Holm K (ed) Die Befragung, vol 6. UTB Francke, Munich, pp 11–213
2. Masdeu JC, Rubino FA (1984) Management of lobar intracerebral hemorrhage: medical or surgical. Neurology (NY) 34:381–383
3. McKissock W, Richardson A, Taylor J (1961) Primary intracerebral haemorrhage. A controlled trial of surgical and conservative treatment in 180 unselected cases. Lancet 2:221–226
4. Nath FP, Nicholls D, Fraser RJA (1983) Prognosis in intracerebral haemorrhage. Acta Neurochir (Wien) 67:29–35
5. Paillas JE, Alliez B (1973) Surgical treatment of spontaneous intracerebral hemorrhage. J Neurosurg 39:145–151
6. Portenoy RK, Lipton RB, Berger AR, Lesser ML, Lantos G (1987) Intracerebral haemorrhage: a model for the prediction of outcome. J Neurol Neurosurg Psychiatry 50:976–979
7. Zuccarello M, Andrioli G, Trincia G, Pardatscher K (1983) Spontaneous intracerebral hematomas. Aspects of treatment. Zentralbl Neurochir 44:209–213

Intracerebral Hemorrhage. A Clinical Presentation of Dural Arteriovenous Fistulas of the Anterior Cranial Fossa: Diagnosis and Microneurosurgical Treatment

B. Huffmann[1], A. Harders[1], L. Mayfrank[1], G. Laborde[1], J. M. Gilsbach[1], and J. Reul[2]

Introduction

Approximately 10%–15% of intracranial arteriovenous malformations originate from arteries that supply the dura mater [13, 27]. Mostly they drain into the transverse, sigmoid, or cavernous sinuses. Patients often have benign symptomatology with headache or pulsatile tinnitus [2]. About 50 cases of dural arteriovenous fistulas (DAVFs) involving the base of the anterior cranial fossa which have been published so far seem to form a distinct subgroup with an unusually high incidence of intracranial hemorrhage [1, 7, 8, 10, 12, 14–19, 22, 28, 31–35, 37, 40, 41]. We report on eight further patients.

Patients and Methods

The clinical, radiological, and surgical features of eight patients with DAVFs of the anterior cranial fossa treated in our department since 1988 are summarized in Table 1. All patients underwent plain computed tomographic (CT) scanning and selective bilateral angiography of the internal and external carotid arteries. In three patients, enhanced CT scans and in four patients transcranial Doppler sonographies (TCDs) were performed. Surgical elimination of the DAVFs was carried out in four patients. Intraoperative Doppler studies confirmed complete fistula obliteration in all four cases. Postoperative angiography was not performed.

Results

All patients were male, ranging in age from 23 to 79 years, with a mean age of 56 years. Three patients presented with an acute intracerebral hemorrhage (ICH). Two of them showed the classic clinical presentation of a frontal lobe hematoma. The third one was found to have a parietal ICH quite a distance from the frontal DAVF.

---

[1] Neurochirurgische Klinik, Klinikum der RWTH Aachen, Pauwelsstraße 30, W-5100 Aachen, FRG.
[2] Klinik für Radiologische Diagnostik, Klinikum der RWTH Aachen, Pauwelsstraße 30, W- 5100 Aachen, FRG.

Advances in Neurosurgery, Vol. 21
R. Lorenz, M. Klinger, M. Brock (Eds.)

Table 1. Clinical and radiographic features of eight patients with anterior fossa DAVFs

Patient no.	Age	Sex	History	Presentation	Contrast CT	TCD (velocity)	AS	VD	AD	Treatment	Outcome
1	23	m	–	ICH, seizure	Not performed	Not performed	AEA	BVR	–	Spontaneous obliteration	No new symptoms
2	35	m	Repeated seizures, trauma	Headache, seizure	Enhancement	Increased	AEA (bilateral) MMA	SSS BVR	–	Surgery	Unilateral anosmia
3	55	m	Repeated cerebral hemorrhages	Acute parietal hemorrhage	Not performed	Not performed	AEA (bilateral)	SSS BVR	–	Surgery	No new symptoms
4	56	m	–	Stroke	Not performed	Increased	AEA	SSS	–	–	
5	65	m	ICH years ago, headache, trauma	Seizure	Enhancement	Not performed	AEA (bilateral) IMA MMA	SSS	Yes	Surgery	No new symptoms
6	66	m	Headache for months	Headache	Not performed	Increased	AEA	SSS	–	Surgery	No new symptoms
7	72	m	–	ICH, obtundation	Not performed	Not performed	ACA	SSS	Yes	–	
8	79	m	Headache for months	Headache	Enhancement	Increased	AEA (bilateral) IMA	BVR SSS	–	–	

DAVFs, Dural arteriovenous fistulas; CT, computed tomography; TCD, transcranial Doppler sonography performed in the anterior segment of the circle of Willis; AS, arterial supply; VD, venous drainage; AD, aneurysmatic dilatation; m, male; ICH, intracerebral hemorrhage; AEA, anterior ethmoidal artery; MMA, middle meningeal artery; IMA, internal maxillary artery; SSS, superior sagittal sinus; BVR, basal vein of Rosenthal.

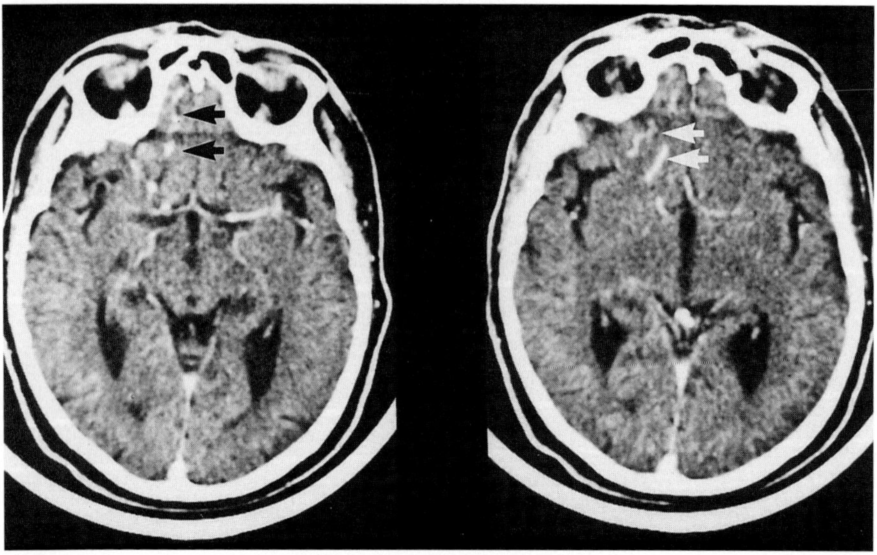

Fig. 1. Two successive contrast CT scans show frontobasal enhanced areas (*arrows*), coinciding with a dilated tortus draining vein

In the other patients, neurological and radiographic examinations were performed because of generalized seizures (two patients), nonspecific headaches (two patients), and a basal ganglia stroke (one patient). In the latter patient, the frontal DAVF was an incidental finding not related to the stroke. One patient with a generalized seizure was found to have a frontobasal hypodense lesion on CT consistent with a former hemorrhage.

On contrast CT scan, small frontobasal enhanced areas, suggestive of vascular structures, were seen in three cases without an acute ICH (Fig. 1). Selective angiography proved that the enhancement coincided with dilated draining veins.

Four patients investigated by TCD displayed increased flow velocities in the anterior segment of the circle of Willis.

In all cases the angiogram demonstrated the DAVF located on the cribriform plate in the region of the foramen caecum along the base of the anterior cranial fossa (Fig. 2). In seven patients, the main feeding arteries were unilaterally or bilaterally enlarged ethmoidal branches of the ophthalmic artery. The internal maxillary artery participated with additional feeders in one case, the middle meningeal artery in another one, and both together in a third. In one patient the primary source of arterial supply was a branch of the anterior cerebral artery.

The draining vessels mostly consisted of superficial cortical or pial veins with drainage into the superior sagittal sinus. Additionally, in four cases, subfrontal veins drained towards the basal vein of Rosenthal, which was in one patient the main venous drainage. The draining vein consisted of a dilated vascular sac in two cases, one near the cribriform plate and one near the superior sagittal sinus. Both patients had a history of ICH.

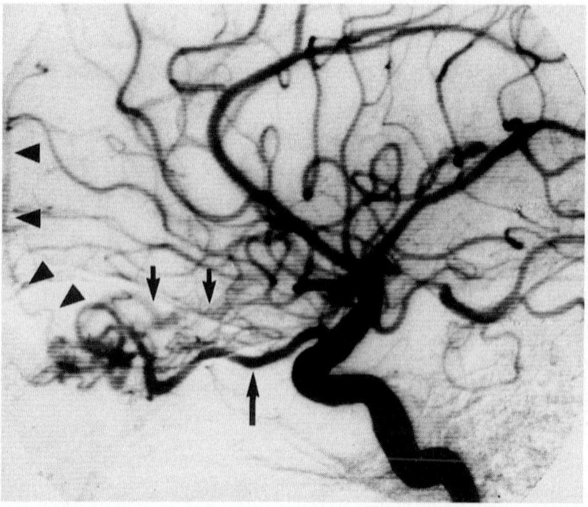

Fig. 2. Left internal carotid angiography demonstrating a DAVF in the anterior cranial fossa. Lateral projection. Ophthalmic artery is large (*large arrow*). Ethmoidal branches are also hypertrophic and feed the dural AVF. A cortical vein (*arrowheads*) drains towards the superior sagittal sinus, a subfrontal vein (*small arrows*) drains via the basal vein of Rosenthal

In one patient the angiography demonstrated additional large arteriovenous malformations involving the parietal and temporal lobe (patient no. 7).

Surgery was carried out in four patients. A 23-year-old patient showed a spontaneous obliteration of the fistula during angiography. Surgical intervention was not considered to be indicated in the patient with multiple arteriovenous malformations. Two patients refused operative treatment.

At surgery we preferred a right-sided high-frontal craniotomy approximately 3 cm before bregma and an interhemispheric approach in front of the genu corporis callosi in order to obtain a good view perpendicular to the floor of the anterior cranial fossa and to the cribriform plate. Intraoperative Doppler sonography revealed in all cases an increased flow velocity in the fistula. Once the fistula was coagulated near the cribriform plate, the dilated pial or cortical vein collapsed. Complete obliteration was proven by Doppler examination. The patients recovered without new deficits from surgery with the exception of the first patient, operated on in 1988, who exhibited a postoperative unilateral anosmia.

Discussion

The mean age at onset of symptoms in our patients was 56 years. This corresponds with the age of patients reported in the literature, as does the strong male predominance [25, 38]. DAVFs can present with a wide clinical spectrum of signs and symptoms depending on their location, size, and venous drainage [3, 21, 24, 39].

Only two of our eight patients presented with a classical frontal ICH. Martin et al. [25] described five out of eight patients with a frontal lobe hematoma and a large venous aneurysm or varix at the venous side of the fistula. Two of our patients also presented with aneurysmatically dilated veins and ICHs. So the presence of long varicose draining veins might increase the risk of an ICH [13, 30]. DAVFs of the anterior cranial fossa can also cause remote hematomas (patient no. 3) [5, 25], perhaps because of elevated venous pressure or venous thrombosis. On the other hand, DAVFs had been found incidentally in two patients suffering from headache and in the patient with cerebral stroke. TCD study as well as contrast CT scan were useful in detecting those lesions although angiography is essential to prove them [6, 9, 26]. The previously reported angiographic findings are quite similar to ours. Frontal DAVFs usually involve the dura in the region of the cribriform plate. Bilateral arteriograms of the carotid arteries should be performed [37] because bilateral ethmoidal arteries can contribute to the arterial supply of DAVFs. Angiography of the external carotid arteries is necessary to demonstrate additional feeders from distal branches of, for instance, the internal maxillary artery and the middle meningeal artery.

As there are no prospective studies regarding the natural history of frontal DAVFs, the real risk of bleeding of such lesions is unknown. However, 60%–80% of reported cases presented with an often massive and life-threatening ICH [25]. Although single cases with spontaneous thrombosis or regression of DAVFs have been observed (patient no. 1) [4, 11, 31, 38], treatment with the aim of exclusion of the DAVF should be performed. At present, surgical elimination of the DAVF is the treatment of choice to prevent further hemorrhages [20]. Endovascular techniques can also decrease or eliminate the arteriovenous shunt. Yet in cases with multiple feeders, interventional techniques are probably less successful than surgery in obliterating all arterial feeders or the fistula itself [38].

At surgery we preferred a high-frontal parasagittal craniotomy to a frontobasal trepanation because the frontal sinuses do not have to be opened using this approach and a straight view of the fistula can be obtained.

In conclusion, DAVFs of the anterior cranial fossa should be included in the differential diagnosis of intracerebral frontal hematomas particularly in elderly men and should be eliminated surgically in order to prevent (re)bleeding events.

References

1. Abumiya T, Kamiyama H, Murata J, Nunomura M, Chono Y, Kobayashi N, Abe H, Saito H, Miyasaka K, Abe S (1987) Dural arteriovenous malformation with uncommon draining veins in the anterior fossa. Case report. Neurol Med Chir (Tokyo) 27:1195–1200
2. Aminoff MJ, Kendall BE (1973) Asymptomatic dural vascular anomalies. Br J Radiol 46:662–667
3. Awad IA, Little JR, Akrawi WP, Ahl J (1990) Intracranial dural arteriovenous malformations: factors predisposing to an aggressive neurological course. J Neurosurg 72:839–850

4. Bitoh S, Sasaki S (1979) Spontaneous cure of dural arteriovenous malformation in the posterior fossa. Surg Neurol 12:111–114
5. Bitoh S, Nakagawa H, Arita N, Fujiwara M (1981) Dural arteriovenous malformation in the anterior fossa. Case report. Neurol Med Chir (Tokyo) 21:131–134
6. Chesna EJ, Naheedy MH, Azar-Kia B (1984) CT demonstration of dural arteriovenous malformation. Comput Radiol 8:49–52
7. Dardenne GJ (1978) Dural arteriovenous anomaly fed by ethmoidal arteries. Surg Neurol 10:384–388
8. Driesen W, Elies W (1972) Über drei Fälle intrakranieller arteriovenöser Mißbildungen mit arterieller Versorgung aus der Arteria ethmoidea anterior. Neurochirurgia (Stuttg) 15:178–181
9. Grady MS, Pobereskin L (1987) Arteriovenous malformations of the dura mater. Surg Neurol 28:135–140
10. Handa J, Shimizu Y (1973) Dural arteriovenous anomaly supplied by anterior falcine artery. Neuroradiology 6:212–214
11. Hansen JH, Søgaard I (1976) Spontaneous regression of an extra- and intracranial arteriovenous malformation. Case report. J Neurosurg 45:338–341
12. Hayashi T, Tokunaga T, Matsuo M (1986) Dural arteriovenous malformation in the anterior fossa with subarachnoid hemorrhage. Kurume Med J 33:187–191
13. Houser OW, Baker HL, Rhoton AL, Okazaki H (1972) Intracranial dural arteriovenous malformations. Neuroradiology 105:55–64
14. Ishimitsu H, Nishimoto K, Harada Y, Miyata I, Matsumi N, Namba S (1986) Dural arteriovenous malformation of the anterior cranial fossa. Case report. Neurol Med Chir 26:822–828
15. Ito J, Imamura H, Kobayashi K, Tsuchida T, Soto S (1983) Dural arteriovenous malformations of the base of the anterior cranial fossa. Neuroradiology 24:149–154
16. Katayama Y, Tsubokawa T, Moriyasu N, Kotani A (1980) Dural arteriovenous malformation in the anterior cranial fossa. Neurol Surg 8:1079–1085
17. Kidooka M, Nakasu S, Nakasu Y, Handa J (1982) Dural arteriovenous malformation in the anterior cranial fossa: report of a case. Nippon Geka Hokan 51:1040–1046
18. Kobayashi H, Hayashi M, Noguchi Y, Tsuji T, Handa Y, Caner HH (1988) Dural arteriovenous malformations in the anterior cranial fossa. Surg Neurol 30:396–401
19. Koga H, Fujii K, Momosaki N, Kishikawa T (1987) Dural arteriovenous malformations in the anterior cranial fossa. Case report. Neurol Med Chir (Tokyo) 27:144–149
20. Kosnitz EJ, Hunt WE, Miller CA (1974) Dural arteriovenous malformations. J Neurosurg 40:322–329
21. Lasjaunias P, Chiu M, Brugge KT, Toua A, Hurth M, Berenstein M (1986) Neurological manifestations of intracranial dural arteriovenous malformations. J Neurosurg 64:724–730
22. Lepoire J, Montaut J, Bouchot M, Laxenaire M (1963) Anévrismes artério-veineux intrafrontaux vascularisés par l'artère ethmoïdale antérieure. A propos de trois observations. Neurochirurgia (Stuttg) 9:159–166
23. Magidson MA, Weinberg PE (1976) Spontaneous closure of a dural arteriovenous malformation. Surg Neurol 6:107–110
24. Malik GM, Pearse JE, Ausman JI, Mehta B (1984) Dural arteriovenous malformations and intracranial hemorrhage. Neurosurgery 15:332–339
25. Martin NA, King WA, Wilson CB, Nutik S, Carter LP, Spetzler RF (1990) Management of dural arteriovenous malformations of the anterior cranial fossa. J Neurosurg 72:692–697
26. Miyasaka K, Tabei H, Nomura M, Sagimoto S, Aida T, Abe H, Tsuru M (1980) Computerized tomography findings in dural arteriovenous malformations. J Neurosurg 53:698–702
27. Newton TH, Cronqvist S (1969) Involvement of dural arteries in intracranial arteriovenous malformations. Radiology 93:1071–1078

28. Notari F, Casasco A, Mani J, Alachkar F, Theron J, Houtteville J, Toumi K (1988) Anterior ethmoidal dural fistulae. 3 new cases. J Radiol 69:663–669
29. Ikada T, Matsuda M, Handa J (1988) Association of cerebral aneurysm and dural arteriovenous malformation in the anterior cranial fossa: a case report. No Shinkei Geka 16:903–906
30. Olutola PS, Eliam M, Molot M (1983) Spontaneous regression of a dural arteriovenous malformation. Neurosurgery 12:687–690
31. Picard L, Bracard S, Moret J, Per A, Giaccobe HL, Roland J (1987) Spontaneous dural arteriovenous fistula. Semin Intervent Radiol 4:219–241
32. Pollock JA, Newton TH (1968) The anterior falx artery: normal and pathologic anatomy. Radiology 91:1089–1095
33. Pradat P, Doyon D, Navarro-Artiles G, Raymond JP (1968) Anévrisme artérioveineux sous-dural de la gouttière olfactive. Neurochirurgia (Stuttg) 14:923–930
34. Tanaka K, Yonekawa Y, Miyake H (1991) Dural arteriovenous malformation in the anterior cranial fossa: report of a case. Surg Neurol 36:221–225
35. Terarda T, Kikuchi H, Karasawa J, Nagata I (1984) Intracerebral arteriovenous malformations fed by the anterior ethmoidal artery: case report. Neurosurgery 14:578–582
36. Tiyaworabun S, Vonofukos P, Lorenz R (1986) Intracerebral arteriovenous malformation fed by both ethmoidal arteries. Surg Neurol 26:375–382
37. Tokunaga T, Hayashi T, Shojimi K, Utsunomigi H, Matsuo M (1986) Dural arteriovenous malformation of the anterior fossa with subarachnoid hemorrhage. No Shinkei Geka 14:1391–1395
38. Van Halbach V, Higashida RT, Hieshima GB, Wilson CB, Barnwell SL, Dowd CF (1990) Dural arteriovenous fistulas supplied by ethmoidal arteries. Neurosurgery 26:816–823
39. Viñuela F, Fox AJ, Pelz DM, Drake CG (1986) Unusual clinical manifestations of dural arteriovenous malformations. J Neurosurg 64:554–558
40. Waga S, Fujimoto K, Morikawa A, Morooka Y, Okada M (1977) Dural arteriovenous malformation in the anterior fossa. Surg Neurol 8:356–358
41. Winter A, Yeager H, Bastidas J (1974) Cerebral vascular hemorrhage. A new surgical approach. Vasc Surg 8:95–106

Monitoring of Jugular Venous Oxygen Saturation in Patients with Intracerebral Hematomas

A. Unterberg[1], A. von Helden[1], G.-H. Schneider[1], and W. L. Lanksch[1]

Introduction

Perioperative treatment of patients with intracerebral hematomas is still a challenge in neurosurgical intensive care medicine. These patients often present with a chronically elevated blood pressure, and it might be surmised that regulation of cerebral blood flow is altered in these patients. Titration of arterial blood pressure is a special problem in these cases since normalization or lowering of blood pressure is essential to prevent rebleeding. As in other acute cerebral lesions, such as severe head injury, monitoring of cerebral blood flow is an unfulfilled request, especially in unconscious patients. Recently, monitoring of jugular venous oxygen saturation enabled at least an estimate of the quality of cerebral blood flow [1–3, 5]. This monitoring is performed by a fiberoptic catheter which is positioned in the jugular venous bulb [2]. Desaturation of cerebrovenous blood indicates an increased cerebral oxygen metabolism or a decreased cerebral blood flow [1, 3–5, 6]. Cerebrovenous oxygen saturation below 55% indicates a critically decreased cerebral blood flow desaturation below 50% definitely indicates cerebral ischemia [1, 3, 6].

In this study, jugular venous oxygen saturation ($SJVO_2$) was monitored in patients who were unconscious due to an intracerebral hematoma. Cerebrovenous oxygen saturation was monitored before, during, and after an operation. Special focus was put on episodes of desaturation, their frequency, and causes. Moreover, it was studied how hypo- and hypercarbia, i.e., hyper- or hypoventilation, affect cerebral oxygenation and whether "cerebral autoregulation" is preserved, i.e., maintenance of oxygen saturation during alterations in arterial blood pressure.

Material and Methods

In 16 patients who were unconscious due to an intracerebral hematoma, $SJVO_2$, intracranial pressure, arterial blood pressure, and cerebral perfusion pressure were continuously monitored. The Glasgow Coma Score of these patients was between 4 and 8, the median was 6. Patients' age was between 36 and 82 years, mean age was 57 years. Cerebrovenous oximetry was performed for 1–9 days (mean duration: 4.2 days).

---

[1] Abteilung für Neurochirurgie, Universitätsklinikum Rudolf Virchow, Freie Universität Berlin, Augustenburger Platz 1, W-1000 Berlin 65, FRG.

Advances in Neurosurgery, Vol. 21
R. Lorenz, M. Klinger, M. Brock (Eds.)

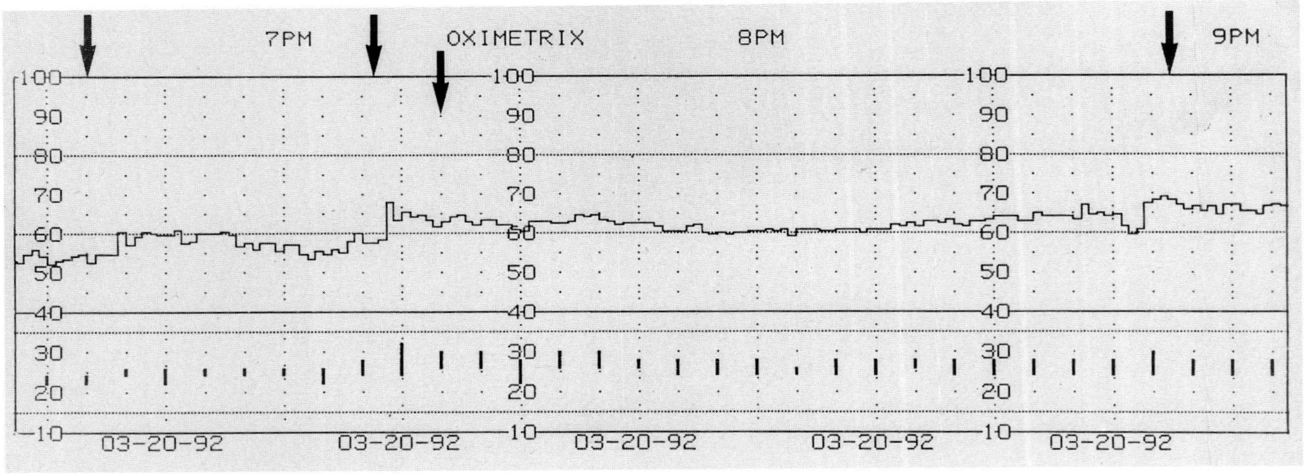

Fig. 1. Continuous tracing of $SJVO_2$ in a patient before and during evacuation of an intracerebral hematoma. Initially $SJVO_2$ was between 50% and 55%. Following trephination, $SJVO_2$ increased slowly into a normal range

Hypo- or hypercarbia were induced by changes in ventilation. Autoregulation was tested by lowering blood pressure with intravenous urapidil.

Results and Discussion

Preoperatively, $SJVO_2$ was between 55% and 50%, indicating a critically reduced cerebral blood flow. Figure 1 depicts an original tracing of $SJVO_2$ before and during evacuation of an intracerebral hematoma. Immediately after trephination, oxygen saturation increases to above 60%. During the following evacuation of the hematoma, oxygen saturation slowly increased further (Fig. 1).

After the operation, oxygen saturation in the jugular bulb was brought into a normal range, i.e., above 55% in all patients. Normal $SJVO_2$ is 69 ± 4% [2, 6]. There were, however, episodes of desaturation in the following course. These are defined as saturation values below 50% for more than 15 min [3]. During these episodes, cerebral blood flow is definitely insufficient. Forty-eight episodes of spontaneous desaturation were observed during 67 days of monitoring in the 16 patients studied. The episodes occurred in all patients. In most instances, an insufficient cerebral perfusion pressure was the cause for such an episode. Figure 2 gives an example where elevation of arterial blood pressure, i.e., increasing cerebral perfusion pressure, normalized $SJVO_2$. Next, hyperventilation was an important reason for these episodes. They were mainly observed during the first 2 days after evacuation of the hematomas.

The effect of hyperventilation (hypocarbia) was studied in eight patients. Arterial PCO_2 was decreased from 35 to 28 mmHg. This maneuver led to a decrease in oxygen saturation, indicating a diminished cerebral blood flow. In six patients,

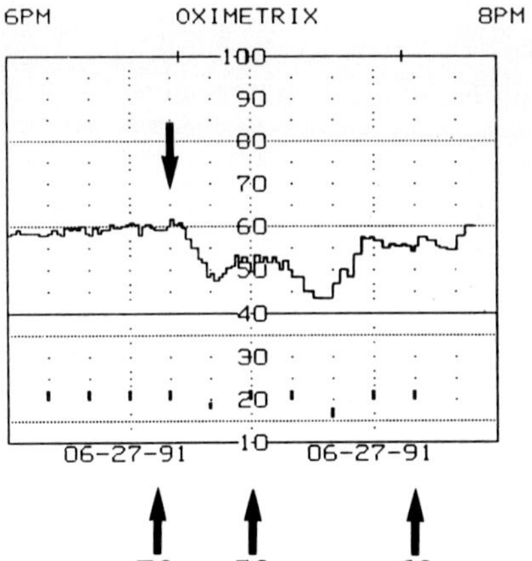

CPP	72	53	68	
MAP	84	68	78	**[mmHg]**
ICP	12	15	10	

Fig. 2. Desaturation episode $SJVO_2$ < 50% for more than 15 min) in a patient following evacuation of an intracerebral hematoma. This episode indicates an insufficient oxygenation of the brain. It was treated by increasing arterial blood pressure

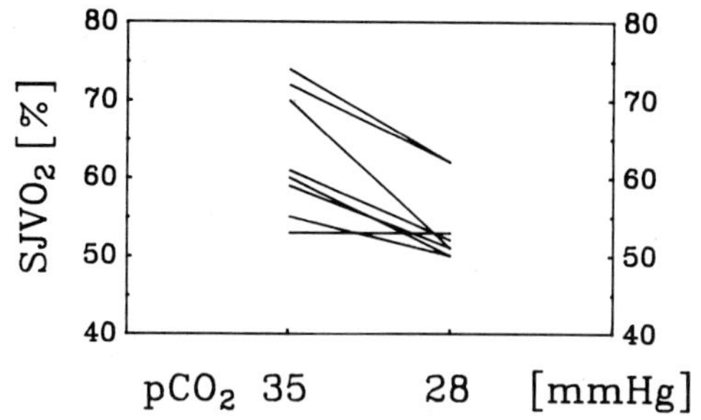

Fig. 3. Effect of moderate hyperventilation (from 35 to 28 mmHg) and $SJVO_2$ in nine patients with intracerebral hematomas. In all patients $SJVO_2$ decreased due to hypocarbia. In some patients moderate hyperventilation even caused a critical reduction in oxygen saturation (< 55%), i.e., cerebral blood flow

oxygen saturation was even critically decreased to 50%–53% (Fig. 3). This is a strong hint that even moderate hyperventilation might be harmful in these patients.

In normal patients with intact cerebral autoregulation, hyper- and hypotension within certain limits (mean arterial blood pressure, MABP, 70–160 mmHg) does not alter cerebral blood flow and thus cerebrovenous oxygen saturation. In nine patients, MABP was decreased from a mean of 100 mmHg to 80 mmHg by i.v. infusion of urapidil. In eight patients, this maneuver caused a decrease of oxygen saturation, in five patients $SJVO_2$ even decreased into the critical range of 50%–55% (see Fig. 4). This demonstrates that autoregulation is disturbed and that a cerebral perfusion pressure of 70 or even 80 mmHg might be too low to maintain a sufficient cerebral perfusion.

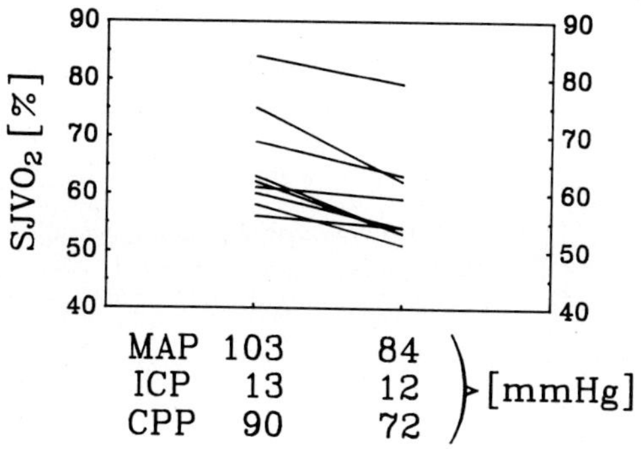

Fig. 4. Effect of a moderately decreased arterial blood pressure (by i.v. infusion of urapidil) on cerebrovenous oxygen saturation. If autoregulation is intact, there is no change in cerebrovenous oxygenation. In patients with intracerebral hematomas, however, $SJVO_2$ fell, in some patients even into the critical range of 50%–55%, though cerebral perfusion pressure was always above 60 mmHg

Summary and Conclusions

Measurement of $SJVO_2$ enables a continuous monitoring of cerebral oxygenation. In unconscious patients with an intracerebral hematoma, cerebral oxygenation is critically diminished before the operation. Evacuation of the hematoma leads to normalization of cerebral oxygenation. In the following course, there are, however, episodes of spontaneous desaturation which can often be prevented or counteracted. An insufficient cerebral perfusion pressure and hypocarbia were the most obvious reasons for these episodes.

Therefore it is advisable to tailor and control hyperventilation. Moreover, it became obvious that arterial normotension is often insufficient to provide a normal cerebral oxygenation.

It is to be hoped that recognition and therapy of episodes of secondary cerebral ischemia will ameliorate the outcome of affected patients.

Acknowledgement. The editorial assistance of Ms. I. Brookes is highly appreciated.

References

1. Andrews PJD, Piper IR, Dearden NM, Miller JD (1990) Secondary insults during intrahospital transport of head-injured patients. Lancet 335:327–330
2. Cruz J, Miner ME, Allen SJ, Alves WM, Gennarelli TA (1990) Continuous monitoring of cerebral oxygenation in acute brain injury: Injection of mannitol during hyperventilation. J Neurosurg 73:725–730
3. Prakash S, Robertson CS, Narayan RK, Grossman RG, Hayes C (1992) Transient jugular venous oxygen desaturation and neurological outcome in patients with severe head-injury. J Neurosurg 76:398A
4. Robertson C, Narayan RK, Gokasean ZL, Pahwa R, Grossman RG, Caram P, Allen E (1989) Cerebral anteriovenous oxygen difference as an estimate of cerebral blood flow in comatose patients. J Neurosurg 70:222–230
5. Unterberg A, Gethmann J, von Helden A, Schneider GH, Lanksch WR (1992) Treatment of cerebral vasospasm with hypervolemia and hypertension. In: Piscol K, Klinger M, Brock M (eds) Advances in neurosurgery, vol 20. Springer, Berlin Heidelberg New York, pp 198–201
6. Unterberg A, von Helden A, Schneider GH, Lanksch WR (1992) Combined monitoring of ICP and cerebrovenous oxygen saturation (CVOS) to estimate cerebral blood flow. In: Avezaat C et al. (eds) ICP IX. Springer, Berlin Heidelberg New York

Lysis of Intraventricular and Intracerebral Hematomas with Tissue Plasminogen Activator

L. Mayfrank[1], B. Lippitz[1], K. Schmieder[1],
G. Laborde[1], A. Harders[1], and J. M. Gilsbach[1]

Introduction

Recent experimental studies [2, 3, 14] as well as clinical investigations [4, 11, 15, 17] have demonstrated the efficacy of intrathecally administered tissue plasminogen activator (rtPA) in lysing subarachnoid hematomas. Encouraged by these results, we performed local fibrinolytic therapy with rtPA in eight patients with severe intraventricular hemorrhage (IVH) and three patients with large intracerebral hematomas.

Patients

Patients with IVH

Patient Population. The clinical characteristics of the eight patients with IVH are summarized in Table 1. All patients were admitted within 24 h of hemorrhage. On admission, the level of consciousness was severely depressed in all of them. In each patient, computed tomographic (CT) scans revealed hemorrhage extending into all ventricular chambers. Seven patients had, additionally, an intracerebral hematoma in the caudate nucleus or thalamus with a mean diameter of 2.6 cm. Pathological ventricular dilatation was found in six cases. Patients with intracranial vascular malformations were not included in this study.

Treatment. Ventricular drainage of one or both lateral ventricles was performed in each patient within 24 h of hemorrhage. Fibrinolytic therapy was started within 24 h of the onset of symptoms in six cases, and in two further cases after 48 h and 5 days, respectively. A total of 2–5 mg rtPA was injected through the ventricular catheter, which was then closed for 45 min and reopened for drainage against a gradient of 0–10 cm. Injection of rtPA was repeated one to six times at intervals of 6–19 h until CT scans demonstrated a substantial reduction of intraventricular blood.

Post-treatment Course. CT obtained daily showed a marked reduction of intraventricular blood and a reduction of ventricular dilatation within 24–48 h of the onset

[1] Neurochirurgische Klinik, Klinikum der RWTH Aachen, Pauwelsstr. 30, W-5100 Aachen, FRG.

Advances in Neurosurgery, Vol. 21
R. Lorenz, M. Klinger, M. Brock (Eds.)

Table 1. Summary of clinical data of eight patients with IVH

Patient no.	Consciousness level				Ventricular dilatation	ICH diameter (cm)	Ventricular drainage (days)	Fibrinolytic therapy with rtPA		
	Age (years)	Sex	Initial (GCS)	After therapy (GCS)				Started[a]	Single doses (mg)	Total dose (mg)
1	78	M	5	12	Yes	1.5	10	< 24 h	3	3
2	50	M	6	12	Yes	2.5	5	< 24 h	2–3	8
3	79	M	12	12	No	2.5	10	5 days	5	15
4	57	F	5	13	Yes	2.5	5	< 24 h	2–3	13
5	59	M	8	13	Yes	3.5	6	< 24 h	3–5	8
6	80	F	12	12	No	3.5	3	< 24 h	5	20
7	63	M	4	5	Yes	2.5	9	48 h	3–5	11
8	60	F	4	12	Yes	None	8	< 24 h	5	15
Mean values			7.0	11.4		2.6	7			11.6

[a] Time from onset of symptoms to first injection of rtPA. ICH intracerebral hematoma.

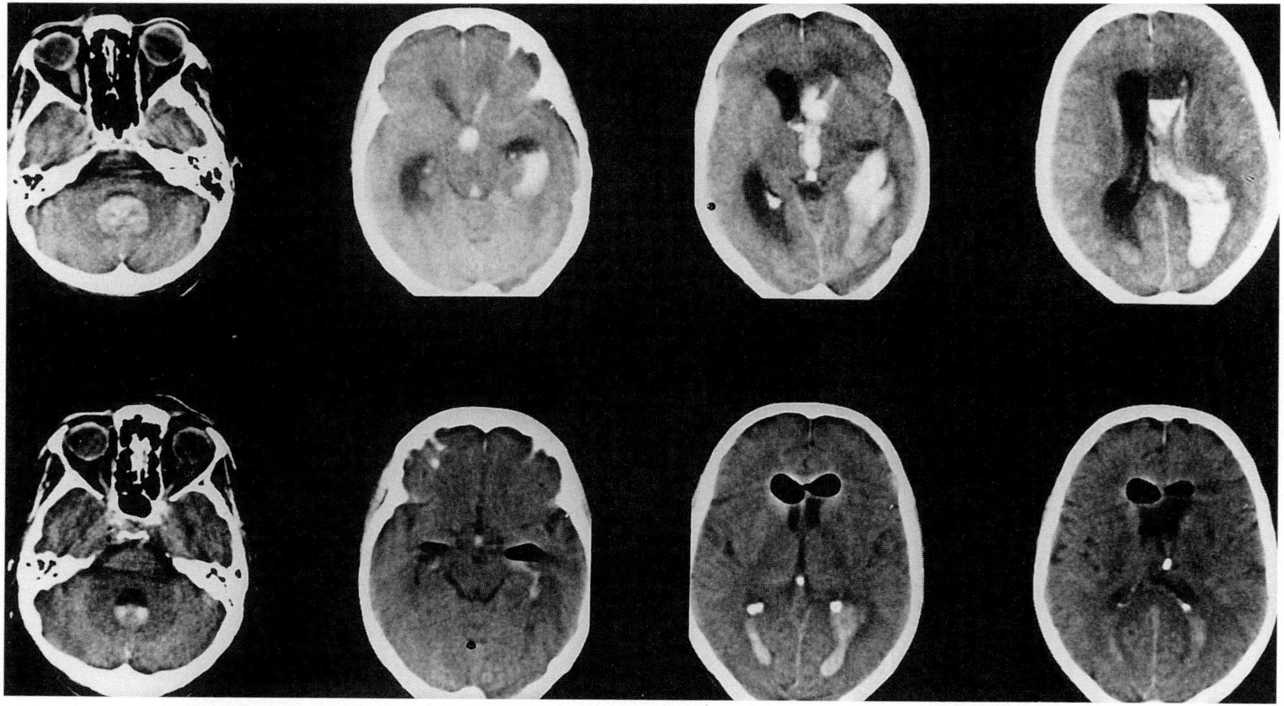

Fig. 1. Patient no. 8. Pretreatment CT (*above*) 4 h after the onset of symptoms shows severe IVH and ventricular enlargement, CT performed 48 h later (*below*), after treatment by ventricular drainage and three intraventricular injections of 5 mg rtPA, respectively: most of the intraventricular blood has been removed, ventricles are almost of normal size

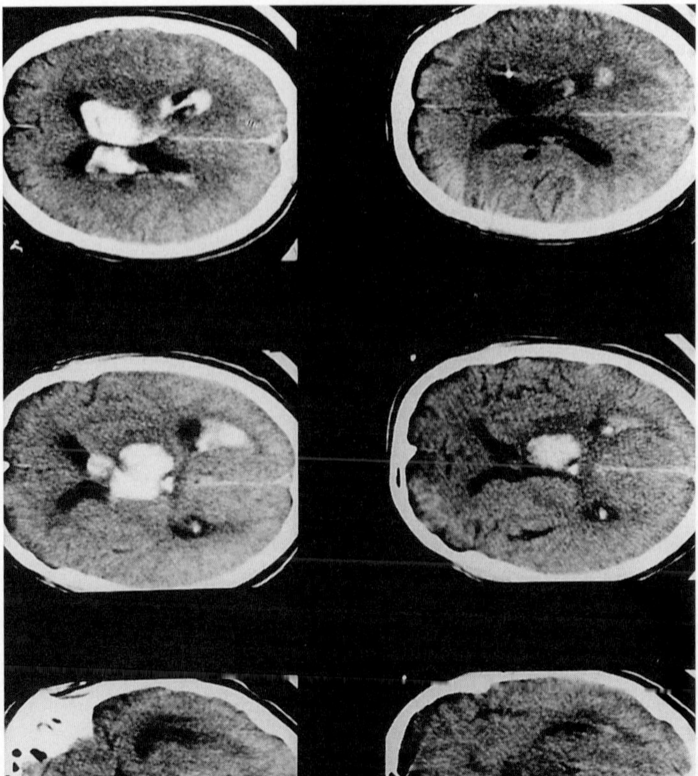

Fig. 2. Patient no. 7. *Above*, CT performed 48 h after the hemorrhage and after treatment by ventricular drainage, but without fibrinolytic therapy. Almost no reduction of intraventricular blood could be detected. *Below*, CT 48 h later, after injection of a total dose of 11 mg rtPA, shows reduction of the amount of intraventricular blood and decrease of ventricular dilatation

of rtPA treatment in all cases. Representative examples are shown in Figs. 1 and 2. Resorption of accompanying intracerebral hematomas did not seem to be improved by intraventricular rtPA injection. After elimination of most of the intraventricular blood, the ventricular catheter was temporarily closed and removed if intraventricular pressure remained normal for 24 h and subsequent CT gave no evidence of ventricular enlargement. It was possible to remove the ventricular drainage after 3–10 days in all patients. During the observation period (mean duration 15 days;

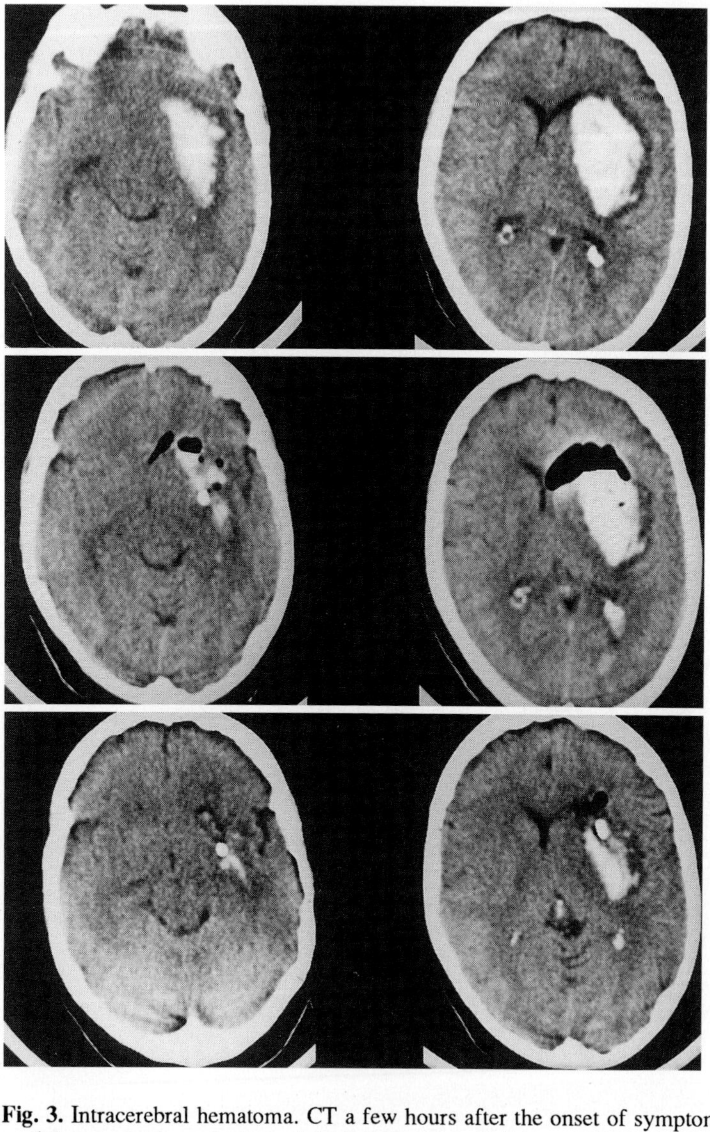

Fig. 3. Intracerebral hematoma. CT a few hours after the onset of symptoms (*above*), after partial stereotactic aspiration of the hematoma (*middle*), and 48 h later after injection of a total dose of 6 mg rtPA into the cavity of the hematoma (*below*)

range 4–26 days) all patients survived, and the mean Glasgow Coma Score rose from 7 (pretreatment) to 11 (post-treatment). No complications related to the rtPA treatment were observed.

Patients with Intracerebral Hematomas

This series included three patients ranging in age from 58 to 64 years with large intracerebral hematomas located in the basal ganglia and the internal capsule. Angiography did not reveal vascular malformations in any of the patients. Before treatment, all of them suffered from severely depressed consciousness levels and hemiparesis. Therapy consisted of stereotactic puncture and partial evacuation of the hematoma, performed within 24 h of hemorrhage. Thereafter, a CT scan was performed. Fibrinolytic therapy was started 1, 17, and 19 h after the end of stereotactic surgery, respectively. A total of 3 mg rtPA was injected through a silicone catheter placed intraoperatively into the residual hematoma. If considered necessary, rtPA injection was repeated. The total rtPA dose administered was 3, 6, and 9 mg, respectively. Follow-up CT scans showed rapid reduction of the residual hematoma after administration of rtPA in two patients. One case is demonstrated in Fig. 3. In the third patient, however, a slight increase of hematoma volume was observed after the first injection of rtPA. In this particular case, fibrinolytic therapy had been started very early, only 1 h after the stereotactic puncture.

Discussion

The prognosis in patients with IVH is directly related to the amount of intraventricular blood, the degree of ventricular dilatation on early CT scans, and to the pretreatment level of consciousness [1, 6, 7, 10, 12, 13]. The mortality rate in patients such as those treated by us, with severe hemorrhages extending into all ventricular chambers and with a high incidence of ventricular dilatation, has been reported to be higher than 80% [1, 6, 7, 12, 13]. Increased intracranial pressure and ventricular enlargement may result from space occupying clotted blood as well as from obstruction of cerebrospinal (CSF) fluid flow at the foramen of Monro, the aqueduct of Sylvius, or the fourth ventricle. Simple external ventricular drainage is of little benefit in patients with severe IVH as the catheters quickly become obstructed by clotted blood [5, 7]; furthermore, ventricular drains have no effect on solid clots within the ventricles.

The most important result of our study on IVH is the ability of rtPA to lyse clots within the ventricular spaces. A considerable reduction of intraventricular blood was observed as early as 24–48 h after the first injection of rtPA. This is much faster than what would be expected for spontaneous hematoma dissolution. During the treatment period, the ventricular catheters never became obstructed by clotted blood. Thus, continuous drainage of bloody CSF and rapid reduction of intracranial pressure and of ventricular dilatation could be achieved in every patient.

Survival rate and clinical improvement during the early post-treatment period were very good compared to the reported prognosis for severe IVH as cited above. Evaluation of long-term results of a larger series is now in progress.

To our knowledge, there has so far been only one case report on lysis of intraventricular hematoma with rtPA [5]. The authors described a case of severe IVH from a ruptured aneurysm. They observed a rapid reduction of hematoma volume and normalization of ventricular size and intracranial pressure. In one reported series of six patients with severe IVH [16], fibrinolysis was performed with intraventricular infusion of urokinase. Rapid elimination of intraventricular blood, a good clinical outcome of the treatment group, and lack of complications related to fibrinolysis were the main results of this study.

In summary, our results and the studies cited above prove that ventricular drainage and fibrinolysis result in rapid hematoma dissolution and normalization of intracranial pressure and ventricular size, and indicate that this method may improve the prognosis of severe IVH. The range of rtPA doses used in our study proved to be highly effective without causing apparent side effects.

Stereotactic hematoma evacuation has been introduced during recent years for the treatment of IVH as an alternative to traditional craniotomy. Injection of fibrinolytic agents such as urokinase into the cavity of the hematoma has proven to be useful for lysis and subsequent aspiration of solid clots [8, 9]. Our preliminary experience in three cases with large basal ganglia hemorrhages treated by stereotactic puncture and stereotactic drainage of the hematoma after injection of rtPA into the cavity indicates that rtPA may be efficient in lysing intracerebral clots. In one patient, in whom the first injection of rtPA was performed very early (1 h) after the stereotactic operation, CT after the first rtPA dose revealed a slight increase of hematoma volume compared to the immediate postoperative CT. Larger series of patients are necessary in order to assess the efficacy and safety of rtPA in the therapy of intracerebral hematomas.

References

1. De Weerd AW (1979) The prognosis of intraventricular hemorrhage. J Neurol 222:45–51
2. Findlay JM, Weir BKA, Gordon P, Grace M, Baughman R (1989) Safety and efficacy of intrathecal thrombolytic therapy in a primate model of cerebral vasospasm. Neurosurgery 24:491–498
3. Findlay JM, Weir BKA, Kanamaru K, Grace M, Baughman R (1990) The effect of timing of intrathecal fibrinolytic therapy on cerebral vasospasm in a primate model of subarachnoid hemorrhage. Neurosurgery 26:201–206
4. Findlay JM, Weir BKA, Kassell NF, Disney LB, Grace MGA (1991) Intracisternal recombinant tissue plasminogen activator after aneurysmal subarachnoid hemorrhage. J Neurosurg 75:181–188
5. Findlay JM, Weir BKA, Stollery DE (1991) Lysis of intraventricular hematoma with tissue plasminogen activator. J Neurosurg 74:803–807
6. Graeb DA, Robertson WD, Lapointe JS, Nugent RA, Harrison PB (1982) Computed tomographic diagnosis of intraventricular hemorrhage. Radiology 143:91–96

7. Little JR, Blomquist GA Jr, Ethier R (1977) Intraventricular hemorrhage in adults. Surg Neurol 8:143–149
8. Matsumoto K, Hondo H (1984) CT-guided stereotaxic evacuation of hypertensive intracerebral hematomas. J Neurosurg 61:440–448
9. Mohadjer M, Eggert R, May J, Mayfrank L (1990) CT-guided stereotactic fibrinolysis of spontaneous and hypertensive cerebellar hemorrhage: long-term results. J Neurosurg 73:217–222
10. Mohr G, Ferguson G, Khan M, Malloy D, Watts R, Benoit B, Weir B (1983) Intraventricular hemorrhage from ruptured aneurysm. J Neurosurg 58:482–487
11. Öhman J, Servo A, Heiskanen O (1991) Effect of intrathecal fibrinolytic therapy on clot lysis and vasospasm in patients with aneurysmal subarachnoid hemorrhage. J Neurosurg 75:197–201
12. Pia HW (1972) The surgical treatment of intracerebral and intraventricular haematomas. Acta Neurochir (Wien) 27:149–164
13. Ruscalleda J, Peiró A (1986) Prognostic factors in intraparenchymatous hematoma with ventricular hemorrhage. Neuroradiology 28:34–37
14. Seifert V, Eisert WG, Stolke D, Goetz C (1989) Efficacy of single intracisternal bolus injection of recombinant tissue plasminogen activator to prevent delayed cerebral vasospasm after experimental subarachnoid hemorrhage. Neurosurgery 25:590–598
15. Stolke D, Seifert V (1992) Single intracisternal bolus of recombinant tissue plasminogen activator in patients with aneurysmal subarachnoid hemorrhage: preliminary assessment of efficacy and safety in an open clinical study. Neurosurgery 30:877–881
16. Todo T, Usui M, Takakura K (1991) Treatment of severe intraventricular hemorrhage by intraventricular infusion of urokinase. J Neurosurg 74:81–86
17. Zabramski JM, Spetzler RF, Lee KS, Papadopoulos SM, Bovill E, Zimmermann RS, Bederson JB (1991) Phase I trial of tissue plasminogen activator for the prevention of vasospasm in patients with aneurysmal subarachnoid hemorrhage. J Neurosurg 75:189–196

Prognostic Value of Initial Median Nerve Somatosensory and Brain Stem Auditory Evoked Potentials in Patients with Spontaneous Intracerebral Hemorrhage

M. S. von Haken[1], H. P. Adams[2], and K. Rieke[2]

Introduction

Median nerve somatosensory evoked potentials (MSSEP) and brain stem auditory evoked potentials (BAEP) provide essential information to the clinician. A close relationship between evoked potential (EP) waveform and specific anatomic lesions could be demonstrated. Beside specificity and their ability to reveal conduction defects, exactly EPs are very resistant to alterations by anything other than structural pathology in the somatosensory pathway. Commonly used drugs in intensive care medicine and anesthesia (except volatile anesthetic agents) do not affect EPs [6]. Neurologic examination is often limited since the majority of these patients are noncompliant, having been pretreated with analgosedative drugs or in coma.

Our study was initiated to establish whether BAEPs and MSSEPs are an objective diagnostic and prognostic tool in the primary treatment of patients with spontaneous intracerebral hemorrhage (SIH). Therefore we examined our patients with SIH using MSSEPs and BAEPs and correlated EPs with clinical outcome.

Clinical Material and Methods

From April 1988 to February 1992 110 patients with SIH, admitted to either the neurosurgical or the neurologic intensive care unit at our institution, were examined using MSSEPs and BAEPs within the first 48 h after hemorrhage. Patients with vascular malformations, secondary hemorrhagic infarcts, SIH located in the brain stem, and hemorrhage secondary to a tumor or trauma were excluded from the study. The study population therefore consisted of 61 patients. The 30 female and 31 male patients ranged in age from 18 to 75 years (mean 55 years, median 59 years). The duration of treatment varied from 1 to 64 days (mean 16 days, median 13 days). In 17 cases the hemorrhage was located in the cerebellum, in 22 a lobe of the cerebrum was affected, and in 22 patients the thalamus or the basal ganglia. All patients were rated using the Glasgow Outcome Scale (GOS) at the time of dis-

[1] Neurochirurgische Klinik, Universität Heidelberg, Im Neuenheimer Feld 400, W-6900 Heidelberg, FRG.
[2] Abteilung Neurologie, Universität Heidelberg, Im Neuenheimer Feld 400, W-6900 Heidelberg, FRG.

Advances in Neurosurgery, Vol. 21
R. Lorenz, M. Klinger, M. Brock (Eds.)

charge from our hospital and the Barthel Index [2] after 6 months or more. For statistical analysis grades of outcome from coma were classified into three groups:

- Group I – patients with good recovery (patients who regain the ability to conduct a normal life or, if a preexisting disability exists, to resume the previous level of activity) and moderate disability (patients who achieve independence in their daily lives, but retain either physical or mental limitations that preclude the resumption of their previous level of function).
- Group II – patients with severe disability (patients who regain at least some cognitive function but depend on others for daily support).
- Group III – patients in a vegetative state (patients who awake, but give no sign of cognitive awareness) or with no recovery (patients who remain in coma until death).

Ranking of EPs was done according to normal, unilaterally by normal, or bilaterally pathologic EPs. Latencies, amplitudes, and side differences were evaluated. Limits for ranking were as follows: BAEP – interpeak latency I–III < 2.50 ms, III–V < 2.20 ms, I–V < 4.44 ms; MSSEP – interpeak latency N13–N20 < 6.30 ms, amplitude N20/P25 > 1.10 μV, amplitude difference N20/P25 < 47.6%.

Limits were established by testing 30 normal controls with the same stimulus and recording parameters, which is mandatory [1]. For statistical analysis of our results we used Fisher's exact test and the contingency coefficient.

Results

Localization of Hemorrhage Versus Outcome of Patients

Results are demonstrated in Table 1. As expected, infratentorial lesions had the most favorable outcome, while data for hemorrhage in a lobar localization or in the basal ganglia/thalamus did not reveal any differences.

Table 1. Localization of hemorrhage by outcome. Fisher's exact test of independence: $p = 0.00603$, contingency coefficient: 0.367

Outcome (GOS) \ Localization	Cerebellum (*n*)	Lobi cerebri (*n*)	Thalamus/ basal ganglia (*n*)	Total (*n*)
Good or fair (I)	11	4	7	22
Poor (II)	4	10	9	23
Vegetative/dead (III)	2	8	6	16
Total	17	22	22	61

Table 2. MSSEP ranking by outcome. Fisher's exact test of independence: $p = 0.000000328$, contingency coefficient: 0.551

MSSEP ranking / Outcome (GOS)	Normal (n)	Unilaterally (n)	Bilaterally abnormal (n)	Total (n)
Good or fair (I)	12	9	1	22
Poor (II)	4	13	6	23
Vegetative/dead (III)	–	4	10	14
Total	16	26	17	59

Outcome of Patients Versus MSSEPs/BAEPs

This is the most important result from our study and is demonstrated in Table 2. It is of note that none of the patients with an initially normal MSSEP had a poor outcome (group 3). On the other hand, there was only one patient with bilaterally pathologic MSSEPs who survived and was graded as having moderate disability. The correlation of the MSSEP result and the outcome of patients was highly significant ($p = 0.000000328$, contingency coefficient 0.551) while BAEP and outcome of patients were not dependent and data were nearly equally distributed ($p = 0.627$, contingency coefficient = 0.218; Table 3).

Outcome Versus Barthel Index

We interviewed all patients after surviving the initial clinical phase (minimum 7, maximum 49 months after hemorrhage) using the Barthel Index to analyze the independency in daily life that patients had gained after they were discharged from hospital. It became evident that only a few patients died after having survived the

Table 3. BAEP ranking by outcome. Fisher's exact test of independence: $p = 0.627$, contingency coefficient: 0.218

BAEP ranking / Outcome (GOS) (n)	Normal	Unilaterally normal (n)	Bilaterally abnormal (n)	Total (n)
Good or fair (I)	9	4	7	20
Poor (II)	7	3	8	18
Vegetative/dead (III)	3	4	8	15
Total	19	11	23	53

acute stage of illness. The cumulative mortality equals the average mortality of the normal population [5, 7]. The correlation of MSSEPs and Barthel Index ($p = 0.000000384$, contingency coefficient = 0.564) was nearly identical to the outcome results at the time of discharge of patients and MSSEP. Outcome, judged by GOS and results from the Barthel Index analysis were clearly correlated ($p = 0.0000000108$, contingency coefficient = 0.627).

Statistical analysis neither showed a correlation between MSSEP and BAEP results, nor did it confirm an intraventricular hemorrhage by computed tomography (CT).

Conclusion

MSSEP and BAEP studies have proven useful in a number of disorders as diagnostic and prognostic tools. The neurologic examination of patients who have suffered an SIH is, at times, difficult and unreliable. EPs provide a noninvasive, reproducible, and objective method to evaluate these patients. They can be used to establish objective evidence of an abnormality when clinical signs and symptoms in these patients are equivocal. This makes therapeutic decisions easier since we always have a tool at our disposal to estimate the later prognosis of the patient.

We found MSSEPs to be clearly correlated with the early and late prognosis of our patients. None of our patients with initially bilateral by normal MSSEPs died or survived in a vegetative state.

In the group with initially bilaterally pathologic MSSEP recordings outcome was poor or vegetative except for one patient. This finding very much corresponds with the literature for outcome of patients from coma and the prognostic relevance of EPs [3, 4].

We could not demonstrate the prognostic value of initial BAEPs in patients with SIH. BAEP changes are caused by compression of the lower midbrain, and therefore these changes can only be expected prior to transtentorial herniation.

For the interpretation of MSSEPs recorded within the first 48 h after hemorrhage, the absence of N19–P22 bilaterally remains one of the best prognostic parameters. In these patients clinical outcome will be a persistent vegetative state at best.

References

1. American EEG Society (1984) Clinical evoked potentials guidelines. Recommended standards for normative studies of evoked potentials, statistical analysis of results, and criteria for clinically significant abnormality J Clin Neurophysiol 1:11–14
2. Barthel D, Mahoney F (1965) Functional evaluation. State Med J 2:61–64
3. Chiappa KH (1990) Evoked potentials in clinical medicine, 2nd edn. Raven, New York, p 424
4. Goldie WD, Chiappa KH, Young RR (1979) Brainstem auditory evoked responses and short-latency somatosensory evoked responses in the evaluation comatose patients. Neurology (Minneap) 29:551

5. Matsumoto N, Whisnant JP, Kurland LT, Okazaki H (1973) Natural history of stroke in Rochester, Minn. 1955 through 1969. Stroke 4:20–29
6. Nuwer MR (1986) Evoked potential monitoring in the operating room, 1st edn. Raven, New York, pp 158–161
7. Whisnant JP (1984) The decline of stroke. Stroke 15:160–168

Computed Tomographic – Stereotactic Evacuation and Fibrinolysis of Spontaneous Intracerebral Hematomas

M. Mohadjer[1]

Introduction

Spontaneous intracerebral hematoma (ICH) has become easier to diagnose as a result of modern diagnostic imaging techniques. A number of generally accepted opinions regarding the age and frequency distribution and the so-called typical courses of the disease and prognoses have had to be revised [1, 8]. The appropriate mode of treatment, however, is still under discussion. Neither conservative therapy nor conventional neurosurgery, even with modern microsurgical methods, has been able to improve the unfavorable course and prognosis of ICH [6, 9]. Since 1985 we have used a different approach which consists of the image-based stereotactic evacuation and fibrinolysis of the ICH.

Surgical Methods

The operation is generally done under local anesthesia. Only in cases where the patient is restless, confused, or suffers respiratory insufficiency is intubation anesthesia necessary.

After a burrhole has been made according to the location of the hematoma, the hematoma is punctured under sterotactic conditions and its contents are partially aspirated – sometimes as much as 30% of the original volume – under continuous irrigation. This allows a rapid reduction of the intracranial pressure without putting additional strain on the patient and without causing a large lesion (Fig. 1). The implantation of a silicone catheter (2 mm outer diameter), if possible in the center of the hematoma cavity, ends the brief procedure. The position of the catheter can be verified by computed tomography (CT) during or after the operation. During the following 24–48 h, 5000–10000 IU urokinase dissolved in 5 ml physiological saline solution can be administered through this catheter to fibrinolyse and evacuate the residual hematoma (Fig. 2).

[1] Abteilung Stereotaxie und Neuronuklearmedizin, Universität Freiburg, Hugstetter Straße 55, W-7800 Freiburg, FRG.

Advances in Neurosurgery, Vol. 21
R. Lorenz, M. Klinger, M. Brock (Eds.)

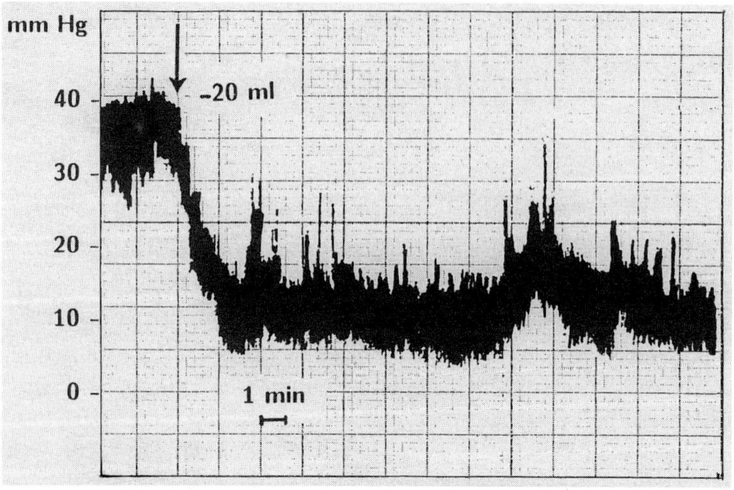

Fig. 1. Increased intracranial pressure rapidly dropped to normal after intraoperative partial aspiration of the hematoma. The pressure level remained almost constant after the placement of continuous suction drainage

Patients

From October 1985 to February 1991, a total of 117 patients (78 men and 39 women, mean age 58.6 and 60.2 years, respectively) were treated for ICH with CT-stereotactic surgery. The most common concomitant conditions and risk factors included cardiovascular insufficiency (32%), obesity (30%), alcohol abuse (29%), renal insufficiency (20%), and diabetes mellitus (15%).

In 39% of the patients the hematomas were located in the lobes, in 38% in the basal ganglia and thalamus. In 17% the lesions were in the cerebellum or brainstem, and in 6% the hematoma was only intraventricular.

The initial state of consciousness of the patients was assessed on the day of admission using the Glasgow Coma Scale. Impaired consciousness as a result of an ICH should be regarded as the sum of all the important clinical parameters relevant for the later course and prognosis. The neurological symptoms were dependent on the location of the hematoma. Accordingly, hemiparesis and hemiplegia were the most frequently seen symptoms, followed by speech disorders and aphasia. Invasion into the ventricle, which was determined in over 60% of the patients, complicates the course and worsens the prognosis [2, 3, 11].

Results

Forty-eight hours after evacuation of the hematoma, the consciousness level improved to normal in all the patients. More than 60% of the patients had regained orientation by this time and showed appropriate reactions. This fast recovery al-

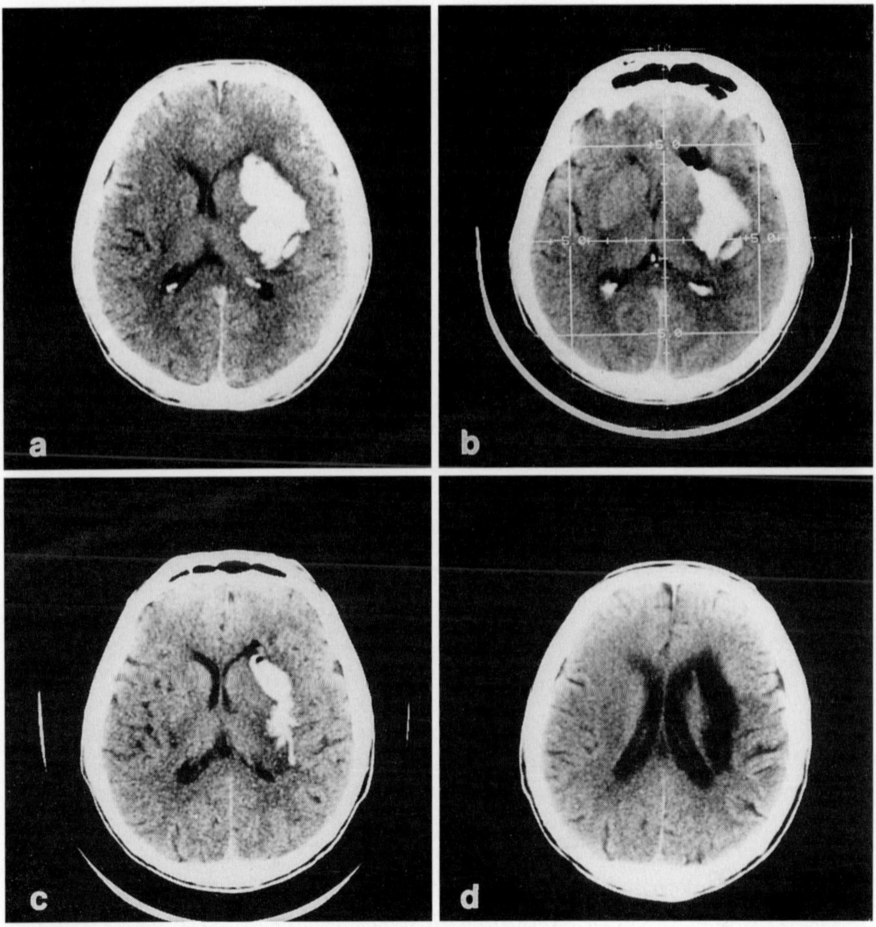

Fig. 2a–d. Hypertensive hemorrhage in left basal ganglia of 55-year-old patient prior to stereotactic puncture (**a**), directly after aspiration of 18 ml blood (**b**), 24 h after two fibrinolysis procedures using 5000 IU urokinase each (**c**), and condition 6 weeks later (**d**)

lowed the patients to move and to resume normal intake of food soon after surgery. It also reduced the elaborate and costly intensive care period.

Within the first 60 days after the operation, 18 patients (15.4%) died, probably as a direct result of the ICH. After a relatively long mean follow-up of 39 months, another ten patients died of diseases unrelated to the ICH. The cumulative mortality was thus 24%. The quality of life of the surviving patients according to the Karnofsky Performance Scale can be rated as good to very good in 54% and moderate in 16%. Only 6% have deteriorated and require continuous care (Table 1).

Table 1. Long-term results after stereotactic partial evacuation and fibrinolysis of spontaneous ICH (mean follow-up period 39 months). October 1985 to February 1991; $n = 117$

Current quality of life according to Karnofsky			
100%–70%	70%–50%	< 50%	
Good to very good	Moderate	Poor	Deceased
(*n*) 63	19	7	28
(%) 54	16	6	24
Mortality within the first 60 days: $n = 18$, 15.4%			

Discussion

Not all patients with ICH require surgical management. Not until the ICH become space-occupying and thus a danger for the patient is surgery necessary. However, despite this seemingly clear-cut indication, differences in judgment exist in terms of both its urgency and management.

The goal of any surgical treatment of ICH is to quickly remove the space-occupying lesion and reduce the intracranial hypertension, especially before the formation of delayed perifocal edema which increases the intracranial pressure even more. Although in the case of superficial hematomas this goal can be effectively reached using conventional neurosurgery, using the method for deep-seated hematomas still carries many risks, despite refined microsurgical techniques. For these deep-seated spontaneous ICH the CT-stereotactic operation represents a new treatment as an alternative to craniotomy [2, 4, 9, 10].

The neurotoxic effect of the fibrinolytic agent urokinase on the parenchyma of the brain and ventricles and in the subarachnoid space has been ruled out by means of light and electron microscopy [5, 7]. No provocation of bleeding has been observed [7]. The CT-guided stereotactic surgical method for ICH carries a low risk, is only minimally invasive, and is precise. Precision is of particular importance since the center of the hematoma should be reached for the fibrinolysis. However, the good results obtained can only be considered a trend at this point and require confirmation in prospective and randomized studies with clearly defined selection criteria, as well as standardized follow-up observation and documentation. Table 2 lists the selection and exclusion criteria recommended for use in indicating CT-stereotactic evacuation and fibrinolysis of ICH.

In addition to the selection and exclusion criteria, follow-up observations should also be documented using a standardized and uniform system. Not until prospective studies conducted according to these rules have been evaluated can the optimal treatment for ICH of different types and locations be determined.

Table 2. Selection and exclusion criteria for indicating CT-stereotactic evacuation and fibrinolysis of spontaneous intracerebral hematomas

Selection criteria

1. Current level of consciousness according to Glasgow Coma Scale > 6
2. Size of space-occupying lesion
   Mean diameter of hematoma > 30 mm or, volume of hematoma > 20 ml
3. Patients with ventricular involvement as special group

Exclusion criteria

1. Severe concomitant or previous disorder: cardiovascular decompensation, clotting disorder, metabolic dysfunction, etc.
2. Brainstem compression
3. Hematoma in brainstem
4. Hematocephalus: complete ventricular tamponade, according to Graeb et al. [2]

References

1. Gänshirt H, Keuler R (1980) Intracerebrale Blutungen. Ursachen, Klinik, Verlauf, Spätprognosen. Nervenarzt 51:201–206
2. Graeb DA, Robertson WD, Lapointe JS, Nugent RA, Harrison PB (1982), Computed tomographic diagnostics of intraventricular hemorrhage – etiology and prognosis. Radiology 143:91–96
3. Jellinger K (1980) Pathology and aetiology of ICH. In: Pia HW, Langmaid C, Zierski J (eds) Spontaneous intracerebral haematomas. Advances in diagnosis and therapy. Springer, Berlin Heidelberg New York, pp 130–135
4. Matsomoto K, Hondo M (1984) CT-guided stereotaxic evacuation of hypertensive intracerebral hematomas. J Neurosurgery 61:440–448
5. Mohadjer M, Anagnastopoulos J, Eggert HR, May J (1988) The effect of urokinase on the central nervous system – animal experimental study. Haemostasis 18 Suppl 2:81
6. Mohadjer M, Ruh E, Hiltl DM, Neumüller M, Mundinger F (1988) CT-stereotactic evacuation and fibrinolysis of hypertensive intracranial haematomas. Fibrinolysis 2:43–48
7. Mohadjer M, Eggert HR, May J, Mayfrank L (1990) CT-guided stereotactic fibrinolysis of spontaneous and hypertensive cerebellar hemorrhage – long-term results. J Neurosurg 73:217–222
8. Müke R, Heienbrok KW, Kühne D (1978) Spontane intracerebrale Hämatome. Neue Gesichtspunkte seit Einführung der Computertomographie. Zentralbl Neurochir 39:135–144
9. Niizuma H, Suzuki J (1988) Stereotactic aspiration of putaminal hemorrhage using a double track aspiration technique. Neurosurgery 22:432–436
10. Niizuma H, Shimizu Y, Yonemitsu T, Nakassato N, Suzuki J (1989) Results of stereotactic aspiration in 175 cases of putaminal hemorrhage. Neurosurgery 24:814–819
11. Weerd AW (1980) The prognosis of intraventricular hemorrhage. J Neurol 222:46–51

Spontaneous Intracerebral Hemorrhages in Childhood

J. Behnke[1], I. Grohmann[2], U. Stephani[2], B. Rama[1], and E. Markakis[1]

Introduction

The nature and distribution of intracranial hemorrhages in 56 children including premature infants, mature infants, and pediatric patients under 17 years of age are presented in this study. The different etiology of the hemorrhages and the different diagnostic and therapeutic regimes in respect of operative indications are also discussed.

Patients

In the time from 1986 to 1988, 35 premature infants suffering from spontaneous intracranial hemorrhages and in the time from 1986 and 1991 nine mature infants and 12 pediatric patients aged 3–17 years were treated at the University of Göttingen.

Group 1: Premature Infants (*n* = 35)

All of these premature infants suffered from periventricular-intraventricular hemorrhages. The known pathogenesis of periventricular-intraventricular hemorrhages is related to intravascular, vascular, and extravascular factors [1]. The neuropathology is characterized by bleeding into the subependymal germinal matrix with subsequent rupture into the lateral ventricle.

Ultrasound scanning of the head was utilized as a diagnostic method to identify periventricular-intraventricular hemorrhages. The grading was done according to Papile et al. [2].

The following parameters were evaluated: the rate of premature infants with periventricular-intraventricular hemorrhage depending on their gestational age, the distribution of these premature infants according to their gestational age, their mortality depending on their gestation age, and the grade of hemorrhage, the rela-

---

[1] Neurochirurgische Klinik, Universität Göttingen, Robert-Koch-Straße 40, W-3400 Göttingen, FRG.
[2] Abteilung Pädiatrische Neurochirurgie, Universität Göttingen, Robert-Koch-Straße 40, W-3400 Göttingen, FRG.

Advances in Neurosurgery, Vol. 21
R. Lorenz, M. Klinger, M. Brock (Eds.)

tion between grade of hemorrhage and gestational age, the operative indication, and the relation between outcome and grade of hemorrhage.

Group 2: Mature Infants ($n = 9$)

Between 1986 and 1991 nine mature infants suffering from intracranial hemorrhages were treated in the pediatric department of the University of Göttingen. First all hemorrhages were diagnosed by ultrasound scanning of the head; only those infants with intracranial hemorrhages differing from the typical picture of periventricular-intraventricular hemorrhage underwent a further diagnostic regime (blood coagulation analysis; nuclear magnetic resonance, NMR; and/or angiography depending on the localization and character of the bleeding). The indication for neurosurgical intervention and the outcome of all of these infants are described below.

Group 3: Pediatric Patients Aged 3–17 Years ($n = 12$)

Between 1986 and 1991 12 pediatric patients were treated at the University of Göttingen. In all patients we intended to clear the bleeding by means of the full neuroradiological spectrum including cranial computer tomography (CCT), NMR, and – should the occasion arise – also angiography. In patients presenting in a bad neurological condition NMR and angiography were not done ($n = 2$) before emergency operation.

Results

Group 1: Premature Infants

Between 1986 and 1988 415 premature infants were treated in the pediatric department of the University of Göttingen; 35 of them had a periventricular-intraventricular hemorrhage (8.4%). There were 11 premature infants with periventricular-intraventricular hemorrhages in the group of 25 infants born before the 28th week of gestation (44%), 11 in the group of 45 (24%) born at the 28th/29th weeks, seven of 65 (11%) born at the 30th/31st weeks, five of 107 (5%) born at the 32nd/33rd weeks, and one of 131 (1%) born at the 34th/35th weeks. None of the 42 premature infants born at the 36th week had a periventricular-intraventricular hemorrhage. Eleven (31%) of the premature infants had a gestational age below the 28th/29th weeks, eleven (31%) had a gestational age of the 28th/29th weeks, seven (20%) had a gestational age of the 30th/31st weeks, five (14%) had a gestational age of the 32nd/33rd weeks, and one (3%) had a gestational age of the 34th/35th weeks. A total of 77% of the immature infants suffering from periventricular-intraventricular hemorrhages had a grade I or II hemorrhage; the remaining infants had a grade III or IV hemorrhage. We found grade III and IV hemorrhages only up to the 30th/31st weeks of gestation, but we did also find grade I and II hemorrhages in older premature infants.

All the infants suffering from periventricular-intraventricular grade I hemorrhages survived, but two of the 14 with grade II (14%), one of the three (33%) with grade III, and all of the premature infants suffering from grade IV periventricular-intraventricular hemorrhages died. Looking at the mortality depending on the gestational age, three of the 11 born before the 28th week (27%), four of the 11 born at the 28th/29th weeks, and one of the seven (14%) born at the 30th/31st weeks died; the remaining infants born after the 31st week survived.

Half of the infants suffering from grade I hemorrhages and 43% of the infants suffering from grade II hemorrhages had a normal neurological development. Six of the 35 premature infants suffering from periventricular-intraventricular hemorrhages developed a hydrocephalus requiring treatment, but only in three cases was a shunt necessary.

Group 2: Mature Infants ($n = 9$)

The hemorrhages were localized as below:

- One grade II periventricular-intraventricular hemorrhage (1st day)
- Two grade III periventricular-intraventricular hemorrhages (1st day)
- One intraventricular hemorrhage with tamponade of the ventricles (7th day)
- One intraventricular hemorrhage caused by coagulation disorder (1st day)
- One gross intraventricular hemorrhage, primarily suspected to be a tumor (intrauterine)
- One hemorrhage of the posterior fossa caused by coagulopathy (1st day)
- Two intraparenchymatous hemorrhages:
  One HbS heterozygote (1st month)
  One vitamin K deficiency (1st month)

The three infants suffering from periventricular-intraventricular hemorrhages were examined by ultrasound scanning of the head. The infants developed normally without any neurosurgical intervention. The 7-day-old infants with exclusive tamponade of ventricles required ventricular drainage for 3 days because of severe bradycardia. Despite a typical onset of the bleeding, an angiomatous malformation could be excluded by NMR. The infant developed normally without any further neurosurgical intervention.

The infant with diffuse coagulopathy and multiple intracranial bleedings was operated on. In addition to the ultrasound scanning, a CCT was performed before evacuation of the space-occupying subdural hematoma. However, the infant died as a result of the multiple bleedings.

The infant suffering from a gross intraventricular mass suspected to be a tumor underwent NMR and was operated on. Intraoperatively gross intraventricular bleeding was found and was partly resected. In the further course the infant required a shunt.

The infant suffering from space-occupying bleeding into the posterior fossa had a good outcome without operation. Angiography did not show any angiomatous malformation. The two infants suffering from intraparenchymatous bleedings underwent also angiographical diagnosis which proved to be normal. The infants had a good outcome without further neurosurgical intervention.

Group 3: Pediatric Patients Aged 3–17 years

Five hemorrhages were supratentorial, six were multiple hemorrhages and in one child they were supra- and infratentorial. In eight of the 12 children we found angiomatous malformations, two children suffering from supratentorial hemorrhages had coagulation disorders without any operative indications. In two of the three infratentorial hemorrhages we did not find any angiomatous malformation intraoperatively. Two required acute operative decompression because of their bad neurological condition. They died in the early postoperative course. All the other patients we operated on had no postoperative deterioration. We operated on most of the children after their first bleeding, but three patients were presented to us after their third bleeding. We operated on two of these children with a good outcome; one girl with eight bleedings has not been operated on yet because of her parents' refusal.

Conclusion

In the group of premature infants the only diagnostic regime is the ultrasound scanning of the head and the only neurosurgical function is treating the hydrocephalus if necessary. We prefer first to implant a Rickham capsula and perform the connection to a permanent shunting system when the infant has put on weight and the fluid is clean.

In the mature infants the management is the same as in the premature infants if the bleedings are comparable to the periventricular-intraventricular hemorrhages. If there is any deviation in respect to their localization or the time of onset, we plan further neuroradiological diagnosis. If there is no acute indication for an operative intervention, we wait until the infant is in a better condition.

In the group of older pediatric patients, we perform the whole spectrum of neuroradiological diagnosis after the first hemorrhage, remembering that the preoperative condition does not allow any delay.

References

1. Volpe JJ (1989) Intraventricular hemorrhage in the premature infant. Ann Neurol 25:3–11
2. Papile LA, Burstein J, Burstein R, Koffler H (1978) Incidence and evolution of subependymal and intraventricular hemorrhage: a study of infants with birth weights less than 1500 gm. J Pediatr 92:529–534

Therapy and Prognosis in Spontaneous Cerebellar Hematomas

U. Neubauer[1] and B. Schwenk[1]

Introduction

Cerebellar hematomas threaten patients in a twofold way: first, by the local mass in the posterior fossa which may cause a significant brain stem compression and, second, by the concomitant hydrocephalus in many patients with increased intracranial pressure (ICP) in the supratentorial space [4, 5, 8] (Fig. 1). For the treatment of cerebellar hematomas we have three options: (a) evacuation of the hematoma by a posterior fossa approach [1–3], (b) CSF drainage by a frontal burr hole to control the hydrocephalus and ICP [6, 10], and (c) conservative treatment only. Criteria for the decision as to how to treat the individual patient may be the size of the hematoma [9] and the patient's clinical condition [7].

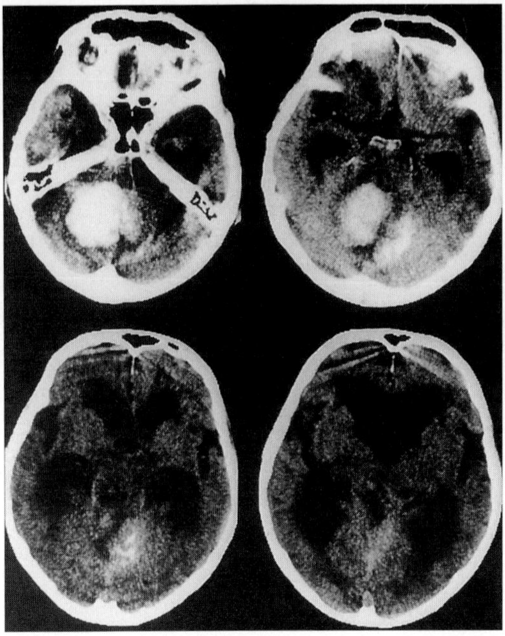

Fig. 1. CT scan in cerebellar hematoma. Hyperdense mass in the left cerebellar hemisphere and vermis with occlusive hydrocephalus

[1] Neurochirurgische Klinik, Universität Erlangen-Nürnberg, Schwabachanlage 6, W-8520 Erlangen, FRG.

Advances in Neurosurgery, Vol. 21
R. Lorenz, M. Klinger, M. Brock (Eds.)

Here we report our results in a retrospective study of 37 consecutive patients with cerebellar hematomas treated in our Department between 1986 and 1991. A total of 31 patients had a history of arterial hypertension; patients with vascular malformations or tumors were excluded. Three patients were on anticoagulant therapy. While other authors recommend operating in all cases [3], our attitude is to observe patients who are fully alert and to operate in all patients with reduced level of consciousness or secondary deterioration.

Results

Of our 37 patients 21 had direct evacuation of the hematoma, 10 were treated by CSF drainage only, and 6 were treated conservatively. Twelve of our patients died, which means an overall mortality rate of 32% (Table 1). The main factor in mortality was a low score on the Glasgow coma scale (GCS) prior to operation. In 22 patients with a score between 3 and 5 the mortality was 50%. Only one patient with a score of 6–8 died (25%) and none with a score of 9 or more. In patients with a poor preoperative condition the best results were achieved by direct operation of the hematoma. In addition to mortality, the quality of survival was also strongly influenced by the preoperative condition (Table 2).

The hydrocephalus in patients with cerebellar hematomas may be interpreted as an indicator for brain stem compression leading to obstruction of the CSF pathways but also acts itself by the increased intracranial pressure. In our series we found an effect of the hydrocephalus both on the GCS and on mortality. From 25 patients with hydrocephalus 10 died (40%), in contrast to only 17% in the group without hydrocephalus (2 out of 12). Of the patients with hydrocephalus 68% had a GCS of 3–5 but only 42% of those without hydrocephalus. The higher mortality rate in patients with hydrocephalus is only partially due to the higher rate of a low GCS. Analyzing only the 22 patients with a GCS of 3–5 we still find a higher mortality in patients with hydrocephalus (53%) compared to those without hydrocephalus (40%).

Finally a major factor influencing outcome was the size of the hematoma (Fig. 2). With increasing size we found more patients with a low GCS, while small cere-

Table 1. Mortality in spontaneous cerebellar hematomas

		Evacuation of hematoma		Ventricular drainage		No operation	
GCS	*n*	*n*	%	*n*	%	*n*	%
3–5	22	6/15	40	4/6	66	1/1	100
6–8	4	1/4	25	0		0	
9–15	11	0/2	0	0/4	0	0/5	0
Total	37	7/21	32	4/10	40	1/6	16

Table 2. Preoperative Glasgow coma score and final outcome

GCS	*n*	Died	V	SD	MD	G
3–5	22	11	0	1	5	5
6–8	4	1	0	0	2	1
9–15	11	0	0	0	4	7
Total	37	12 (32%)	0	1 (2.7%)	11 (29%)	13 (35%)

V, Vegetative; SD, severely disabled; MD, moderately disabled; G, good.

bellar hematomas generally had clinically a higher score. However, even huge hematomas of more than 25 ml may be well tolerated.

Concerning mortality the critical volume in our series was 15 ml or a diameter of 3 cm. No patient with a hematoma smaller than 3 cm died, but 50% of those with larger hematomas did so.

In conclusion, in all cases of cerebellar hematomas with a GCS lower than 9 and/or hematoma larger than 3 cm in diameter the hematoma should be evacuated. In patients with a GCS of 9 or better and a hematoma below 3 cm the patient may be watched closely and operated on promptly if deterioration occurs.

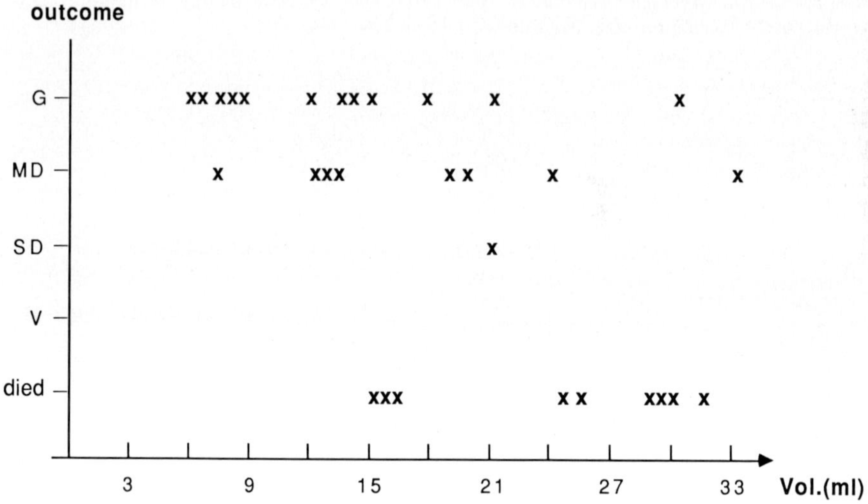

Fig. 2. Size of hematoma and outcome. With increasing size the final outcome becomes worse. *G*, Good; *MD*, moderately disabled; *SD*, severely disabled; *V*, vegetative

References

1. Auer LM, Auer T, Sayama I (1986) Indications for surgical treatment of cerebellar haemorrhage and infarction. Acta Neurochir (Wien) 79:74–79
2. Billy C, Boissonot L, Bataille B, Gil R, Neau J, Lefevre J (198...) Hématomes circonstricts parenchymateux non traumatiques de al fosse postérieure. Semin Hôp Paris 64(25):1665–1672
3. Calliauw L, Dehaene I (1980) Cerebellar haematomas: operative treatment. In: Pia H, Langmaid B, Zierski J (eds) Spontaneous intracerebral hematomas: advances in diagnosis and therapy. Springer, Berlin Heidelberg New York, pp 365–366
4. Dinsdale H (1964) Spontaneous hemorrhage in the posterior fossa. Arch Neurol 10:200–217
5. Hoop RG van der, Vermeulen M, Gijn J van (1988) Cerebellar hemorrhage: diagnosis and treatment. Surg Neurol 29:6–10
6. Firsching R, Frowein RA, Thun F (1987) Intracerebellar haematoma: eleven traumatic and non-traumatic cases and a review of the literature. Neurochirurgia (Stuttg) 30:182–185
7. Klinger M, Kunze S (1980) Cerebellar haematomas: operative treatment. In: Pia H, Langmaid B, Zierski J (eds) Spontaneous intracerebral hematomas: advances in diagnosis and therapy. Springer Berlin Heidelberg New York pp 358–365
8. Ott KH, Kase CS, Ojemann RG, Mohr JP (1974) Cerebellar hemorrhage: diagnosis and treatment. Arch Neurol 31:160–167
9. Sano K, Yoshida S (1980) Cerebellar haematomas: indications and prognosis In: Pia H, Langmaid B, Zierski J (eds) Spontaneous intracerebral hematomas: advances in diagnosis and therapy. Springer Berlin Heidelberg New York pp 348–356
10. Seelig JM, Selhorst JS, Young HF, Lipper M (1981) Ventriculostomy for hydrocephalus in cerebellar hemorrhage. Neurology 31:1537–1540

Spontaneous Cerebellar Hemorrhage: Acute Management and Prognosis*

D. Rosenthal[1], G. Marquardt[1], and T. Sievert[1]

Introduction

Although spontaneous cerebellar hematomas only represent 1%–13% [12] of all intracerebral hemorrhages, their reported mortality rate varies between 50% and 80% [7]. With the introduction of computed tomography (CT) as a diagnostic tool, diagnosis and localization can be done very early. Since then, and using different therapeutic approaches, a higher rate of survivors has been achieved. Despite this fact the management of this affection is still controversial and different procedures such as conservative treatment, ventricular drainage, and direct or stereotactic clot evacuation have been advocated [1, 10, 13–16]. We have reviewed our cases in an attempt to clarify the management and improve the outcome of these patients.

Patients and Methods

In a 10-year period (1980–1990) 398 consecutive patients presenting with acute primary intracerebral hemorrhage were admitted to our department. All patients were explored neurologically, had a CT scan and, as far as the clinical condition allowed it, angiographical examination on admission. The size of the hematoma was measured volumetrically [18]. Special attention was paid to the form of the quadrigeminal cisterns, the presence of intraventricular hemorrhage, and the size of the lateral ventricles (Fig. 1).

Patients with traumatic, aneurysmal, angioma, or tumor bleedings as well as pontine hemorrhages were excluded from the study. Treatment was decided according to the clinical and radiological findings. Outcome was assessed using a four-grade scale, divided into *good* if the patient returned to normal life with no or slight neurological deficits, *poor* if the patient did not return to normal activities because of a moderate to severe deficit, *vegetative* if the patient was in an apallic condition, and *dead*.

---

* Dedicated to Prof. Dr. Dr. h.c. R. Lorenz on his 60th birthday.

[1] Klinik für Neurochirurgie, Johann-Wolfgang-Goethe-Universität, Schleusenweg 2–16, W-6000 Frankfurt am Main 71, FRG.

Advances in Neurosurgery, Vol. 21
R. Lorenz, M. Klinger, M. Brock (Eds.)

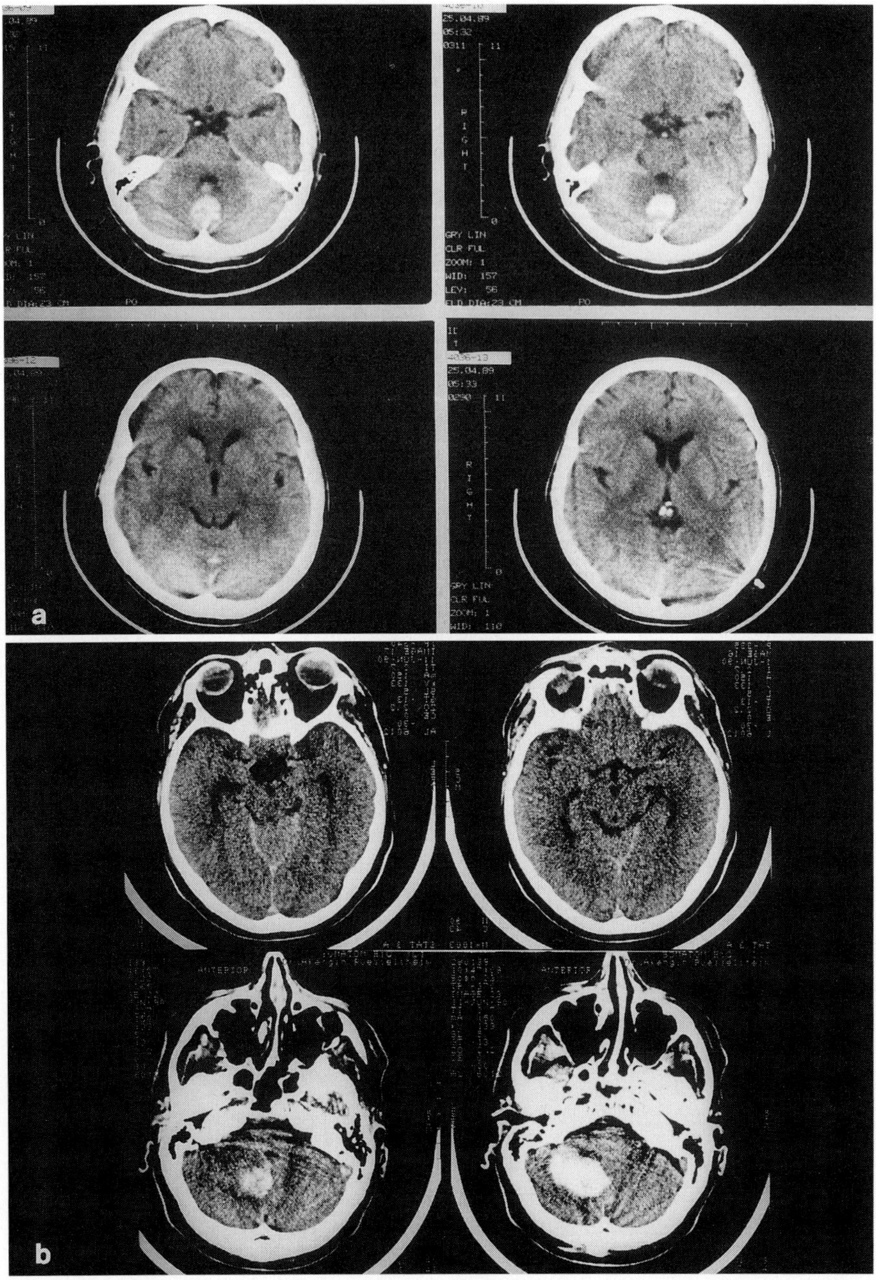

Fig. 1a–c. Typical findings in grade I (**a**), grade II (**b**) and grade III (**c**) patients

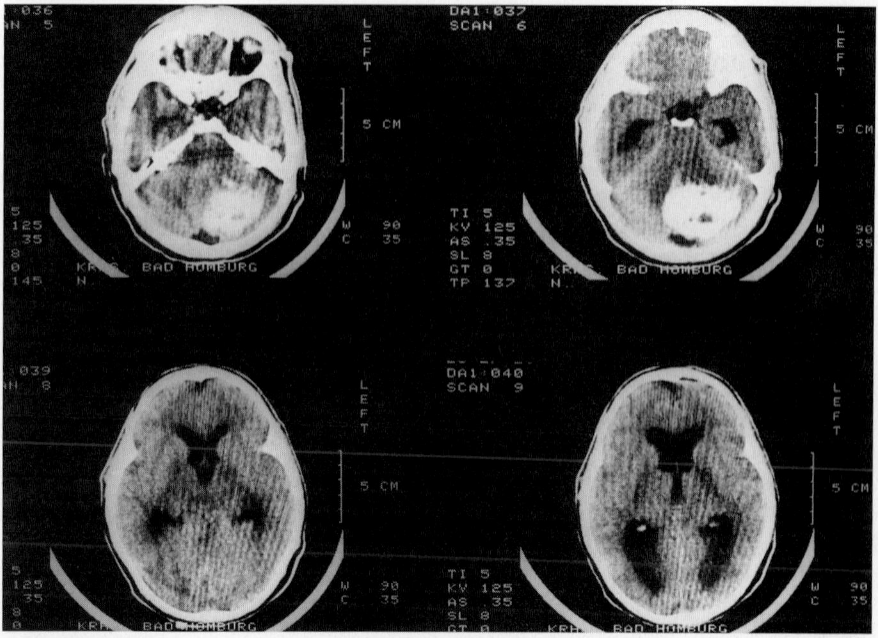

Results

Sixty-six patients presented with cerebellar hemorrhage, but only 44 (66%) met the previously established criteria for inclusion in this study. These included 19 females (43%) and 25 males (57%) with a mean age of 53.9 years (range 12–82), 28 (63%) of them being between 50 and 70 years old.

Among the predisposing factors arterial hypertension was the most frequent, with 22 cases (50%), nine patients (20%) had cardiovascular disorders, four patients (9%) had diabetes mellitus, seven patients (16%) were taking anticoagulants, and two patients (5%) had renal disorders. Onset of symptoms was acute in 38 pa-

Table 1. Clinical symptoms on admission

Clinical symptom	Cases (*n*)	(%)
Headache	40	91
Nausea and vomiting	33	75
Loss of consciousness	20	45
Dizziness	12	27
Ataxia	5	11
Dysarthria	2	5

Table 2. Neurological signs on admission

Neurological sign	No. of cases
Level of consciousness	
Alert	14
Stuporous	10
Comatose	20
Absent corneal response	17
Conj. eye deviation	12
Babinski response	11
Nystagmus	8
Miosis	8
Hemiparesis	6
Ataxia	5
Dilated fixed pupils	2
Decerebration	2
Respiratory disturbances	2

tients (83%); the clinical symptoms and neurological signs on admission are listed on Tables 1 and 2.

Patients in a comatose condition were admitted at a mean time of 20.35 h after onset of symptoms; alert or somnolent cases arrived in our department 30.25 h after becoming symptomatic.

A CT scan was performed preoperatively in all cases (Table 3). Angiography was done preoperatively in 24 patients (54%) who were either alert or somnolent; in contrast, only eight (18%) comatose patients were examined preoperatively and three after surgery. According to their clinical condition and radiological findings the patients were divided into three different categories (Table 4). Fourteen patients (32%) were classified as grade I, ten as grade II (23%) and 20 as grade III (45%). Treatment comprised conservative therapy, external ventricular drainage only, craniotomy and direct hematoma evacuation or a combination of the last two

Table 3. CT findings

	Grade I	Grade II	Grade III
Mean size (cm^3)	8.5	17.8	28.5
Location			
Left	7	5	8
Right	5	4	8
Vermis	2	1	4
Hydrocephalus	6	5	16
Basal cisterns (compressed)	–	3	16
Intraventricular Hemorrhage	1	1	10

Table 4. Initial clinical and radiological grading system

Grade I	Alert Basal cisterns normal Hematoma volume up to 10 cm^3
Grade II	Stuporous Basal cisterns compressed Hematoma volume between 10 and 20 cm^3
Grade III	Comatose Basal cisterns absent Hematoma volume bigger than 20 cm^3

Table 5. Relationship between treatment, grading, and outcome

	Grade			Outcome		
	I	II	III	Good	Poor	Dead
1. Conservative	5			5		
2. Ventriculostomy	5			4		1
3. Decompression						
4. Combined (2 + 3)	4			3	1	
1. Conservative						
2. Ventriculostomy		2				2
3. Decompression		5		4	1	
4. Combined (2 + 3)			3	1	1	1
1. Conservative						
2. Ventriculostomy			8		2	6
3. Decompression			4	2		2
4. Combined (2 + 3)			8		5	3

Table 6. Causes of death

Cause	No. of cases
Herniation	7[a]
Pulmonary	
Embolism	2
Pneumonia (sepsis)	2
Adult respiratory distress syndrome	1
Cardiac	
Infarction	1
Valve clotting	1
Bone marrow aplasia	1

[a] One supratentorial bleeding 1 month after treatment.

procedures. Overall results were good in 19 patients (43%) and poor in 10 (23%) and death occurred in 15 cases (34%). Details of the relation between grading, treatment, and outcome are shown in Table 5. Death was directly related to surgery in 12 cases (Table 6), one patient died due to bone marrow aplasia 3 months after discharge, another died of a supratentorial hemorrhage caused by a angioblastoma 7 weeks after decompressive surgery, and the last patient died 1 year after surgery due to clotting of an artificial aortic valve.

Discussion

Although surgical evacuation of hematomas is nowadays widely accepted as the treatment of choice [15] there are still reports of isolated cases where good outcome has been achieved either with conservative treatment [1] or with external ventricular drainage only [3]. The aim must be to recognize early the patient's grading and select the best treatment out of the variety of therapeutic possibilities. Taking the clinical status as well as the hematoma volume and compression of the basal cisterns (both from the CT scan), a fairly good classification can be achieved and used as a treatment guide. Different classifications have been published, most of them dividing the patients according to their clinical state [3, 6, 7, 13, 16] or CT scan findings [11, 15, 17]. Our approach is to make use of both since they complement each other. In our experience a patient grade II, drowsy, with only slight brainstem compression signs but with partial obliteration of the quadrigeminal cisterns and ventricular dilatation, will deteriorate if treated only with external ventricular drainage instead of also evacuating the hematoma, as happened in two of our cases, both with a fatal outcome. Acute diagnosis and treatment are of crucial importance since mortality increases markedly in comatose patients [4, 7, 8, 13, 15], reaching up to 95% in some cases [15]. Although coma and decerebration signs worsen the prognosis, they are not a contraindication for decompression: two of our grade III patients admitted in this condition recovered completely after decompressive surgery. The combination of coma and abolished corneal response is also a prognostically relevant feature (7 out of 15 patients admitted in our series with these signs died), and some authors have suggested that this is a probably irreversible state [11, 12]; however, we and many others encourage aggressive treatment in these cases [4, 7]. In experience, patients may recover and reach a functional life if decompression is performed quickly.

Isolated ventriculostomy is, in our opinion, the treatment of choice for small bleedings without signs of brainstem compression that are due to hemorrhage extension or occlusion of the fourth ventricle leading to occlusive hydrocephalus. In this case, if pressure is high (over 25 cm H_2O) we place the drainage first at about the opening pressure level over the head, reducing the distance at a rate of 5 cm/h until 5 or 10 cm has been reached. Ventriculostomy alone is still being suggested by some authors as the treatment of choice [3, 14]; this may be contraindicated in large hematomas because it does not decompress the brainstem, resulting in a danger of secondary upward herniation [2, 8, 12]. Indeed, results of cases treated in this way have a high mortality rate [8, 12, 16] comparable with that of conservative treatment [6, 15], and even worsening after ventriculostomy has also been reported [12]. Knüpling et al. [5] described deterioration of consciousness after ventriculography in patients with posterior fossa pathology which improved after direct brainstem decompression, or died if decompression did not occur. In the last group microcirculation disturbances were demonstrated in the mesencephalopontine area as a sign of upward herniation. Taking into account the results achieved in this study, we suggest direct brainstem decompression, if necessary combined with external ventricular drainage, in patients of grades II and III.

There is general agreement that hematomas with a diameter greater than 3 cm are related to occlusive hydrocephalus [6], tight posterior fossa [17], obliteration of the quadrigeminal cisterns [15], or intraventricular hemorrhage [13] and should be evacuated. Looking at the anatomy, the total volume of the posterior fossa is 160 cm^3 and the total volume of the cerebellum is 140 cm^3 [9]. That is why mass-occupying lesions of about 9 cm^3 (calculated from a hemorrhage of 3 cm) exceed the compensatory capacity of the posterior fossa and lead to brainstem compression.

Taneda et al. [15] demonstrated that hematoma size is a determinant of severity of brainstem compression or a predictor of outcome only at the extreme end of the volume range (when compensation is exhausted). This correlates with our findings in four grade I patients where decompressive surgery had to be done because of clinical deterioration although the hematoma volume was under 10 cm^3. Using hematoma size as the only parameter can lead to wrong surgical indications, as shown in the report of Bogousslavsky et al. of two cases of large spontaneous cerebellar haemorrhage treated conservatively with good results, probably because both patients (75 and 80 years of age) had marked cerebellar atrophy and were able to compensate the mass effect caused by the hemorrhage [1].

With the aid of this grading the main goals of treatment of spontaneous cerebellar hemorrhage (detection and removal of brainstem compression and obstructive hydrocephalus) can be matched, helping to improve outcome and reduce morbidity and mortality.

References

1. Bogousslavsky J, Regli F, Jeanrenaud X (1984) Benign outcome in unoperated large cerebellar haemorrhage. Report of 2 cases. Acta Neurochir 73:59–65
2. Brillman J (1979) Acute hydrocephalus and death one month after nonsurgical treatment for acute cerebellar hemorrhage. J Neurosurg 50:374–376
3. Firsching R, Huber M, Frowein R (1991) Cerebellar haemorrhage: management and prognosis. Neurosurg Rev 14:191–194
4. Heros RC (1982) Cerebellar hemorrhage and infarction. Stroke 13:106–109
5. Knüpling R, Fuchs EC, Stoltenburg G et al. (1979) Chronic and acute transtentorial herniation with tumors of the posterior cranial fossa. Neurochirurgia 22:9–17
6. Little JR, Tubman DE, Ethier R (1978) Cerebellar hemorrhage in adults. Diagnosis by computerized tomography. J Neurosurg 48:575–579

7. Lui TN, Fairholm DJ, Shu TF et al. (1985) Surgical treatment of spontaneous cerebellar hemorrhage. Surg Neurol 23:555–558
8. McKissock W, Richardson A, Walsh L (1960) Spontaneous cerebellar haemorrhage. A study of 34 consecutive cases treated surgically. Brain 83:1–9
9. Mitchell N, Angrist A (1942) Spontaneous cerebellar hemorrhage: Report of 15 cases. Am J Pathol 18:235–253
10. Mohadjer M, Braus DF, Myers A et al. (1992) CT stereotactic fibrinolysis of spontaneous intracerebral hematomas. Neurosurg Rev 15:105–110
11. Ott KH, Kase CS, Ojemann RG et al. (1974) Cerebellar hemorrhage: diagnosis and treatment. A review of 56 cases. Arch Neurol 31:160–167
12. Richardson AE (1972) Spontaneous cerebellar hemorrhage. In: Vinken PJ, Bruyn GW, (eds) Handbook of clinical neurology. Elsevier, New York, pp 54–67
13. Salazar J, Vaquero J, Martinez P et al. (1986) Clinical and CT scan assessment of benign versus fatal spontaneous cerebellar haematomas. Acta Neurochir 79:80–86
14. Shenkin HA, Zavala M (1982) Cerebellar strokes: mortality, surgical indications and results of ventricular drainage. Lancet 2:429–432
15. Taneda M, Hayakawa T, Mogami H (1987) Primary cerebellar hemorrhage. Quadrigeminal cistern obliteration on CT scans as a predictor of outcome. J Neurosurg 67:545–552
16. Waidhauser E, Hamburger C, Marguth F (1990) Neurosurgical management of cerebellar hemorrhage. Neurosurg Rev 13:211–217
17. Weisberg LA (1986) Acute cerebellar hemorrhage and CT evidence of tight posterior fossa. Neurology 36:858–860
18. Zieger A, Vonofakos D, Steudel WI (1984) Nontraumatic intracerebellar hematomas: prognostic value of volumetric evaluation by computed tomography. Surg Neurol 22:491–494

Cerebellar Hematomas: Prognosis and Risk of Upward Transtentorial Herniation

R. Firsching[1] and A. Kleindienst[1]

Cerebellar hematomas are no longer an almost exclusive postmortem finding since the advent of computed tomography (CT) [1, 2]. They are not particularly frequent either.

Patients and Methods

We encountered 44 patients between 1978 and 1992 at our Cologne hospital. Age ranged from 13 to 88. The probable cause of the hematomas was hypertension in 15 patients, a head injury in ten patients, anticoagulation in five patients, and an arteriovenous malformation in one patient. In 13 patients the probable cause remained unclear.

There were four alternatives for treatment; conservative treatment was preferred in eight patients; a ventricular shunt was placed in 28 patients (particular care was taken to maintain a positive intraventricular pressure of approximately 10 cm H_2O); the hematoma was evacuated in five patients; and in three patients it was evacuated in addition to a ventricular shunt.

Results

Mortality was quite variable (Fig. 1), ranging from 12% in the conservative group to 66% in patients in whom the hematoma had been evacuated and a ventricular shunt had been performed.

Mortality was also variable with the initial state of consciousness at the time of admission. In five fully alert patients there was no mortality at all; with clouding of consciousness it was 28%; in coma grade III, i.e., coma with extensor rigidity, mortality reached 87%. Among patients with wide responseless pupils there was no survivor (Fig. 1).

Location was also associated with outcome: mortality was 20% when only the hemispheres were affected, while it was 66% when midline structures were involved.

[1] Klinik für Neurochirurgie der Universität Köln, Joseph-Stelzmann-Straße 9, W-5000 Köln 41, FRG.

Advances in Neurosurgery, Vol. 21
R. Lorenz, M. Klinger, M. Brock (Eds.)

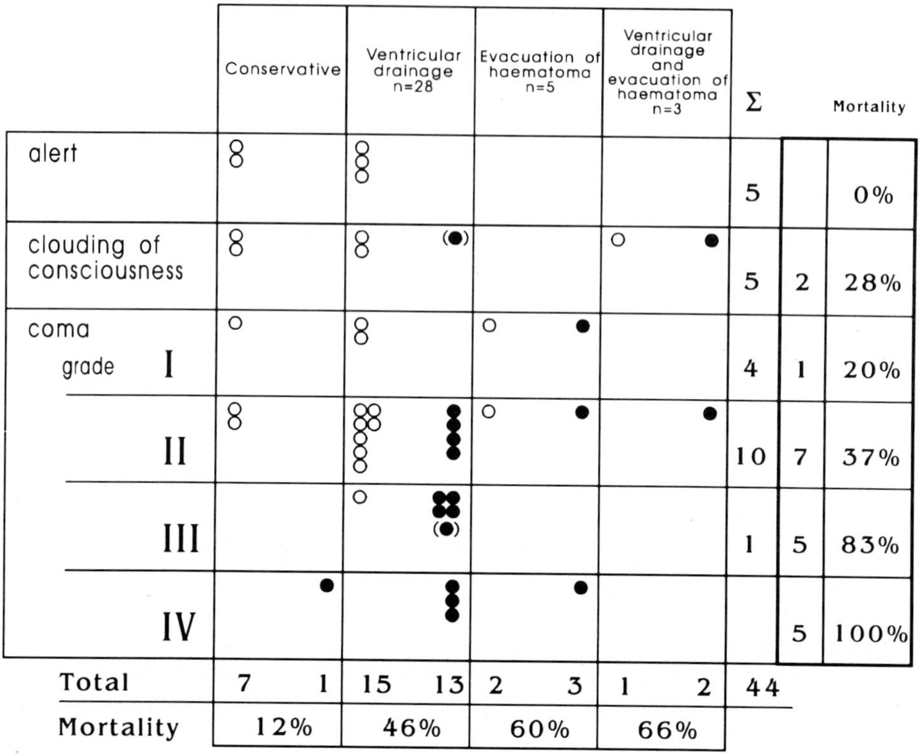

Fig. 1. Synopsis of level of consciousness, type of treatment, and survival. *Open circles*, survivors; *solid circles*, died; *circles in parenthesis*, died of unrelated cause

Evoked potentials were also correlated with outcome (Fig. 2). When a bilaterally normal somatosensory evoked potential (SEP), a brainstem auditory EP (BAEP), or a transcranial magnetic EP (TMEP) was recorded, all patients survived

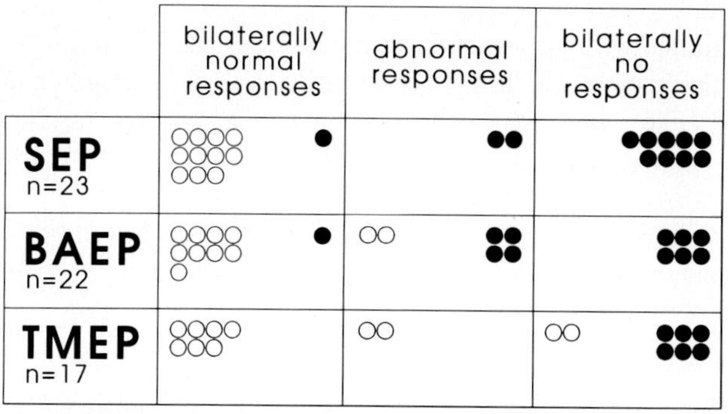

Fig. 2. Presence or absence of evoked potentials as related to outcome. *Open circles*, survivors; *solid circles*, died

		normal as related to age	enlarged as related to age
Intracranial pressure at placement of ventricular shunt	normal		○○○○ ○○○○ ●●
	above < 20 cm H_2O	●●	○○ ●●●●

Fig. 3. Size of ventricles and intracranial pressure as assessed at placement of shunt and relation with outcome. *Open circles*, survivors; *solid circles*, died

with only two exceptions. By contrast, when there were no reproducible responses, all patients except two died.

The most frequently taken measure was the placement of a ventricular shunt. Data on the size of ventricles and on the intraventricular pressure at the time the shunt was inserted are based on subjective assessment rather than on measurements. Only in two patients was the pressure measured and found to be higher than 20 cm H_2O. The relation of intracranial pressure and the size of ventricles was variable (Fig. 3). Enlarged ventricles were found with normal and with increased intracranial pressure. No patient deteriorated in temporal relation with the placement of a shunt.

Autopsy was possible in seven cases. Particular care was taken to find signs of upward transtentorial herniation (Fig. 4). This was the case in two autopsies and only in addition to cerebellar coning, in one of these cases after evacuation of the hematoma, in the other after ventricular drainage and evacuation. In five cases cerebellar coning within the foramen magnum was noted without upward transtentorial herniation after ventricular drainage only.

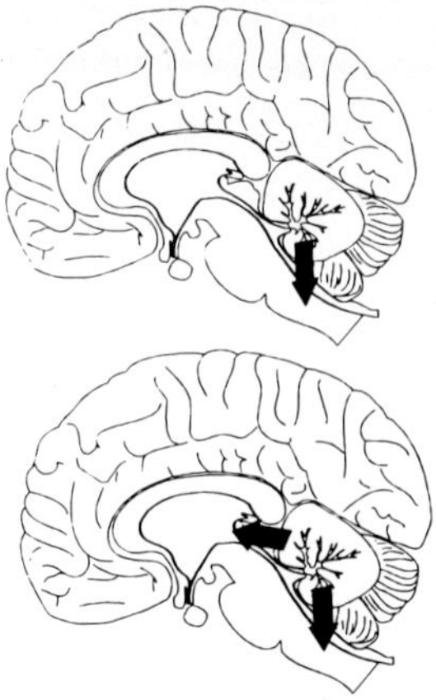

	Ventricular drainage	Evacuation of haematoma	Ventricular drainage and evacuation of haematoma
Coning	XXX XX		
Coning and transtentorial upward herniation		X	X

Fig. 4. Postmortem findings and preceding neurosurgical procedure

Discussion

Management of cerebellar hematomas is controversial [1, 2] and associated with a high mortality. Results from this analysis suggest a high prognostic value of the initial state of consciousness, location of the hematoma, and evoked potentials. Upward transtentorial herniation seems a rare occurrence and not necessarily a phenomenon associated with ventricular drainage.

Ventricular drainage itself appears a safe procedure, as long as ventricles are adequately large and a moderate positive intraventricular pressure is maintained. Evacuation of the hematoma seems warranted in comatose patients and in deteriorating patients with clouding of consciousness.

References

1. Firsching R, Frowein RA, Thun F (1987) Intracerebellar haematoma: 11 traumatic and non-traumatic cases and review of the literature. Neurochirurgia (Stuttg) 30:182–185
2. Firsching R, Huber M, Frowein RA (1991) Cerebellar haematoma: management and prognosis. Neurosurg Rev 14:191–194

Posterior Fossa Haematomas Secondary to Occult Angiomatous Malformation (Cavernomas)

L. Symon[1]

Although Luschka [2] in 1854 gave a description of what appears to have been an intracranial cavernoma, the first clear description of the entity was in 1928 by Walter Dandy [1]. The true frequency of symptomatic cavernomas remains hard to establish, but they are uncommon and probably represent only some 5%–13% of all CNS vascular anomalies, and estimates for the proposition below the tentorium vary from 10% to 23%. This report deals with our findings in 13 cases of brainstem haematoma related to confirmed cavernoma in 9 and probable cavernoma in the others, 12 lying within the brainstem and 1 in the superior vermis of the cerebellum. All were managed by direct microsurgical approach with evacuation of the haematoma and, in the majority of instances, verification of abnormal vessels consistent with cavernoma within the wall [5].

Characteristics of Cavernoma

Cavernoma is substantially a diagnosis nowadays based on magnetic resonance imaging (MRI). While the tumour itself consists of a well-defined purple or dark red lesion, the vascular spaces often visible to the naked eye form a honeycomb of unequal blood-filled spaces with no abnormally large feeding arteries or veins draining the lesion. This accounts for the largely negative findings at angiography.

The discovery of these lesions usually attends an episode of brainstem dysfunction consistent with an acute haemorrhage. Computed tomography (CT) characteristically shows a moderately hyperdense nodule with occasional modest contrast uptake, and calcification is observed in up to 33% of cases. MRI not only displays the lesion but gives evidence of current or previous haemorrhage. The nodule itself may show up as a multi-signal lesion with associated haemorrhage appearing either as high or low signal intensity depending upon its exact age. Older absorbed haemorrhages leave haemosiderin deposits in the gliotic border surrounding the lesion, and these show up particularly well on T2-weighted high-field imaging.

While angiography shows no abnormal circulation, we have found in two of our patients a co-existent but completely separate cerebellar venous anomaly, the so-called venous malformation, an association recently noticed by others [3].

---

[1] Gough-Cooper Department of Neurological Surgery, Institute of Neurology, The National Hospital, Queen Square, London WC1N 3BG, UK.

Advances in Neurosurgery, Vol. 21
R. Lorenz, M. Klinger, M. Brock (Eds.)

Clinical Findings

The best illustration of clinical findings is the description of a typical case: a 22-year-old woman who had four episodes of transient diplopia at the age of 4 years, at 9 years with sudden onset of hemiparesis which lasted for 6 weeks, and at 20 years, a left facial weakness, right hemiparesis and right hemisensory disturbance. She was found to have sixth and seventh cranial nerve palsies and CT and MRI revealed the cavernoma. Angiography was normal. A fourth acute episode occurred 19 months after the third, with sudden exacerbation of her facial palsy, loss of sensation on that side of the face, recurrence of the diplopia, and decreased power in the shoulder muscles on the left side. CT again showed a region of high density with calcification in the left pons. MRI revealed on T1- and T2-weighted sequences a well-defined multi-signal intensity lesion in the central and left pons surrounded by a rim of hypodensity which clearly indicated previous haemorrhage.

Surgical Approach

The surgical approach depends on the location of the cavernoma. In general the cavernoma should be approached from the nearest surface pial or ependymal. Thus in the case described above the approach was made through the lateral aspect of the pons. In other cases, a mid-line approach through the fourth ventricle has been used, the floor of the fourth ventricle being opened over any evident area of discolouration, care being taken to avoid the acoustic striae and the abducent colliculus. Identification of the seventh nerve nucleus is possible by direct stimulation of the floor of the fourth ventricle recording from the facial musculature, and it is also possible to determine the situation of the hypoglossal nuclei, provided recording is made in the tongue musculature.

Discussion

The overall lateral history of cavernomas remains ill defined. In cases which present with recurrent episodes of haemorrhage over many years there is little argument that such lesions are best excised if possible. It is less easy to advise surgery where there has been a single episode of haemorrhage with complete neurological recovery. Operation in the brainstem in the complete absence of neurological deficit requires careful consideration. Steiner [4] has recently indicated his view that cavernomas are not suitable for stereotactic radiosurgery. Stereotactic aspiration of the haematoma alone without removal of the causative lesion is of no value, and direct exploration is in our view best.

Modern techniques of microscopic neurosurgery render what might have seemed an impossible task some years ago quite feasible now, and in our own cases while there has been a transient exacerbation of neurological deficit in 3 of the 13, progressive improvement has thereafter occurred in all, with no recorded further haemorrhage in a follow-up extending from 6 months to 5 years.

References

1. Dandy WE (1928) Venous abnormalities and angiomas of the brain. Arch Surg 17:715–793
2. Luschka H (1854) Blutgeschwulst des Gehirns. Virchows Arch Path Anat 6:458–470
3. Rigamonti D, Spetzler R, Medina M, Rigamonti K, Geckle D, Pappas C (1990) Cerebral venous malformations. J Neurosurg 73:560–564
4. Steiner L, Lindquist, Steiner M. (1992) Radiosurgery In: Advances and technical standards in neurosurgery, vol 19. Springer, Berlin Heidelberg New York (in press)
5. Symon L, Jackowski A, Bills D (1991) Surgical treatment of pontomedullary cavernomas. Br J Neurosurg 5:339–347

Brainstem Hematomas Caused by Vascular Malformations: Results of Microsurgical Therapy

N. Klug[1], T. Betten[1] and G. Hildebrandt[1]

Arteriovenous malformations involving the posterior fossa represent treacherous lesions not only because of their propensity to hemorrhage but also because of the vital structures when located in a small confined space like the brainstem.

Because of the common use of magnetic resonance (MR) imaging [1, 6, 7, 12] intrinsic cavernous malformations of the brainstem are detected as another source of hemorrhage with increasing frequency. In such areas these lesions present a growing challenge to the neurosurgeon [2, 3, 8, 13, 14] who has to weigh the risks of a recurrent bleeding or growth [7, 10] of a brainstem cavernoma against its low bleeding rate in other CNS locations [1, 7].

To help clarify these issues, ten patients presenting with brainstem hematomas were reviewed to evaluate the results of microsurgical treatment aimed at the prevention of progressive morbidity.

Patients and Methods

The review included the historical, clinical, radiographic, neuromonitoring, and intraoperative data of ten patients with new or recurrent hemorrhages intrinsic to the brainstem (Table 1). The follow-up period ranged from 3 months to 4 years. In those in whom a definite pathological diagnosis was not obtained, highly characteristic MR images of cavernomas were deemed to be reliable, e.g., an inhomogeneous hyperintense signal surrounded by a hypointense ring on the T_2-weighted sequence [1, 6].

The neurological findings were classified into long tract and/or nuclear signs, obtained at basal state, 4–6 weeks postoperatively, and at the latest follow-up (Table 1). The surgical approach was chosen according to the relation of the lesion to the pial surface in order to minimize traumatization of eloquent nervous tissue, e.g., foci within the cerebellar peduncle and lateral pons were reached via the infratentorial supracerebellar approach [4] (Fig. 1). Intraoperative neuromonitoring, including somatosensory and brainstem evoked potentials, was applied in each case. Ultrasonography (Kontron) with a conventional transducer (5–7.5 MHz) was used in conjunction with a small metal clip to determine the shortest distance

[1] Neurochirurgische Klinik, Universität Köln, Joseph-Stelzmann-Straße 9, W-5000 Köln 41, FRG.

Advances in Neurosurgery, Vol. 21
R. Lorenz, M. Klinger, M. Brock (Eds.)

Table 1. Clinical data of ten patients presenting with brainstem hematomas

Patient no.	Age[a] (years)	Sex	Bleeding episodes (*n*)	Location	Time since last hemorrhage evacuation (months)	Surgical approach	Complete removal	Pathology	Recurrent bleeding postop-eratively	Follow-up (months)
1	32	m	2	Pons	3	Vermis and 4th ventricle	–	Atrioventricular malformation[b]	–	22
2	42	f	2	Midbrain	1	Vermis and 4th ventricle	–	Cavernoma	–	48
3	33	m	3	Pons	2	Supracerebellar, infratentorial	+	Cavernoma[b]	–	12
4	44	f	3	Pons	7	Supracerebellar, infratentorial	–	Cavernoma	–	9
5	38	m	2	Pons	1	Vermis and 4th ventricle	+	Cavernoma[b]	–	3
6	40	m	3	Pons	3	Vermis and 4th ventricle	–	Cavernoma[b]	–	2
7	6	m	1	Pons	1	Cerebellopontine angle	–	Cavernoma[b]	–	4
8	36	m	1	Pons	6	Vermis and 4th ventricle	+	Cavernoma	–	10
9	33	f	1	Midbrain	3	Subtemporal	+	Cavernoma	–	3
10	43	f	1	Pons	2	Cerebellopontine angle	–	Cavernoma	–	7

[a] Age at diagnosis. [b] Verified by histology.

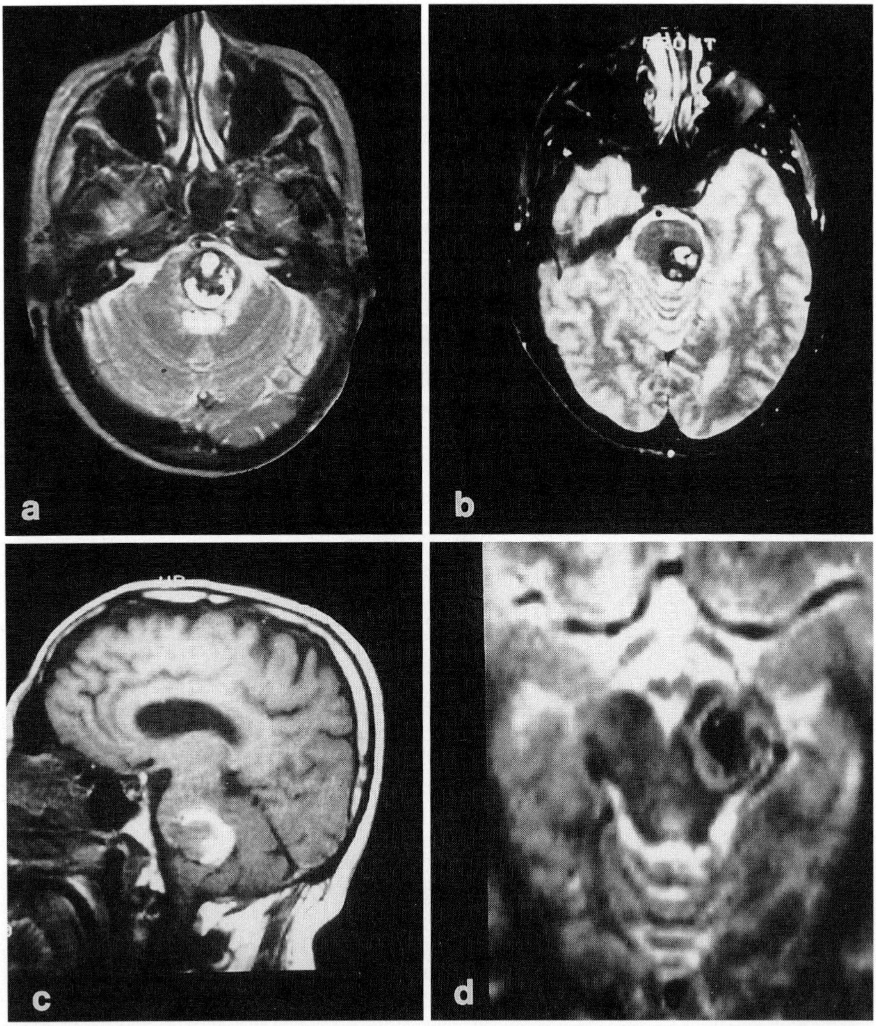

Fig. 1a–d. Preoperative MR images of cases 10 (**a**), 3 (**b**), 5 (**c**), and 9 (**d**). The cavernomas were removed by the transvermian, transventricular approach (case 5), via cerebellopontine angle (case 10), by the supracerebellar, infratentorial (case 3), or the subtemporal approach (case 9)

between the lesion and pial incision in cases 4, 6, 9, and 10. Cavernomas were removed bit by bit using an ultrasound aspirator, forceps, and bipolar coagulation.

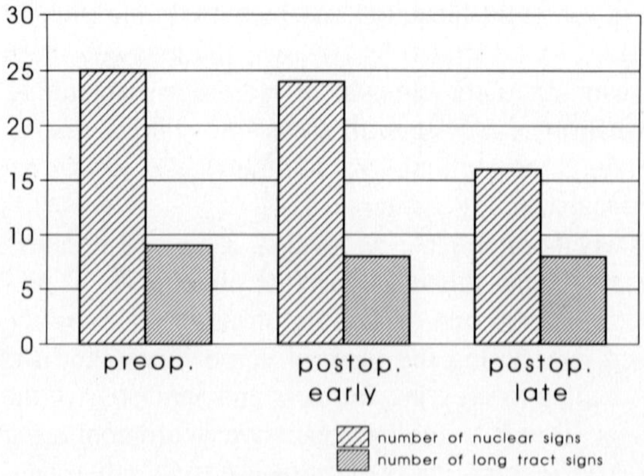

Fig. 2. Pre- and postoperative neurological signs after evacuation of brainstem hematomas ($n = 10$): *early*, 4–6 weeks postoperatively; *late*, latest follow-up

Results

A total number of 19 symptomatic episodes associated with progressive morbidity formed the indication for surgical treatment with different intervals between last hemorrhage and evacuation (Table 1). According to postoperative MR images, total removal of the underlying vascular malformations was performed in only four cases (Table 1). It was felt that complete resection in cases 1, 2, 4, 6, 7, and 10 was prevented by the firm and fibrotic surrounding nervous tissue containing dense fibrillary gliosis and extensive calcification [10].

This rendered the finding of a cleavage plane difficult. Nevertheless, no recurrent hemorrhage was observed during follow up (Table 1). Figure 2 outlines that the neurological performance had improved at the latest follow-up when compared with baseline findings.

In no case was an association of a cavernoma with a venous malformation observed intraoperatively [9, 14]. Cases 1–4, 6, and 7 experienced a psychoorganic syndrome lasting up to 2 weeks postoperatively which consisted of hyperactivity, depression, or cognitive impairment. No serious alterations of somatosensory or brainstem evoked potentials were recorded intraoperatively, despite occasional and transient neurological dysfunction during the immediate postoperative period (days 1–7).

Discussion

Using clinical evaluation, neuromonitoring, morphological data provided by anatomical landmarks [5], MR studies [12], intraoperative ultrasound localization techniques and different surgical corridors including combined approaches [11] the distance between pial incision and surface of a vascular brainstem malformation can be minimized. This strategy results in an acceptable morbidity in the early postoperative phase, prevention of recurrent bleeding, and increased neurological performance at late follow-up (Fig. 2) as is shown by our own findings and those of others [2, 13, 14]. Potential candidates for removal of brainstem hematomas with underlying vascular malformations are those with accessible lesions, associated with growth, symptomatic single or multiple gross hemorrhages and/or repeated episodes of distressing or incapacitating symptoms [14].

An unresolved issue remains whether complete removal of a brainstem cavernoma is feasible in every instance, whether this is an absolute prerequisite to prevent progressive neurological deterioration, and the timing of surgery aiming the optimal period between increased risk during the peak of acute illness and the point when cleavage planes are lost due to evolving firmness and adhesions of the perifocal nervous tissue. Moreover, in our hands intraoperative neuromonitoring turned out to have little predictive value concerning additional postoperative neurological deficits in the immediate postoperative period. It remains to be shown whether the intraoperative identification of various nuclei under the floor of the rhomboid fossa by electrophysiological means results in a better operative outcome.

References

1. Del Curling O, Kelly D, Elster AD, Craven TE (1991) An analysis of the natural history of cavernous angiomas. J Neurosurg 75:702–708
2. Fahlbusch R, Strauss C, Huk W, Röckelein G, Kömpf D, Ruprecht KW (1990) Surgical removal of pontomesencephalic cavernous hemangiomas. Neurosurgery 26:449–457
3. Hahn M, Aschoff A, Kunze S (1991) 667 histologically verified cavernous hemangiomas of the CNS: review of localization, symptoms, and signs, diagnosis, and results of operative treatment. In: Bock W-J, Brock M, Klinger M (eds) Advances in neurosurgery, vol 19. Springer, Berlin Heidelberg New York, pp 122–126
4. Laborde G, Gilsbach JM, Harders A, Seeger W (1992) Experience with the infratentorial supracerebellar approach in lesions of the quadrigeminal region, posterior third ventricle, culmen cerebelli and cerebellar peduncle. Acta Neurochir (Wien) 114:136–138
5. Lang J, Ohmachi N, Lang J (1991) Anatomical landmarks of the rhomboid fossa (floor of the 4th ventricle), its length and its width. Acta Neurochir (Wien) 113:84–90
6. Requena I, Arias M, López-Ibor L, Pereiro I, Barba A, Alonso A, Moután E (1991) Cavernomas of the central nervous system: clinical and neuroimaging manifestations in 47 patients. J Neurol Neurosurg Psychiatry 54:590–594
7. Robinson JB, Awad IA, Little JR (1991) Natural history of the cavernous angioma. J Neurosurg 75:709–714
8. Sakai N, Yamada M, Tanigawara T, Asano Y, Andoh T, Tanabe Y, Takada M (1991) Surgical treatment of cavernous angioma involving the brainstem and review of the literature. Acta Neurochir (Wien) 113:138–143
9. Sasaki O, Tanaka R, Kolke T, Koide A, Kolzumi T, Ogawa H (1991) Excision of cavernous angioma with preservation of coexisting venous angioma. J Neurosurg 75:461–464
10. Scott RM, Barnes P, Kupsky W, Adelman LS (1992) Cavernous angiomas of the central nervous system in children. J Neurosurg 76:38–46
11. Spetzler R, Daspit CP, Pappas CTE (1992) The combined supra- and infratentorial approach for lesions of the petrous and clival regions: experience with 46 cases. J Neurosurg 76:588–599

12. Wowra B, Layer G, Schad LR, Ullrich B, Semmler W, Aschoff A, Kiessling M, Kunze S (1991) Three-dimensional time-of-flight MR angiography and the surgical indication in brain stem cavernomas. Acta Neurochir (Wien) 112:77–82
13. Yoshimoto T, Suzuki J (1986) Radical surgery on cavernous angioma of the brain stem. Surg Neurol 26:72–78
14. Zimmermann RS, Spetzler RF, Lee KS, Zabramski JM, Hargraves RW (1991) Cavernous malformations of the brain stem. J Neurosurg 75:32–39

Spontaneous Intracerebral Hematomas: Considerations in Atypical Presentations

M. Westphal[1], D. Winkler[1], N. Freckmann[1], J. Freitag[2], and H. D. Herrmann[2]

Spontaneous intracerebral hematomas may present with a wide range of clinical symptoms and neuroradiological appearances. Upon presentation of a patient with an intracerebral hemorrhage (ICH) it needs to be decided whether there is time or necessity for further diagnostic procedures after the initial computed tomographic (CT) scan, which is still the most frequently used diagnostic tool. Apart from the clinical decision as to how urgently an evacuation of the clot needs to be undertaken, the decision for or against further diagnostic procedures has to be made if no underlying disease is known and the CT presentation is different from the typical ICH occurring in hypertensive patients.

In this context we present a series of 245 ICHs seen in the past 6 years and try to relate the diagnosis to the frequency of atypical presentations associated with intracerebral vascular disease and the specific neuroradiological features. In 29 cases, the clot was due to an aneurysmal rupture; 27 cases were associated with a cerebrovascular malformation; and in seven cases tumor was the cause of the bleeding. It is apparent from this analysis that in a high percentage an atypical ICH will be due to a neurosurgically treatable disease. The rate is 25% in this series. Therefore, whenever time (the clinical condition of the patient) and departmental organization permit, an angiography should be carried out. In this respect, special attention was focused on atypical presentations of clots. This was arbitrarily defined to be present when the clot was peripheral, was in connection with the sylvian fissure or other cerebrospinal fluid (CSF) cisternal spaces. Furthermore, lobar hematomas were considered atypical as were hemorrhages seen without mass effect and with clinical symptoms which were inappropriately insignificant in comparison to the size of the clot. This arbitrary definition will exclude most ICHs due to hypertension. The decision for further diagnostic procedures is based on clues from the patient's medical history. Arteriovenous malformations (AVM) as well as cavernous hemangiomas are frequently associated with seizures. An aneurysmal ICH, which may well occur without subarachnoid hemorrhage (SAH) (Fig. 1), is often due to a second aneurysmal rupture, and upon scrutinous interview of the patient or the relatives, a history of a previous SAH may be extracted. The lack of blood in the subarachnoid space complicates the distinction from

[1] Abteilung Neurochirurgie, Universitätskrankenhaus Eppendorf, Martinistraße 52, W-2000 Hamburg 20, FRG.
[2] Abteilung Neuroradiologie, Universitätskrankenhaus Eppendorf, Martinistraße 52, W-2000 Hamburg 20, FRG.

Advances in Neurosurgery, Vol. 21
R. Lorenz, M. Klinger, M. Brock (Eds.)

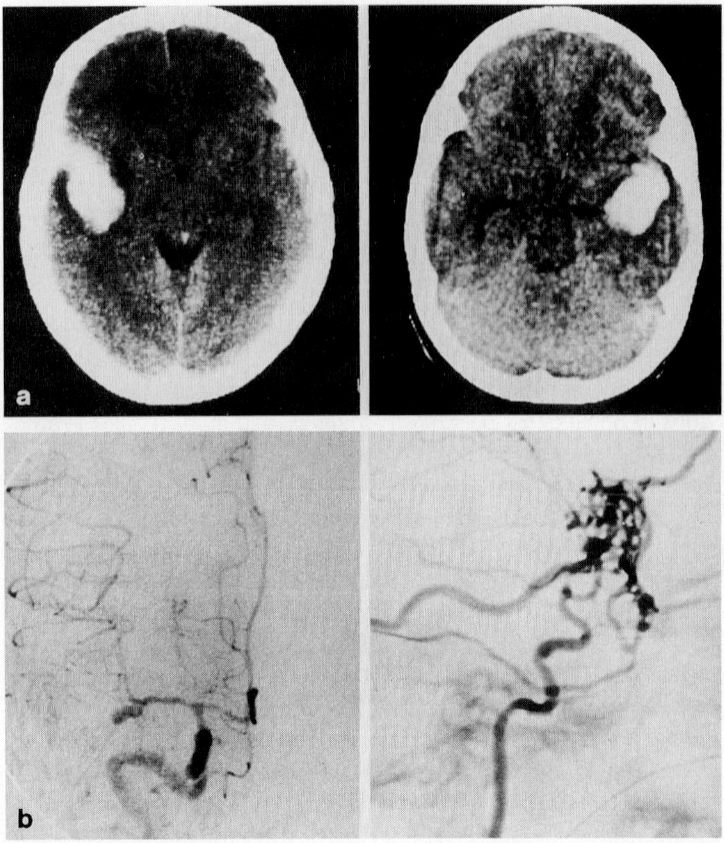

Fig. 1a, b. Two temporal hematomas with close anatomical relationship with the sylvian fissure which were due either to an aneurysm (**a**) or to an AVM (**b**)

hematomas of other causes such as AVM (Fig. 1). Finally dural fistulas are often associated with a pulsatile bruit.

Histological examination was only inconsequentially performed. Two patients had amyloid angiopathy and one of these presented with several successive hemorrhages in different anatomical locations, which is in agreement with the reported high frequency of multiple ICH in these patients [7]. Only in seven cases was a tumor the cause of an ICH. It was interesting though that three of the tumors were oligodendrogliomas, which in our series seem to have a tendency to hemorrhage more than the other histological types of tumor.

Table 1. Intracerebral hematomas and underlying disease; disease association with ICH

Disease	Clot (n)	Total in series (n)
Aneurysm	106	663
AVM	26	176
Cavernoma	11	35
Dural fistula	15	89
	158	963

To support our findings, we also used another approach and determined the rate of ICH in our series of aneurysms, AVMs, cavernomas, and dural fistulas (Tables 1, 2). Of 663 aneurysms seen in our department and documented over the past 7 years, 106 were accompanied by an intracerebral clot. Patients with an AVM had a clot in 26 of 176 cases. Cavernomas were also frequently associated with an acute clot or evidence of a previous clot (11/35) which, however, was only rarely the reason for an immediate operation. Among 89 cranial dural AVMs, 13 either presented with a hemorrhage or had a hemorrhage in their past history. It was observed that the risk of hemorrhage is close to 70% in the presence of a cortical venous drainage of the type seen in the carotid-cavernous sinus fistula shown in Fig. 2 and reported in the literature [1, 4]. All of the 13 fistulas associated with ICH had such cortical venous drainage. Among these four disease entities, the rate of intraparenchymal hemorrhage is 16.4%. Other vascular disorders which may be the cause of an acute clot and are revealed in angiography are moyamoya disease or venous thrombosis.

Neuroradiologically, cavernomas often present with a clot which appears irrelevant to the surrounding brain [10]. Angiography is usually negative and, together with a history of seizures, the diagnosis of a cavernoma is more likely than anything else. It has been stated in recent series [2, 11] that the risk of cavernomas bleeding is very low and this is especially true for a rebleeding, which is the main threat to patients with either aneurysm or AVM. Thus magnetic resonance imaging should be performed to further secure the diagnosis and distinguish from an ICH

Table 2. Cause of intracerebral hemorrhage in 245 surgical cases

Cause	Total in series (n)
Aneurysm (n)	29
AVM/cavernoma (n)	27
Tumor (n)	7
– Glioblastoma	3
– Oligodendroglioma	3
– Sarcoma	1

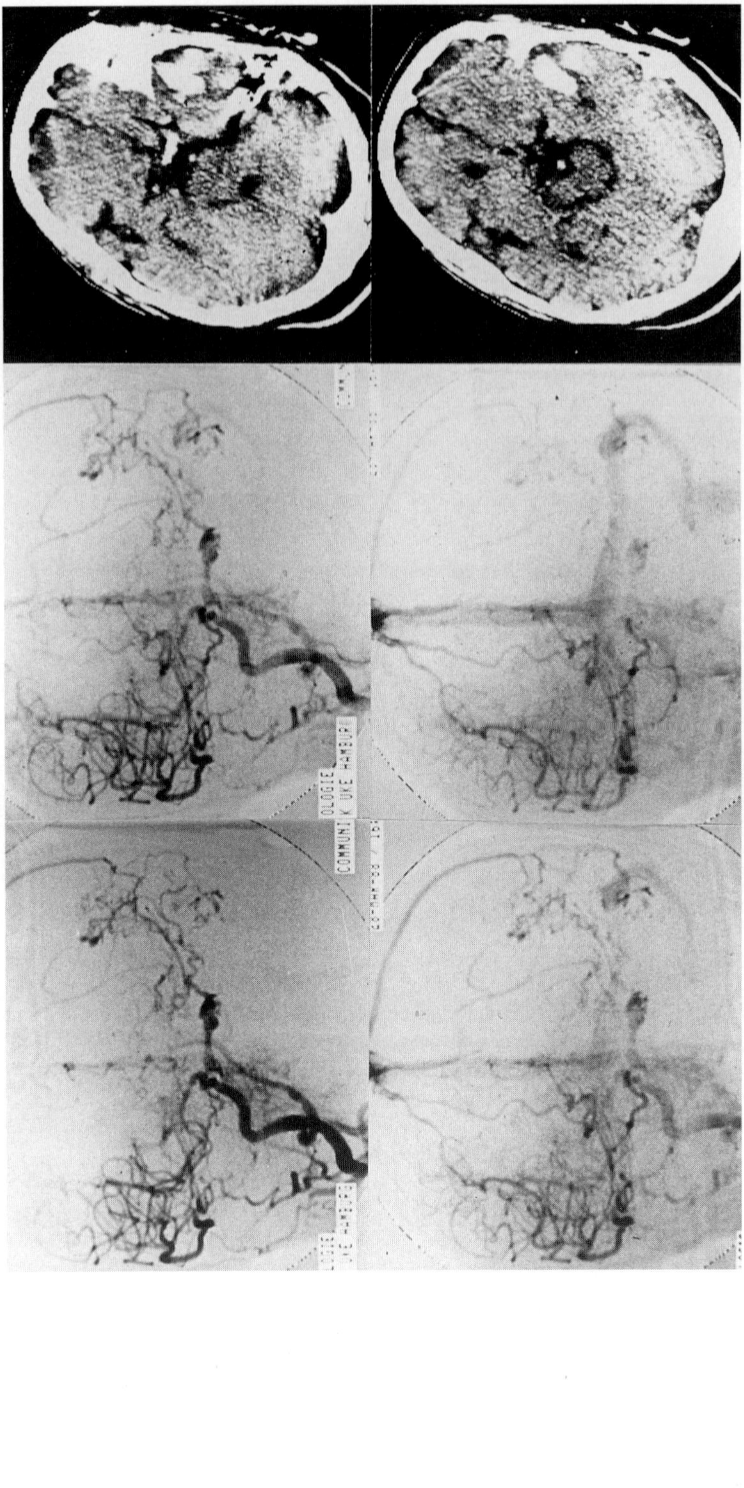

Fig. 2. Right-sided temporobasal hematoma due to a carotid-cavernous fistula on the left side, draining to the contralateral side via the intercavernous sinus and then through a cortical vein to the superior saggital sinus

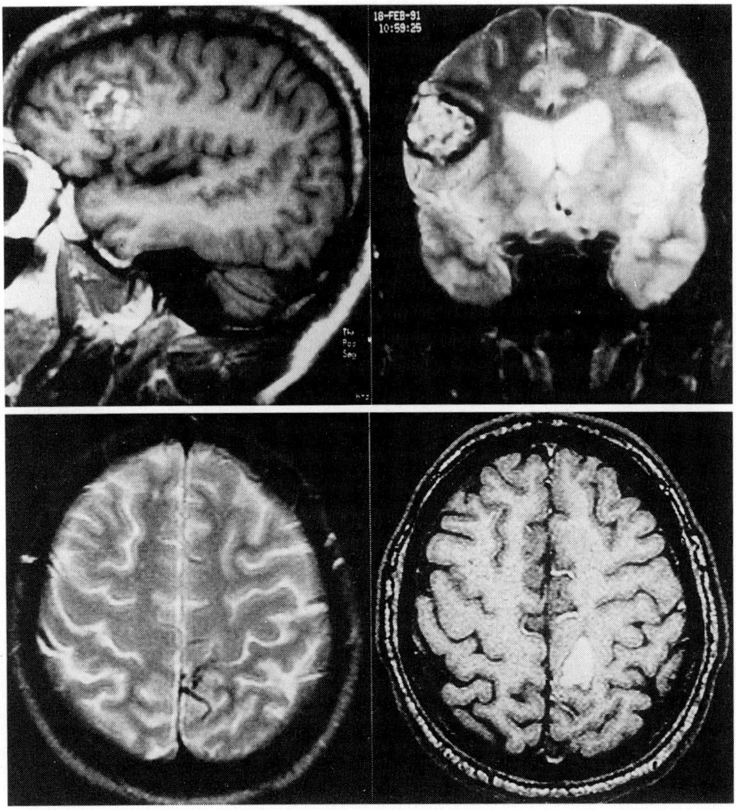

Fig. 3a, b. Two typical cases of "inert" small intracerebral clots. In one patient, the remnants of a recent frontolateral, superficial hemorrhage are still visible but also a thick ring of deposited hemosiderin indicating frequent earlier bleedings at this site due to a cavernous hemangioma (**a**). In the other case, two images, 6 weeks apart, show the resolution of a small inert hemorrhage in the left parietal region close to the cortex with no signs of hemosiderin at the time of bleeding and very little later, which is seen on another lower cut which is not shown. The tubular structure seen on both images already indicates that the hemorrhage was due to an AVM which had bled for the first time

due to an AVM (Fig. 3). When the decision is made to evacuate the clot or to remove the lesion, it is permissible to wait for the optimal time point, which is in the postacute phase in which the hematoma has liquified and drainage of the fluid during the procedure easily provides further space for removal with least traumatization.

It is concluded that an angiography should be performed whenever time permits and a lesion is atypical for hypertensive hemorrhage or no coagulopathy due to leukemia, liver disease, or medical anticoagulation is known to be present. This information is essential because, according to the literature [5, 8], the rate of anticoagulation in ICH is about 14% when trauma, tumor, or aneurysm are excluded.

Prior angiography allows the choice between therapeutic options, among which interventional neuroradiological measures are to be considered and, in the case of dural fistulas, should be preferred to surgical intervention. In the presence of an aneurysm, an approach would need to be selected which allows the exposure of the main arterial trunks in case of a rupture of the aneurysm during evacuation of the clot.

Upon presentation of an ICH, the decision about the immediate necessity of surgical intervention is made in accordance with the established rules [3, 9]. Careful analysis of the CT in respect to the size of the clot, its location, and its impact on the surrounding brain, together with the medical history of the patient then provide further clues for possible underlying causes and will improve management of intracerebral hematoma by allowing the selection of the appropriate surgical or neuroradiological treatment option and strategy. It is to be expected that atypical ICH will become more frequent due to acquired immunodeficiency syndrome and substance abuse [6].

References

1. Awad IA, Little JR, Akrawi WP, Ahl J (1990) Intracranial dural arteriovenous malformations: factors predisposing to an aggressive neurological course. J Neurosurg 72:839–850
2. Del Curling O, Kelly DL, Elster AD, Craveb TE (1991) An analysis of the natural history of cavernous angiomas. J Neurosurg 75:702–708
3. Herrmann HD, Arnold H (1986) Operationsindikationen bei spontanen intracraniellen Blutungen. Nervenheilkunde 5:130–134
4. Hiramatsu K, Utsumi S, Kyoi K, Sakaki T, Tada T, Iwasaki S, Kichikawa K (1991) Intracerebral hemorrhage in carotid-cavernous fistula. Neuroradiology 33:67–69
5. Kase CS, Robinson RK, Stein RW, DeWitt LD, Hier DB, Harp DL, Williams JP, Caplan LR, Mohr JP (1985) Anticoagulant-related intracerebral hemorrhage. Neurology (NY) 35:943–948
6. Klonoff DC, Andrews BT, Obana WG (1989) Stroke associated with cocaine use. Arch Neurol 46:989–993
7. Leblanc R, Preul M, Robitaille Y, Villemure J-G, Pokrupa R (1991) Surgical considerations in cerebral amyloid angiopathy. Neurosurgery 29:712–718
8. Radberg JA, Olsson JE, Radberg CT (1991) Prognostic parameters in spontaneous intracerebral hematomas with special reference to anticoagulant treatment. Stroke 22:517–576
9. Tsementis SA (1985) Surgical management of intracerebral hematomas. Neurosurgery 16:562–572
10. Westphal M, Winkler D, Nowak G, Schwachenwald R, Arnold H, Herrmann HD (1991) Cerebral cavernous hemangiomas: treatment and surgical decisions. Adv Neurosurg 19:110–115
11. Zimmermann RS, Spetzler RF, Lee KS, Zabramski JM, Hargraves RW (1991) Cavernous malformations of the brain. J Neurosurg 75:32–39

Morbidity and Mortality of Patients with Spontaneous Intracerebral Hematoma

J. Nadstawek[1], J. Zentner[2], U. Ruta[1], S. Albrecht[1], and B. Kaden[2]

Introduction

Spontaneous intracerebral hemorrhage accounts for about 10% of all strokes and is associated with high morbidity and mortality [4, 6, 10]. The initial level of consciousness, hemorrhage size, and intraventricular extension of blood have proven to be accurate predictors of outcome [2, 5, 8]. Predisposing factors are hypertension, treatment with anticoagulants, alcoholism, and coronary heart disease, all affecting cerebral vasculature [1, 3, 5, 9]. However, the influence of these factors on the course of the disease has not been established so far in the literature. Therefore, this study was designed to clarify whether risk factors predisposing to spontaneous intracerebral hemorrhage are important with respect to the prognosis of these patients.

Patients and Methods

This retrospective study included 242 patients, aged 10–80 years, with computed tomography verified spontaneous intracerebral hematomas who were treated in the intensive care unit (ICU) of the Department of Neurosurgery, University of Bonn, between 1982 and 1990. There were 101 women and 141 men. The average age was 54 years. Patients with hemorrhage resulting from trauma, brain tumor, or vascular malformation were excluded. Data analyzed in particular were those of medical history and current diagnoses with special regard to risk factors predisposing to intracerebral hemorrhage such as hypertension, diabetes, coronary heart disease, treatment with anticoagulants, and alcoholism. Patients were divided into to groups depending on the presence or absence of these risk factors as evaluated on the basis of current findings and the patients' histories and/or information from their relatives. The course of disease and outcome was assessed using a modified Glasgow Outcome Scale (GOS) [7] and evaluated for both groups. Observation time was at least 2 months after initial treatment. Data collection and evaluation were computerized (dBase III+). The nonparametric test of statistical significance was the Mann-Whitney *U* test.

[1] Institut für Anästhesiolgie, Universität Bonn, Sigmund-Freud-Straße 25, W-5300 Bonn 1, FRG.
[2] Neurochirurgische Klinik, Universität Bonn, Sigmund-Freud-Straße 25, W-5300 Bonn 1, FRG.

Advances in Neurosurgery, Vol. 21
R. Lorenz, M. Klinger, M. Brock (Eds.)

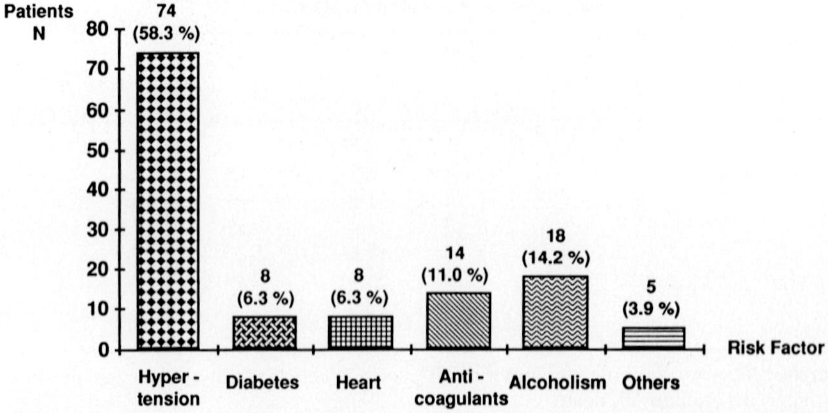

Fig. 1. Frequency of different risk factors predisposing to spontaneous intracerebral hemorrhage in 127 patients

Results

Of the 242 patients, 127 (52.5%) had risk factors predisposing to intracerebral hemorrhage. The most frequent condition was hypertension, found in 74 patients (58.3%). Of the remaining patients, 8 (6.3%) suffered each from coronary heart disease or diabetes mellitus; 14 (11.0%) were treated with anticoagulants. Alcoholism was observed in 18 (14.2%) patients. Five patients (3.9%) had other risk factors such as hepatopathy or renal disorders (Fig. 1).

The average duration of stay in the ICU was 9.6 days. Patients with risk factors had to be treated in the ICU for an average of 14 days as opposed to 7 days for patients without risk factors (Fig. 2); this difference is statistically significant.

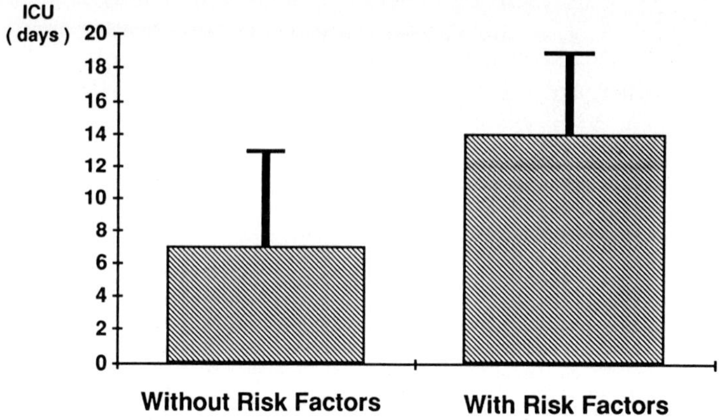

Fig. 2. Duration of treatment in the ICU of patients with and without risk factors

Table 1. Outcome (GOS) of patients with and without risk factors

	Without risk factors		With risk factors		Total	
GOS	*n*	%	*n*	%	*n*	%
I	3	2.6	1	0.8	4	1.7
II	10	8.6	8	6.3	18	7.4
III	11	9.6	15	11.8	26	10.7
IV	18	15.7	17	13.4	35	14.5
V	4	3.5	16	12.6	20	8.3
VI	69	60.0	70	55.1	139	57.4
Total	115	47.5	127	52.5	242	100.0

I, Complete recovery; II, moderate disability; III, considerable disability; IV, severe disability; V, vegetative status. VI, death.

The outcome of our patients with and without risk factors predisposing to intracerebral hemorrhage is presented in Table 1. Ninety-six (60.0%) of the patients without and 70 (55.1%) with risk factors died. The others survived with outcome scores from I to V. Among these there were 4 patients (3.5%) without and 16 (12.6%) with risk factors who survived in a vegetative status (GOS V); this difference is statistically significant. The remaining patients, showing outcome scores between I and IV, were distributed nearly equally in the two groups.

The cerebral situation was the main problem influencing course of disease in the ICU in 34 patients (29.6%) without and in 38 (29.9%) with risk factors. Internal medical problems were the principal disorders in 18 patients (15.6%) without and in 35 (27.6%) patients with risk factors (Table 2).

Discussion

Many reports address epidemiologic, pathophysiologic, and therapeutic aspects of spontaneous intracerebral hemorrhage [2, 5, 6, 9, 10]. There is general agreement that several factors such as hypertension, diabetes, coronary heart disease, treatment with anticoagulants, and alcoholism may predispose to hemorrhage [1, 3, 4]. To our knowledge, no report exists addressing their influence on the course of dis-

Table 2. Main disorders in patients with and without risk factors

	Without risk factors (*n* = 115)		With risk factors (*n* = 127)		Total (*n* = 242)	
Main disorders	*n*	%	*n*	%	*n*	%
Cerebral	34	29.6	38	29.9	72	29.8
Internal medical	18	15.6	35	27.6	53	21.9

ease. Therefore, this study was designed to clarify whether these risk factors are important with respect to the prognosis of these patients.

Our results show that the duration of stay in the ICU correlates strongly with the presence or absence of risk factors (14 versus 7 days on average). Moreover, internal medical disorders were the predominant problem in 15.6% of the patients without but in 27.6% of the patients with risk factors. In general, we did not find significant differences in the groups regarding outcome. However, it is remarkable that only 3.5% of the patients without but 12.6% of those with risk factors survived in vegetative status. This difference is statistically significant.

The total mortality rate (57.4%) of our patients was higher than that reported in the recent literature, where numbers ranging around 35% are reported [5, 9]. This results from our selection of patients since we considered only patients primarily treated in the ICU; obviously these patients were in a relatively bad condition. Therefore, our figures in terms of mortality and morbidity are not representative for all patients with spontaneous intracerebral hemorrhage seen in our institution.

A major problem of this study is that the criteria for assignment of patients to one or the other group (with or without risk factors) were based mainly on the history obtained from patients and/or their relatives. It can be assumed that these data are unreliable to some extent. Some of our patients assigned to the group without risk factors may have had distinct internal medical disorders that remained obscure. However, in our opinion it is very difficult or even impossible to evaluate unknown risk factors at the time when severe impact on the life resulting from the hemorrhage itself interferes with preexisting disorders.

In conclusion, risk factors predisposing to intracerebral hemorrhage may influence the course of the disease and, at least in part, the outcome. Therefore it seems essential to include these risk factors in prognostic evaluation and decision making for adequate treatment (surgical versus conservative) of patients with spontaneous intracerebral hemorrhage.

References

1. Brott T, Thalinger K, Hertzberg V (1986) Hypertension as a risk factor for spontaneous intracerebral hemorrhage. Stroke 17:1078–1083
2. Bolander HG, Kourtopoulos H, Liliequist B, Wittboldt S (1983) Treatment of spontaneous intracerebral haemorrhage. A retrospective analysis of 74 consecutive cases with special reference to computer tomographic data. Acta Neurochir 67:19–28
3. Calandre L, Arnal C, Fernandez Ortega J (1986) Risk factors for spontaneous cerebral hematomas. Case-control study. Stroke 17:1126–1128
4. Garraway WM, Whisnant JP, Furlan AJ, Phillips LH, Kurland LT, O'Fallon WM (1979) The declining incidence of stroke. New Engl J Med 300:449–452
5. Helweg-Larsen S, Sommer W, Strange P, Lester J, Boysen G (1984) Prognosis for patients treated conservatively for spontaneous intracerebral hematomas. Stroke 15:1045–1048
6. McKissok W, Richardson A, Taylor J (1961) Primary intracerebral hemorrhage: a controlled trial of surgical and conservative treatment in 180 unselected cases. Lancet II:221–226

7. Nadstawek J, Böker DK, Hausmann D, Wassmann H, van Roost D (1989) Neurological and neuropsychological of prolonged comatose patients. In: Bartko D, Gerstenbrand F, Turcani P (eds) Neurology in Europe. Libbey, London, pp 393–397
8. Portenoy RK, Lipton RB, Berger AR, Lesser ML, Lantos G (1987) Intracerebral hemorrhage: a model for the prediction of outcome. J Neurol Neurosurg Psychiatry 50:976–979
9. Schütz H, Bödecker RH, Damian M, Krack P, Dorndorf W (1990) Age-related spontaneous intracerebral hematoma in a German community. Stroke 21:1412–1418
10. Weisberg LA (1979) Computerized tomography in intracranial hemorrhage. Arch Neurol 36:422–426

Stereotactic Evacuation and Local Fibrinolysis of Spontaneous Intracerebral Hematomas

K. D. Lerch[1], D. Schäfer[1], and J. Uelzen[1]

Introduction

Since introduction of computerized tomography (CT) by Hounsfield in 1974 [4] soft tissue differentiation in the imaging of brain lesions has become self-evident; the differential diagnosis of the origin of stroke – infarction versus hemorrhage or versus hemorrhagic infarction – can be made immediately after the onset of the uniform symptomatology indicating a clinical entity. However, having obtained the concrete diagnosis of spontaneous intracerebral hematoma (ICH) the discussion as to what kind of treatment would be the best – conservative or operative – still remains controversial [3, 12].

The main problem is that nobody knows whether a patient with spontaneous ICH in the basal ganglia who is primarily in a good condition and for whom a conservative mode is adopted may remain in that stable condition or may deteriorate later, so that the decision for conventional open surgery might increase the risk of this tendency to deteriorate with the well-known poor results; on the other hand, open surgery traumatizes the surrounding brain structures and tends to fix or even to increase the preoperative neurological deficit so that no surgeon wants to make the decision for surgery when the patient is still in a good condition. In this dilemma the stereotactic evacuation of hematomas through a small burr hole, or even by percutaneous trephination which was first described by Backlund and von Holst [1], offers a true therapeutic alternative. Through a special evacuation canula (hematoma evacuator), designed on the principle of an Archimedes screw, up to 50% of the volume of a hematoma could be removed [8].

The operative procedure proved to be less traumatic than open surgery, especially where deep-seated hemorrhages were concerned. With technical modifications [13] and the introduction of local fibrinolysis using urocinase [9, 11] it is now possible to liquefy remaining blood clots and to remove up to 80%–90% of an ICH.

[1] Neurochirurgische Klinik der Städtischen Kliniken, Münsterstraße 240, W-4600 Dortmund 1, FRG.

Advances in Neurosurgery, Vol. 21
R. Lorenz, M. Klinger, M. Brock (Eds.)

Materials and Methods

Patients

From April 1988 to October 1991 58 patients with spontaneous ICH (34 male and 24 female) underwent stereotactic hematoma evacuation. Eighteen patients presented with lobar hematomas and 40 with hemorrhages in the basal ganglia. Intraventricular rupture, mainly from hemorrhages in the basal ganglia, occurred in 21 cases. Preoperative conventional or digital substraction angiography (DSA) was performed in order to exclude a vascular malformation as the source of bleeding. In cases of a localization and a patient's age which are atypical of a spontaneous hypertensive ICH, an examination by magnetic resonance (MR) was also performed in order to identify angiographically occult angiomas. Patients with extensive brainstem herniation and late midbrain syndrome regularly were not operated stereotactically. Volume of the hematomas ranged from 10 to 113 ml; mean volume was 35 ml. Patients anamnestic data revealed the primary disease and thus also the cause of bleeding: in 26 patients arterial hypertension had been known over several years, five underwent anticoagulative therapy for different reasons, eight were chronic alcoholics, and in six an extensive vascular encephalopathy was found by CT, while 23 cases remained agnogenic.

Study Design

The level of consciousness was documented according to the Glasgow Coma Scale (GCS) [5] and neurological deficits such as hemiparesis, aphasia, and others were documented according to the recommendations of the British Medical Research Council [2]. Before hematoma evacuation and during the first 2 days after operation, neurological examinations were carried out every 8 h accompanied by CT volumetry.

Surgical Procedure

In general the stereotactic evacuation was performed under local anesthesia; in cases of patient intolerance because of confusion and in cases of respiratory obstruction or depressed respiratory function, patients were operated on under neuroleptanalgesia with laryngeal intubation. First of all the basic frame of our Dortmund Microstereotactic System [6] was attached to the patient's skull and then a CT examination was performed under stereotactic conditions. The rectangular (cartesian) coordinates (x, y, z) of the target point were read directly by means of target plates. In additional, coronal and sagittal image reconstructions were made in order to determine a trajectory leading right through the mean axis of the hematoma. The initial volume of the hematoma was measured digitally by the CT

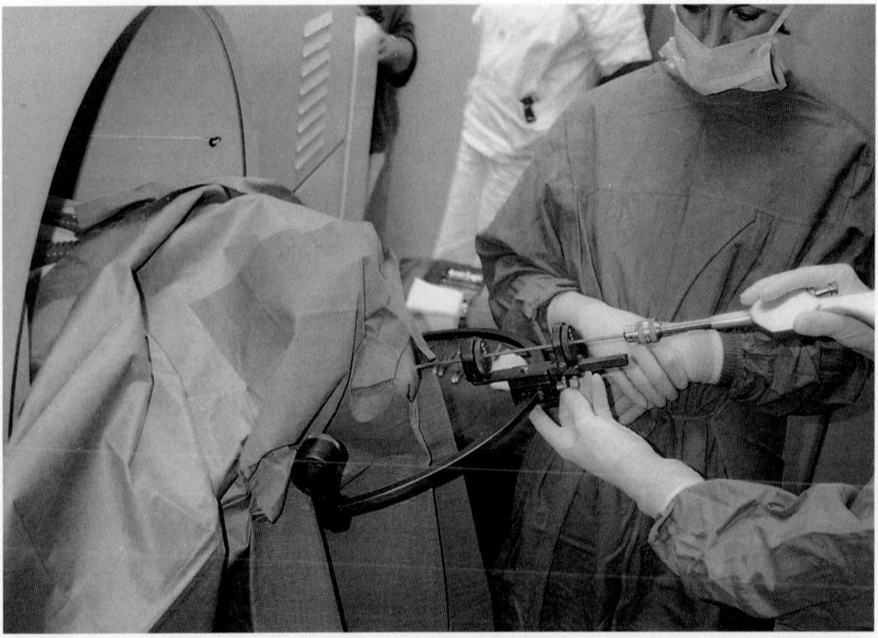

Fig. 1. Performance of stereotactic operation in the gantry of the CT. The couch has been pushed through the aperture to the back of the gantry. Percutaneous trephination with Steinmann's nail

scanner's "region of interest" in order to obtain a basic value for comparison during the postoperative follow- up.

In order to control the success of evacuation immediately intraoperatively under the same positioning and scan level, we aspired to perform the operation directly in the gantry of the CT (Fig. 1).

The approach can be planned according to the Centre-of-Arc principle, or the aiming trajectory can be defined by two points (entry and target points). The next steps are percutaneous trephination with Steinmann's nail (4 mm in diameter) [7], which is driven by a hand or air drill; introduction of an aspiration cannula with a frontal hole or a side window along the aiming trajectory, which corresponds to the mean axis of the hematoma, and stepwise aspiration by manually controlled gentle suction; intracerebral pressure monitoring with the Camino intracranial pressure (ICP) device (Fig. 4). CT examination with volumetry has to be repeated some minutes later in order to exclude rebleeding. If 80%–90% of the hematoma can be removed, the cannula is withdrawn, and the operation is finished. If the residual blood volume is more than 20% of the initial volume, a silicon tube (ventricular catheter) with a multiperforated tip is introduced into the middle of the clot for local fibrinolysis with urokinase. For this purpose, 5000 IU urokinase dissolved in 2 ml saline solution is instilled. After 6 h we aspirate again and control the result

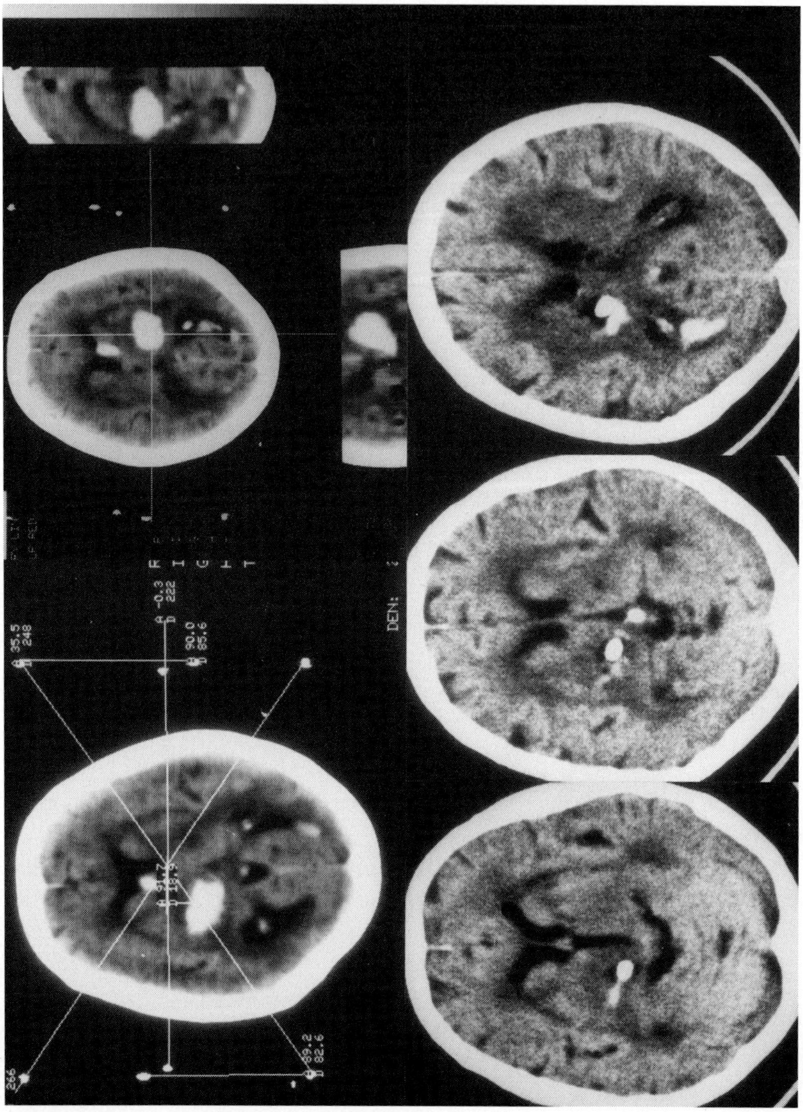

Fig. 2. Intrathalamic hemorrhage. CT-guided definition of the target's coordinates and of the angulation of the entering trajectory representing the mean axis of the hematoma by coronal and sagittal reconstructions. Postoperative CT examination demonstrates complete removal of the ICH; the silicon catheter is still in place

by CT; this sequence is repeated up to six times until the hematoma is almost completely removed (Fig. 2).

Results

The ultimate goal of stereotactic evacuation is to achieve an extensive but subtotal removal of a space-occupying ICH in order to decompress the surrounding recuperative brain tissue, thus favorably influencing the perifocal vasogenic brain edema and the local cerebral blood flow. Aspiration alone was sufficient for almost complete evacuation in eight ganglionic and in four lobar hemorrhages; local fibrinolysis became necessary in 46 cases. The mortality in the postoperative course of 2 weeks was 10% and the operative morbidity 5%. Rebleeding, which occurred in seven cases, was responsible for mortality in two and morbidity in another two cases. The follow-up of patients' consciousness (GCS) and the development of neurological deficit during the postoperative course is shown in Fig. 3 in the case of ganglionic bleedings. The graphics for lobar hemorrhages look quite similar. Focal neurological deficit such as hemiplegia/hemiparesis improved in 46% of cases, and aphasia in 60% of cases. The response curve of perifocal ICP measurements shown in Fig. 4 demonstrates how the pressure is decreased by stepwise aspiration of the hematoma.

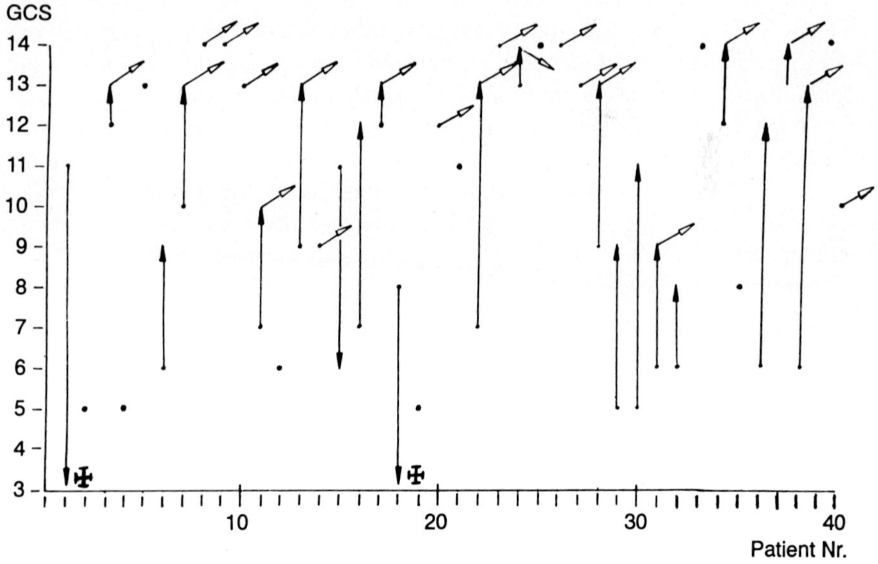

Fig. 3. Development of consciousness evaluated according to the Glasgow Coma Scale (*GCS*) in 40 patients with spontaneous basal ganglionic hematomas from preoperative state (*dots*) to 7 days postoperatively (*black arrows*). *Diagonal arrows*, course of the focal neurological deficit: *upwards*, improvement; *downwards*, deterioration

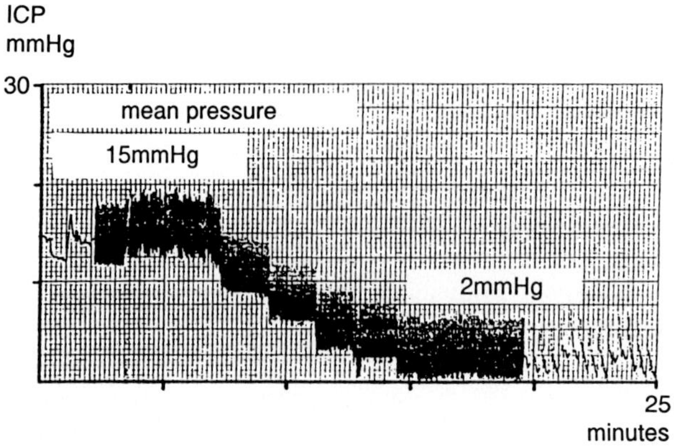

Fig. 4. Monitoring of ICP in frontal subcortical location of the affected hemisphere during stereotactic aspiration of a large putaminal hematoma. The mean pressure decreases from initially 15 mm Hg to 2 mm Hg after aspiration of 25 ml coagulated hematoma in five steps over a period of 15 min

Discussion

Analyzing the lethal factors of spontaneous intracerebral hemorrhage, the volume of the hematoma, the localization, and the extension of the intraventricular rupture are revealed as the most decisive criteria. The critical volume in the case of supratentorial localization amounts to 30 ml; above this value mortality increases dramatically to about four times [14]. Conventional open operative decompression could not produce decisive advantages compared with conservative treatment, especially in the case of ganglionic location. Operatively induced additional brain edema as well as direct damage to brain tissue while penetrating the cortical and subcortical structures with consecutive accentuation of the neurological deficit were reasons given for the unsatisfactory results as far as mortality and morbidity were concerned [3, 12]. Summarizing 13 papers published during the post-CT era [10], conservative treatment revealed a mean mortality of 35% and a mean morbidity of 13%, while open neurosurgical treatment showed a mortality of 30% and an operative morbidity of 17%. The same author reports a mean mortality of 11% and a mean morbidity of 10.7% in his own experience and that of some Japanese study groups in stereotactic evacuation of spontaneous ICH. These results coincide with ours. We are also in almost complete agreement regarding the indications for stereotatic treatment; also we prefer to decompress the hematoma as early as possible! In addition, hematomas with a volume of more than 30 ml which were initially in good condition have been evacuated and liquified in order to avoid a secondary deterioration. We can conclude that the minimal invasive stereotactic evacuation with consecutive local fibrinolysis has become not only a therapeutical alternative but probably the method of choice in treating spontaneous ICH. A prospective multicenter study is now being planned to provide a precise evaluation of this hopeful tendency.

References

1. Backlund EO, von Holst H (1978) Controlled subtotal evacuation of intracerebral hematomas by stereotactic technique. Surg Neurol 9:99–101
2. Delank HW (1985) Neurologie. Enke, Stuttgart, p 22
3. Drake CG, Vinters HV (1985) Intracerebral hemorrhage. In: Plumm F, Pulsinelli W (eds) Cerebrovascular diseases. Raven, New York
4. Hounsfield GN (1973) Computerized transverse axial scanning (tomography). I. Description of system. Br J Radiol 46:1016–1022
5. Jennett B, Teasdale J (1976) Predicting outcome in individual patients after severe head injury. Lancet 1:1031–1034
6. Lerch KD (1992) Development of a new arc-centered stereotactic system with special regard to stereotactically guided microresection of deep-seated lesions. Neurosurgery (in press)
7. Lerch KD (1992) Percutaneous trephination with Kirschner's wire and Steinmann's Mail in stereotactical and ventricular drainage procedures. Neurosurgery (in press)
8. Matsumoto K, Hondo H (1984) Evacuation of hypertensive intracerebral hematomas. J Neurosurg 61:440–448
9. Mohadjer M, Ruh E, Hittl DM, Neumüller H, Mundinger F (1988) CT-stereotactic evacuation and fibrinolysis of hypertensive intracranial hematoma. Fibrinolysis 2:43–48
10. Mohadjer M, Braus DF, Krauss JK, Milios E, Birg W, Mundinger F (1990) CT-stereotaktische Entleerung und Fibrinolyse der spontanen, vorwiegend hypertensiven intrakraniellen Massenblutungen – Langzeitergebnisse. Jahrb Neurochir 189–201
11. Nizuma H, Shimizu Y, Yonemitsu T, Nakazato N, Suzuki J (1989) Results of stereotactic aspiration in 175 cases of hemorrhage. Neurosurgery 24:814–819
12. Ojemann RG, Heros RC (1983) Progress in cerebrovascular disease: spontaneous brain hemorrhage. Stroke 14:468–475
13. Pan DHC, Lee LS, Chen MS, Manns AG (1986) Modified screw-and-suction technique for stereotactic evacuation of deep intracerebral hematomas. Surg Neurol 25:540–544
14. Schütz HJ (1988) Spontane intrazerebrale Hämatome. Pathophysiologie, Klinik und Therapie. Springer, Berlin Heidelberg New York

Hydrocephalus malresorptivus

The Solved and Unsolved Problems of Hydrocephalus Valves: A Critical Comment

A. Aschoff[1], C. Benesch[1], P. Kremer[1], M. S. von Haken[1], A. Klank[1], M. Osterloh[1] and K. Fruh[1]

Introduction

Four goals should be aimed at with an artificial shunt: (1) The intraventricular pressure must be kept within physiological ranges, especially during intracranial pressure (ICP) crises, independent of the body position, coughing, crying of children, external pressure, and flexion and torsion of valve or shunt components. (2) In venous shunting, reflux must be strictly excluded. For peritoneal shunting this aim seems less obligatory. (3) Ideally, a shunt system should offer the possibility of reestablishing shunt independency step by step, or a very close approximation to this. (4) Design, material, and surface of a life-long implant should produce optimum biocompatibility, stability, and durability: In 25 years, a valve must potentially resist a billion opening and closing maneuvers, caused by cardiac actions and breathing. When a valve is pumped, pressure peaks of up to 2000 mmHg, a maximum flow of 2000 ml/h, and a suction before the valve of –330 mmHg occur. Shunts are surrounded by a chemically aggressive milieu and threatened by protein, calcium precipitations, and detritus around the clock.

Does the currently available shunt technology enable the achievement of the outlined goals?

Presently, in the Federal Republic of Germany we have a choice between four technical principles (slit, membrane, ball-in-cone and needle valves), 54 different valve constructions, about 180 pressure ranges and 200 prefixed configurations of valves, tubes, and devices: in other words, at least 500 options. What should we prefer?

The first precondition is accurate function. We can basically measure the hydraulic properties of valves in two ways: Either we produce a definite flow and register the flow *resistance* before the valve or we simulate pressure and measure the resultant *flow*, including the opening and closing points. Both tests can be done with isolated valves or with complete shunt systems and with simulation of horizontal or vertical position.

When we are buying a car, every brochure offers 50–100 data on the performance of the "complete" car (speed, acceleration, size, load, fuel consumption, etc.), as well as data of "isolated" components (power and torque of engine) which were measured in test stands.

---

[1] Neurochirurgische Klinik, Universität Heidelberg, Im Neuenheimer Feld 400, W-6900 Heidelberg, FRG.

Advances in Neurosurgery, Vol. 21
R. Lorenz, M. Klinger, M. Brock (Eds.)

When a neurosurgeon is making a decision on a lifelong implant, with far-reaching consequences for the patient, the valve industry only informs us about the resistance of isolated valves at flows of between 5 and 50 ml/h, according to the ASTM [2]. In vivo flowmeter measurements have documented a shunt-flow between 0.6–116 ml/h [30, 31]. Therefore, the ASTM range is *arbitrarily restricted* and scotomizes typical pediatric flow conditions. Resistance values are abstract and only allow the user a comparison with official specifications, not with physiological data such as CSF production rate. Therefore, the biological consequences, e.g., the specific risk of overdrainage, are not transparent for the users.

Criteria and Methods of Valve Testing

The principles of accurate and reliable valve tests are [4]:

1. Saturated *water content of silicon*, which requires 3–14 days storage under water.
2. Standardized pre-perfusion and *long-term observation*. We have tested 50 valves for 14 days and 24 specimen for 90 days. Most valves show significant changes in the course of time, above all those with slit constructions. These results have been confirmed by other tests of 1–2 weeks [16, 23, 32, 33, 47, 51, 57, 59]. A pre-test procedure and a registration time of some hours (ASTM) are inadaequate.
3. Strict *exclusion of air bubbles*. They can increase the valve resistance by up to 400% and are not excluded in the ASTM-test (open water column!).
4. Exact *temperature* (± 0.5 °C). With the tolerances of ± 2 °C (ASTM), failures of up to 12% are possible.
5. Control of *external pressure* offset, caused by diffuse (hydraulic) tissue pressure and directed (vectorial) pressure, when the patient lies on the valve [3, 4]. The subcutaneous pressure of, usually, 3–5 mmHg increases on touching a soft pillow to 10–20 mmHg. When the valve is exactly centered on a hard board, a pressure of 125 mmHg can occur. With 20 mmHg external pressure, the resistance of antisiphon devices increases about 2000% [34] and of Orbis-Sigma and Heyer-Schulte LPV valves up to 90% [3]. In the ASTM-test the submersion of valves is *not* defined and may vary between 0 and 25 cm. It is evident that systematic failures are unavoidable.
6. Valves are implanted in curved regions, which can have a radius in premature babies of only 40 mm. Some valves are susceptible to deformation (e.g., Heyer-Schulte LPV or mini-inline valves) and even open valve lips (Denver shunt) [3]. These properties during *flexing and torsion* are also neglected by ASTM.
7. Subtests with *increased protein content* [58].
8. Subtests with *pulsed superimpositions* [4, 23, 32, 33, 57].
9. Data or *flow rates* of valves, which neither the ASTM nor most producers offer.
10. *Complete shunts* in typical assemblies, including the opening and closing point [47].
11. Tests with complete shunt systems *in a vertical position* are obligatory to investigate the overdrainage (neglected by ASTM).

12. *Reflux resistance*: Uni shunts and Denver shunts fail in this regard, and Orbis-Sigma valves have problems [3].

In summary, the neurosurgeon must make his decision on the basis of valve data which are *fragmentary, irrelevant for practical use, and not free from methodological failures.*

The accuracy and reliability of most valves is disappointing: Only every third valve of 120 specimens tested was found in acceptable accordance (± 30%) with manufacturer's specification. Similar experiences have been published by many authors [16, 23, 32, 33, 46, 47, 51, 57, 58, 59]. The ball-in-cone constructions often show the best values, the membrane valves vary more, and the slit valves are widely scattered.

Overdrainage and Flow-Control Shunt Technology

The driving forces for shunt flow are pressure differences (ICP vs atrial/peritoneal pressure) and hydrostatic[2] pressure in the upright position [17, 22, 41, 44].

Using an in vitro simulation of a common pressure in a vertical position (30 cmH_2O), nearly all valves show an absolutely unphysiological flow of 50 up to 3450 ml/h, which is 2–170 times more than the normal rate of liquor production (Table 1). Only defective valves, intact Orbis-Sigma valves, and some hydrostatic valves offer a relatively normal flow rate in an upright position.

Indeed, for a correct analysis we should remember that a valve is only *one* of five to six resistance components of a shunt system, which consists of the perforation zone, the distal catheter, valve, sometimes an antisiphondevice, the proximal catheter, and the outlet zone. The resistance of *each* shunt component contributes to the total shunt resistance, and each can vary significantly[3]. In particular, the influence of the silicon tubes is underestimated: the Hagen-Poisseuille equation includes the internal diameter as the fourth exponent. The consequences for shunt flow are dramatic: With a pressure of 30 cmH_2O and a length of 75 cm, a catheter with an internal diameter of 1.3 mm shows a flow rate of 923 ml/h, one of 1.1 mm 442 ml/h, one of 0.8 mm 105 ml/h, and one of 0.6 mm 37 ml/h. Additionally, the flow is directly proportional to the length. The consequence: After opening of a valve, up to 80% of the flow control may be caused *by the tubes, not by the valves*! It is evident that the common internal diameter of 1.1–1.3 mm supports

---

[2] In calculation of hydrostatic pressure confusions are common: Often speculations of 70–80 cmH_2O pressure are made, the distance to the pouch of Douglas. In reality the abdominal space is comparable to a water-filled tank. Therefore, the zero point is at the highest level, subphrenic in an upright and umbilical in a prone position. Obesity or marked tension of the abdominal wall may cause additional pressure. In summary, the peritoneal "siphon" may be similar to the atrial shunt conditions with an effective hydrostatic pressure set-off of 30–40 cmH_2O in adults.

[3] We have often observed that new and explanted distal catheters with lateral slits and closed ends have the properties of *additional valves* sometimes with a higher resistance than the main valve. Similar findings were confirmed by Richard et al. [47].

Table 1. Flow rates of valves without catheter at 30 cmH_2O hydrostatic pressure

Valve[a]	Pressure range[b]	Flow rate[c] (ml/h)
Orbis-Sigma III[d]		0
French-Neurone[d]	Normal	0
Holter-Hausner N[d]		2
French-Neurone[d]	High	5
Orbis-Sigma IV[d]		6
Spitz-Holter[d]	Normal	6
Phoinix[d]	Normal	7
Phoinix[d]	Medium	12
Hakim Lumbar I (vertical)		18 (1367 horizontal)
Orbis-Sigma I		21
Orbis-Sigma II		25
Sophy Hydrostatic I (vertical)		27 (2713 horizontal)
Denver Standard		50
Heyer-Schulte on-off I	High	59
Sophy Hydrostatic II (vertical)		81 (2787 horizontal)
Holter-Hausner Paediatric	Medium	140
Denver	Low	203
Heyer-Schulte LPV	High	261
Spitz-Holter	Medium	240
Chhabra 4-Ball (vertical)		393 (1853 horizontal)
Medos-Hakim Programmable I	200 mmH_2O	436 (1517 with 30 mmH_2O)
Hakim Lumbar II (vertical)		444 (1255 horizontal)
Medos-Hakim Programmable II	180 mmH_2O	454 (1567 with 20 mmH_2O)
Luisa Shunt (Phillipinian Shunt)		556
French-Neurone	Low	570
Holter-Hausner	Medium	575
Heyer-Schulte on-off II	High	598
Sophy-SU-8 II	High (170 mmH_2O)	605 (1800 with 50 mmH_2O)
Medos-Hakim Nonprogrammable	130 mmH_2O	715
Hakim Lumbar III (vertical)		720 (1260 horizontal)
Pudenz-Schulte Medical CSF Flow I	Medium	817
Heyer-Schulte LPV with ASD I	Medium	832[e]
Pudenz-Schulte Medical CSF Flow II	Medium	910
Medos-Hakim Nonprogrammable	100 mmH_2O	970
Heyer-Schulte Burr hole	High	1020
Heyer-Schulte LPV with ASD II	Medium	1134
Sophy-SU-3	High (160 mmH_2O)	1200 (2047 with 50 mmH_2O)
Medos-Hakim Programmable IV	(90 mmH_2O)	1210
Hakim Lumbar III (horizontal)		1260 (720 vertical)
Hakim Lumbar II (horizontal)		1255 (444 vertical)
Hakim Lumbar I (horizontal)		1367 (18 vertical)
Sophy-SU-8 I	High (170 mmH_2O)	1380 (1950 with 50 mmH_2O)
Heyer-Schulte LPV	Medium	1387
Medos-Hakim Programmable III	130 mmH_2O	1389
Hakim-Cordis I	Medium (80–120 mmH_2O)	1500

Table 1 (cont.)

Valve[a]	Pressure range[b]	Flow rate[c] (ml/h)
Pudenz-Schulte Medical Delta	Level II	1554[e]
Pudenz-Schulte Medical Delta	Level I	1632[e] Hakim-Cordis II
Medium (80–120 mmH_2O)	1650	
Heyer-Schulte Burr hole	Low	1750
Sophy-SU-8 II Low	50 mmH_2O	1800 (605 with 170 mmH_2O)
Chhabra 4-Ball (horizontal)		1853 (393 horizontal)
Chhabra 2-Ball (horizontal)		1930 (942 vertical)
Sophy-SU-8 I	Low (50 mmH_2O)	1380 (1950 with 170 mmH_2O)
Codman Unishunt	(50–90 mmH_2O)	1960
Sophy-SU-3	Low (50 mmH_2O)	2047 (1200 with 160 mmH_2O)
Sophy Hydrostatic I (horizontal)		2713 (27 vertical)
Sophy Hydrostatic II (horizontal)		2787 (81 vertical)
Codman Unishunt	90–140 mmH_2O	3450

[a] I, II, III = No. of tested specimens.
[b] Low, medium, normal, high, level I, II, 100, 130 mmH_2O, etc., = official pressure ranges.
[c] Flow-rates of isolated valves: connecting tubes with negligible resistance (3–5 mm internal diameter) –, (distal slit valves, last 5 cm of tube with slits): mean of three measurements.
[d] Obviously defective valves.
[e] Without "siphon": no hanging tube distal to the valve. Prepressure = 30 cmH_2O.

overdrainage. A silicon tube of about 0.8–0.9 mm internal diameter may decrease overdrainage and be sufficiently insusceptible to obstructions.

Many ICP measurements of shunt patients supine and vertical have been published [1, 8, 19, 20, 41]. They agree in stating that two of three shunt patients show spectacularly negative ICPs of up to -30 or -44 cmH_2O in the upright position, most *without* clinical symptoms.

In summary, nearly all traditional shunt systems produce overdrainage in a vertical position [17–19, 22, 38, 43, 45, 53]. In concrete terms: When a patient stands up at 7:00 a.m., with a Unishunt or a simple tube he may develop unphysiological negative ICP 3 min later[4], with a typical ball-in-cone or membrane valves at 7:05 or 7:07, and with a slit valve at 7:15. As long as the patient is upright, the ICP remains negative, relatively independent of the valve type.

To prevent *overdrainage*, hydrostatic, programmable, and variable-resistance valves and antisiphon devices were developed.

Hydrostatic Valves

The hydrostatic valves of Hakim and Chhabra consist of one conventional valve for the supine position and two to four metal balls, which in the vertical position

[4] Calculation: Valves *including* common tubes, normal ventricle size, in which 20 ml CSF loss is sufficient for negative ICP.

Table 2. Flow-rates of hydrostatic valves (30 cmH_2O, without silicon tubes)

Valve	Horizontal flow (ml/h)	Vertical flow (ml/h)
Hakim-Cordis Lumbar I	1367	18
Hakim-Cordis Lumbar II	1255	444
Hakim-Cordis Lumbar III	1260	720
Hakim-Cordis Lumbar IV	1569	943
Hakim-Cordis Lumbar V	1494	1098
Chhabra Z-Flow 2-Ball	1930	942
Chhabra Z-Flow 4-Ball	1853	393
Sophy Hydrostatic I	2713	27
Sophy Hydrostatic II	2787	81

[a] Special version of the Hakim lumbar valve: Only with hydrostatic balls, and without a proximal valve with ball-in-cone and spring.

are progressively recruited to press on a second ball-valve. If the weight of the balls is optimally adapted, these simple constructions can reduce the flow very effectively, the first Hakim lumbar from 1367 to 18 ml/h (Table 2). The other Hakim and Chhabra valves contain balls which are too light and reduce the flow excess only to 393–1098 ml/h. Unfortunately, when patients are walking the balls make ballistic movements, which inactivate this principle. The hydrostatic Sophysa valves function only in a sagittal direction. Lying face down or in a lateral position, paradoxical effects occur [5].

Programmable Valves

Programmable valves were proposed by S. Hakim in 1973 [24] and realized by Sophysa in 1985, by C. Hakim in 1986, and by Hashimoto et al. even more recently [26]. The advantages are evident: We can change the valve resistance percutaneously with respect to the flow rate, "titrate" problematic patients, and even undertake noninvasive therapy of smaller hygromas [6, 14, 15, 36, 37, 39, 56]. In the "low" position we have observed flow rates of 1800–1950 ml/h with Sophy SU 8 valves and with 1517–1567 ml/h Medos-Hakim valves (30 cmH_2O, without tube). In the "high" position, the Sophy valve shows widely scattered flow-rates of between 315 and 1092 ml/h and the Medos-Hakim of 436–840 ml/h. *With* a catheter, a representative Sophy valve shows a drainage of 168 ml/h, compared to 120 ml/h through a Medos-Hakim valve. Confirming these laboratory findings we have observed patients with very high positions (189–200 mmH_2O) presenting subdural hygromas, as well as symptomatic slit ventricles. Programmable valves are an undoubtable progress in shunt therapy, and beneficial for minor overdrainage problems, but they can offer only a *compromise* between vertical and horizontal conditions, which is not sufficient for all patients [56]. Additionally, in

Sophy valves many details should be improved such as the design (voluminous and edged), accuracy and reliability of hydraulic properties, resistance to corrosion, and stability of adjustment, which is susceptible to common magnetic fields and fast movements [5].

Antisiphon Devices

The use of negative pressure in a hanging tube as a high-resistance switch, the antisiphon device (ASD, SCD), seemed a sensible answer to overdrainage problems [44]. Clinical experience has shown a normalization of postural ICP alterations [8, 11] and a decreased incidence of slit-ventricle syndromes [1, 10, 22, 27, 29, 56]. However, serious problems with shunt insufficiency in 5–30% of patients have also been reported, which were not clearly understood [5, 28, 34, 41, 42, 53]. The antisiphon effect is dependent on (1) the length of the hanging tube, (2) the proximal pressure, and (3) the external pressure.

Although some authors have stressed the importance of placement in soft underlying tissue, systematic laboratory investigations of the susceptibility to external pressure have been missing for 17 years after the start of clinical use. Test bench results were first published in 1990 [3, 34]. Recently, da Silva has confirmed our findings in laboratory and animal experiments [13]. The excessive sensitivity to subcutaneous pressure, which is inherent in the principle of antisiphon devices with external switching membranes, is the crucial point of the concept.

In summary, antisiphon devices successfully limit flow in the upright position, but the price is a potential mechanical lability of the shunt system with significant risk, particularly nocturnal shunt obstruction, when the patient is lying on the device.

"Flow-Regulated" Valve (Orbis-Sigma)

The most recent concept is the Orbis-Sigma valve, a so-called "flow-regulated"[5] construction [48]. Two tested valves worked according to the manufacturer's specification, but showed a marked hysteresis, particularly in the main working range [51, 57], insufficient reflux resistance, and a marked increase of resistance when physiological subcutaneous pressure was applied. One valve was fully blocked. The fourth Orbis valve showed an insufficient flow of 5.7 ml/h with 30 cmH_2O. In contrast, during a 90-day long-term perfusion the resistance was nearly zero in five

[5] The terms "flow-control" and "flow-regulated" valve suggest either a flowmeter with an active pump or at least another kind of flow measurement with "smart" regulation. With respect to the reality of physics, the term is misleading: The driving force of Orbis-Sigma valves is (differential or hydrostatic) *pressure*, as in all other passive valves. The only difference is a relatively flat graph of pressure flow properties, similar to slit valves, which is sometimes S-shaped. "Flow-control" and "flow-regulation" are terms of marketing, not of physics, and should be avoided.

subtests and only sufficient in one. This performance may be caused by a ruby pin, which tends to stick to the surrounding ruby disc, particularly in both extreme positions. Schoener et al. also observed an obstructed Orbis-Sigma valve in which the notch on the ruby pin was missing [51]. An inherent risk of the tiny outlet and the filigree mechanism of all valves is an increased susceptibility to obstructions.

The crucial *concept* of the Orbis-Sigma valve is the coupling to CSF production. Except for rare diseases such as plexus papillomas or bilateral plexus hypertrophy the CSF production rate seems to be relatively constant around 20 ml/h or 0.33 ml/min in adults. What is the reality of shunt flow?

Numerous methods have been created for measuring shunt flow in vivo. Cold transfer [10, 35] is inaccurate with valves with temperature-dependent resistance (3%/1 °C). The clearance of isotopes [9, 39] requires an invasive procedure and only shows the shunt flow for 10–20 min. Flow-sensitive MRI sequences [7, 40, 49] are limited in low flow, impossible in a sitting position, and impractical for a 24-h recording. All of these methods are snapshots and cannot show the real-time flow around the clock, during sleep and daily activities.

Hara, Kadowaki, and colleagues produce gas bubbles made by intrashunt telemetric electrolysis and count the running-time of the bubbles using two ultrasonic Doppler probes [25, 30, 31]. The method is the first which is compatible with daily activities, sleep, and 24-h recording results:

1. The flow rates are widely scattered between 0.6 and 116 ml/h.
2. All 19 patients showed significant circadian fluctuations of shunt flow (relation 1:3 to 1:10!).
3. The shunt-flow is maximal, not during the day, in an upright position, but rather during the REM phases and nocturnal ICP crisis, which corresponds well with long-term ICP recordings and is not caused by increased CSF production, but rather by cerebral hyperemia in combination with too low a CSF resorption capacity.

In these situations the rigid flow limitation of an Orbis-Sigma valve, even when it is functioning in accordance with the producer's specifications, must unavoidably lead to underdrainage. In children with low CSF production, or in borderline patients who have a significant residual CSF resorption capacity, the limited flow rate of an Orbis-Sigma valve seems to be enough to drain nocturnal flow peaks. Encouraging results in pediatric patients [12, 21, 48] are in contrast to disappointing experiences in some German [51] and Swedish hospitals, where 80% of the Sigma valves had to be explanted (Ekstedt, personal communication).

In summary, the basic concept as well as the filigree mechanism give rise to problems. The significant decrease in overdrainage may be outweighed by the increased rate of shunt insufficiency.

Conclusions

- Two out of three new valves do not meet the manufacturer's own specifications.
- Some valves are not resistant to reflux, external pressure, flexion, or torsion.
- Shunt resistance (and the resulting shunt flow) is influenced by many factors. Up to 80% of the flow control is caused by the silicon catheters.
- No valve construction has solved the problem of overdrainage when the body is in a vertical position: We only have the choice between differential pressure valves, which produce an unphysiologically negative ICP whenever the patient is upright, or valves with significant new risks for shunt insufficiency caused by mechanical instability.
- All existing valves sustain shunt dependency.

A combination of diameter smaller catheters, an additional hydrostatic offset mechanism resisting the movements of daily life, and the programmable valve technology may reduce the overdrainage risks to a minimum.

References

1. Abe H, Chiba Y, Tokoro K (1991) Effect of anti-siphon device in shunting procedure: Intraventricular pressure during posture changes. In: Matsumoto S, Tamaki N (eds) Hydrocephalus. Pathogenesis and treatment. Springer, Berlin Heidelberg New York, pp 391–398
2. American Society for Testing and Materials (1989) Standard practice for evaluating and specifying implantable shunt assemblies for neurosurgical application. Designation F 647–679
3. Aschoff A, Osterloh M, Kunze S (1990) Longtime-tests of 30 hydrocephalus-valves. 18th annual scientific meeting of the International Society for Pediatric Neurosurgery, Paris, 17–19.9.1990. Childs Nerv Syst 6:282
4. Aschoff A, Osterloh M, Benesch C, Von Haken M, Kremer P, Kunze St (1990) Criteria and methods for testing of hydrocephalus-valves and anti-siphon-devices. Results of 102 tested exemplares. Joint Meeting of the Deutsche und Griechische Gesellschaft für Neurochirurgie, Athens, 14.–17.10.1990
5. Aschoff A, Kremer P, Benesch C, Klank A, Kunze S (1991) Shunt-technology and overdrainage. A critical review of hydrostatic, programmable and variable-resistance-valves and flow-reducing devices. Eur J Pediatr Surg 1 (Suppl I):49–50
6. Benesch C, Aschoff A (1992) Hydrocephalus treatment with the programmable Medos-Hakim valve – laboratory testing and clinical experiences with 70 implantations. Meeting of the Society for Research into Hydrocephalus and Spina Bifida, Mainz, 15–18.7.1992
7. Castillo M, Hudgins PA, Malko JA, Burrow BK, Hoffmann JC (1991) Flow-sensitive MR imaging of ventriculoperitoneal shunts: In vitro findings, clinical applications, and pitfalls. AJNR 12:667–674
8. Chapman PH, Cosman ER, Arnold MA (1990) The relationship between ventricular fluid pressure and body position in normal subjects and subjects with shunt: a telemetric study. Neurosurgery 26:181–189
9. Chervu S, Chervu LR, Vallabhajosyula B, Milstein DM, Shapiro KM, Shulman K, Blaufox MD (1984) Quantitave evaluation of cerebrospinal fluid shunt flow. J Nucl Med 25:91–95

10. Chiba Y, Yuda K (1980) Thermosensitive determination of CSF shunt patency with a pair of small disc thermistors. J Neurosurg 52:700–704
11. Chiba Y, Tokoro K, Abe H (1991) Importance of anti-siphon devices in shunt therapy of pediatric and adolescent hydrocephalus In: Matsumoto S, Tamaki N (eds) Hydrocephalus. Pathogenesis and treatment. Springer, Berlin Heidelberg New York, pp 375–382
12. Cinalli G, Sainte-Rose C, Pierre-Kahn A, Renier D, Hoppe-Hirsch E, Hirsch JF (1992) Analysis of a pediatric series of 523 hydrocephalic patients treated with a CSF flow regulating device. In: Hydrocephalus 92 – consensus conference on pediatric neurosurgery, Assisi, 1992 (abstract p 66). Editrice C.S.H., Milan
13. Da Silva MC, Drake JM (1992) The effect of subcutaneous implantation on anti-siphon device function. Clinical and experimental results. In: Hydrocephalus 92 – consensus conference on pediatric neurosurgery, Assisi, 1992 (abstract p 99). Editrice C.S.H., Milan
14. Dautheribes M, Liguoro D, San Galli F, Kerdiles C, Guerin J (1992) Programmable shunting in various hydrocephalus: a series of 28 cases. In: Hydrocephalus 92 – consensus conference on pediatric neurosurgery, Assisi, 1992 (abstract p 95). Editrice C.S.H., Milan
15. Dietrich U, Lumenta C, Sprick C, Majewski B (1987) Subdural hematoma in a case of hydrocephalus and macrocrania. Experience with a pressure-adjustable valve. Childs Nerv System 3:242–246
16. Ekstedt J, Friden H (1980) Hydrodynamic properties of CSF shunt systems. In: Shulmann K, Marmarou A, Miller JD, Becker DP, Hochwald GM, Brock M (eds) Intracranial pressure IV. Springer, Berlin Heidelberg New York, pp 483–485
17. Faulhaber K, Schmitz P (1978) Overdrainage phenomena in shunt treated hydrocephalus. Acta Neurochirurg 45:89–101
18. Foltz EL, Blanks JP (1988) Symptomatic low intracranial pressure in shunted hydrocephalus. J Neurosurg 68:401–408
19. Fox JD, McCullough DC, Green RC (1973) Effect of cerebrospinal fluid shunts on intracranial pressure and on cerebrospinal fluid dynamics. 2. A new technique of pressure measurements: results and concepts. 3. A concept of hydrocephalus. J Neurol Neurosurg Psychiatr 36:302–312
20. Fox JD, Portnoy HD, Shulte RR (1973) Cerebrospinal fluid shunts: an experimental evaluation of flow rates and pressure values in the anti-siphon valve. Surg Neurol 1:299–302
21. Genitori L, Lena G, Erdincler P, Tavares de Lima F, Achouri M, Choux M (1992) Mechanical and functional complications in shunts. A series of 1244 children and 2845 operations. In: Hydrocephalus 92 – consensus conference on pediatric neurosurgery, Assisi, 1992 (abstract p 63). Editrice C.S.H., Milan
22. Gruber R, Jenny P, Herzog B (1984) Experiences with the antisiphon-device (ASD) in shunt therapy of pediatric hydrocephalus. J Neurosurg 61:156–162
23. Hakim S, Duran de la Roche F, Burton JD (1973) A critical analysis of valve shunts used in the treatment of hydrocephalus. Dev Med Child Neurol 15:230–255
24. Hakim S (1973) Hydraulic and mechanical miss-matching of valve shunts used in the treatment of hydrocephalus: the need for a servo-valve shunt. Dev Med Child Neurol 15:646–653
25. Hara M, Kadowski C, Konishi Y (1983) A new method for measuring CSF flow in shunts. J Neurosurg 58:557–561
26. Hashimoto T, Nakamura N, Kanki T, Shimazu H, Yamakoshi K, Gondoh M, Tamai T (1991) A new shunt system with non-invasive flow rate regulation and pressure measurement. In: Matsumoto S, Tamaki N, (eds) Hydrocephalus. Pathogenesis and treatment. Springer, Berlin Heidelberg New York, pp 422–431
27. Horton DD, Williams G, Pollay M (1991) The effectiveness of a siphon control device in preventing the complications of overshunting. In: Matsumoto S, Tamaki N (eds) Hy-

drocephalus. Pathogenesis and treatment. Springer, Berlin Heidelberg New York, pp 370–374
28. Jaskoska E, MacKinnon AE (1988) Experience with antisiphon devices: successes and complications. Z Kinderchir 43:22–23
29. Jones RFC, Teo C, Currie B, BCT Kwok, VV Nayanar (1991) The antisiphon device: its value in preventing excessive drainage. In: Matsumoto S, Tamaki N (eds) Hydrocephalus. Pathogenesis and treatment. Springer, Berlin Heidelberg New York, pp 383–390
30. Kadowaki C, Hara M, Numoto M, Takekeuchi K (1986) Factors affecting cerebospinal fluid flow in a shunt. Br J Neurosurg 1:467–475
31. Kadowaki C, Hara M, Numoto M, Takekeuchi K (1989) CSF hydrodynamics and CSF flow through a shunt in hydrocephalus. Hoff JT, Betz AL (eds) Intracranial pressure 7. Springer, Berlin Heidelberg New York
32. Keith HD, Watts C (1983) Testing of cerebrospinal fluid shunt systems under dynamic flow conditions. Med Instrum 17:297–302
33. Keith HD, Avula X, Schelich C, Watts C (1981) Investigation of cerebrospinal fluid valves. Final report, Phase II. USPH FDA 223–79–5064, University of Missouri, August 1, 1981
34. Kremer P, Aschoff A, Kunze S (1991) Therapeutical risks of anti-siphon-devices. Eur J Pediatr Surg 1 (Suppl I):47–48
35. Lakke JPWF, Go KG (1968) A simple method to determine patency of ventriculo-atrial shunts in children with hydrocephalus. Neurochirurgia 11:210–216
36. Lumenta CB, N Roosen, Dietrich U (1990) Clinical experience with a pressure-adjustable valve SOPHY in the management of hydrocephalus. Childs Nerv Syst 6:1–6
37. Maitrot D, Valery CA, Boyer P, Kehrli P, Buchheit F (1991) Sophy shunts in the treatment of 130 patients. In: Matsumoto S, Tamaki N (eds) Hydrocephalus. Pathogenesis and treatment. Springer, Berlin Heidelberg New York, pp 399–404
38. Matsumae M, Murakami T, Ueda M, Suzuki Y (1987) Dynamic changes of cerebrospinal fluid shunt in patient's daily life. Shoni no Noshinkei 3:30–34
39. Matsumae M, Sato O, Itoh K, Fukuda T, Suzuki Y (1989) Quantification of cerebrospinal fluid shunt flow rates. Assessment of the programmable pressure valve. Childs Nerv Syst 5:356–360
40. Martin AJ, Drake LM, Lemaire C, Henkelman RM (1989) Cerebrospinal fluid shunts: MR measurement of CSF shunt flow. Radiology 173:243–247
41. McCullough DC (1982) Complications with antisiphon devices in hydrocephalics with ventriculoperitoneal shunts. In: Concepts in paediatric neurosurgery II. Karger, Basel, pp 63–74
42. McCullough DC (1986) Symptomatic progressive ventriculomegaly in hydrocephalus with patent shunt and anti-siphon devices. Neurosurgery 4:617–621
43. Oi S, Matsumoto S (1987) Infantile hydrocephalus and the slit ventricle syndrome in early infancy. Child's Nerv Syst 3:145–150
44. Portnoy HD, Schulte RR, Fox JL (1973) Antisiphon and reversible occlusion valves for shunting in hydrocephalus and preventing post-shunt subdural hematomas. J Neurosurg 38:729–738
45. Pudenz RH, Foltz EL (1991) Hydrocephalus: overdrainage by ventricular shunts. A review and recommendations. Surg Neurol 35:200–212
46. Rayport M, Reiss J (1969) Hydrodynamic properties of certain shunt assemblies for the treatment of hydrocephalus. Part 2: Pressure flow characteristics of the Spitz-Holter, Pudenz-Heyer, and Cordis-Hakim shunt systems. J Neurosurg 30:463–467
47. Richard KE, Block FR, Ackermann CW, Britten E, Steinberg J, Weber M (1989) Untersuchung des Regelverhaltens von Shuntsystemen zur operativen Behandlung des Hydrocephalus. Abschlußbericht zum Forschungsvorhaben RI 328/3–2 der DFG
48. Sainte-Rose C, Hooven MD, Hirsch JF (1987) A new approach in the treatment of hydrocephalus. J Neurosurg 66:213–226

49. Savader SJ, Savader BL, Murtagh FR, Clarke LP, Silbinger ML (1988) MR evaluation of flow in a ventricular shunt phantom with in vivo correlation. J Comp Ass Tomogr 12:765–769
50. Schmitt J, Spring A (1990) Die Therapie des Normaldruckhydrocephalus mit dem transcutan magnetisch verstellbaren Ventil. Neurochirurgia 33 (Suppl I):23–26
51. Schoener WF, Verheggen R, Reparon C, Markakis E (1991) Evaluation of shunt failures by compliance analysis and inspection of shunt valves and shunt materials, using microscopic or scanning electron microscopic techniques. In: Matsumoto S, Tamaki N (eds) Hydrocephalus. Pathogenesis and treatment. Springer, Berlin Heidelberg New York, pp 452–472
52. Seida M, Ito U, Tomida S, Yamazaki S, Inaba Y (1987) Ventriculoperitoneal shunt malfunction with antisiphon device in normal-pressure hydrocephalus: report of three cases. Neurol Med Chir (Tokyo) 27:769–773
53. Serlo W, Saukkonen AL, Heikkinen E, von Wendt L (1989) The incidence and management of the slit ventricle syndrome. Acta Neurochir 99:113–116
54. Sparrow OC (1989) Laboratory performance of single-piece ventriculoperitoneal shunts with distal slit-valve control. J Neurosurg 70:946–953
55. Tokoro K, Chiba Y (1991) Optimum position for an antisiphon device in a cerebrospinal fluid shunt system. Neurosurgery 29:519–525
56. Tokoro K, Chiba Y, Abe H (1991) Pitfalls of the Sophy programmable pressure valve: Is it really better than a conventional valve and an anti-siphon device? In: Matsumoto S, Tamaki N (eds) Hydrocephalus. Pathogenesis and treatment, Springer, Berlin Heidelberg New York, pp 405–421
57. Trost HA, Claussen G, Heissler H, Gaab MR (1991) Testing the hydrocephalus shunt valve: long term bench test results of various new and implanted hydrocephalus shunt valves. The need for a model for testiung shunt valves under physiological conditions. Eur J Pediatr Surg 1 (Suppl I):38–40
58. Van der Veen PH (1972) Hydrodynamics of Holter ventriculo-atrial shunt systems under various conditions. Dev Med Child Neurol 14 (Suppl 27):132–139
59. Whitehouse HE, Czosnyka M, Pickard JD (1992) Shunt audit: a computerized method for testing the performance characteristics of CSF shunts in vitro. In: Hydrocephalus 92 consensus conference, Assisi, April 26–30 1992

External Ventricular Drainage for Treatment of Acute Hydrocephalus After Subarachnoid Hemorrhage

T. Brinker[1], H. G. Höllerhage[1], D. Fotopoulou[1], and C. Götz[1]

Introduction

Acute hydrocephalus after subarachnoid hemorrhage (SAH) parallels the clinical condition of the patient. It can be observed only in a minority of patients in good condition after SAH but in contrast in the majority of those in poor condition [8, 11]. Modern management protocols do not exclude the latter patients from active treatment [1, 2, 10]. In spite of its risks – a rate of infection up to 50% [3, 7, 12] and an increased rate of rebleed [3, 9] – early ventricular drainage after SAH has been suggested to be useful in patients in poor condition [1, 4]. The risks of ventricular drainage were investigated with special regard to those patients in whom it was done even before aneurysmal surgery.

Material and Methods

A total of 237 patients with subarachnoid hemorrhage requiring neurosurgical care for more than 48 h, admitted to the Neurosurgical Department of the Medical School Hannover between 1987 and 1990, constitute the basis of this report. The charts of these patients were reviewed to obtain relevant data such as sex, neurological grade at admission and during clinical course according to Hunt and Hess [5], timing of surgery and ventricular drainage, incidence and effects of rebleeding, infection, and the need for permanent ventriculoperitoneal shunt. Rebleeding was taken into account only in those patients in whom it was proven by computed tomographic (CT) scan. Infection was noted according to the bacteriological and cytological examination of the cerebrospinal fluid (CSF).

Results

Clinical Material and Overall Management. A total of 150 women and 87 men were admitted. The age of the women was 53.3 ± 13.8 years (mean ± standard deviation); the age of the men was 46.6 ± 12.2 years. In 210 cases angiography revealed at least one aneurysm. A total of 160 patients were admitted in good neu-

[1] Neurochirurgische Klinik, Medizinische Hochschule Hannover, Konstanty-Gutschow-Straße 8, W-3000 Hannover 61, FRG.

Advances in Neurosurgery, Vol. 21
R. Lorenz, M. Klinger, M. Brock (Eds.)

Table 1. Timing of ventriculostomy

Group	VS before surgery (n)	VS during and after surgery (n)	Duration of CSF drainage – all cases – (days[a])	Duration of CSF drainage before surgery (days[a])
H&H I–III	14	27	6.9 ± 6.1	6.0 ± 7.3
H&H IV–V	41	9	10.8 ± 7.7	9.9 ± 11.9
Total	55	36	9.8 ± 8.6	8.0 ± 8.5

[a] Mean ± standard deviation.
VS, ventriculostomy; H&M, Hunt and Hess grade.

rological condition (Hunt and Hess grades I–III). In 95 of these patients aneurysmal surgery was performed within 72 h after the SAH; in 43 cases it was done later. A total of 77 patients were admitted in poor neurological condition (Hunt and Hess Grades IV–V). In 34 of these patients aneurysmal surgery was performed within 72 h after the SAH; in 17 cases it was done later. Finally, in 48 patients no surgery was performed because either no aneurysm was found or the patient died prior to surgery.

General Handling of Ventricular Drainage. Ventricular drainage was performed in 91 patients for an average of approximately 7 days in good-grade patients and approximately 11 days in poor-grade patients. Ventriculostomy was done prior to aneurysmal surgery in 55 cases. In these patients ventricular drainage was continued until definitive operative treatment of the ruptured aneurysm for an average of approximately 6 days in patients in good condition and approximately 10 days in patients in poor condition (Table 1). Ventriculostomy was performed preferentially in patients in poor condition: fewer than 20% of initial patients in good condition needed a ventricular drainage, sharply contrasting with the 70% rate of patients in poor condition in whom this treatment was performed. Generally, a drainage gradient of 10–15 cm H_2O was adjusted during continuous CSF drainage. Broad-spectrum antibiotic therapy was started immediately in every patient suspected of infection.

Clinical Effects of Ventricular Drainage. Ventriculostomy for CSF drainage was performed in 41 of those patients who were initially in good condition but who deteriorated within the first days after SAH. Ventriculostomy was done to treat developing hydrocephalus in 26 patients to improve the neurological condition after rebleeding in 12, and to improve neurological condition during symptomatic cerebral vasospasm in three patients. Of 41 initially good-grade patients requiring ventricular drainage, 31 benefitted from the procedure.

Ventricular drainage was performed in 50 of the 77 patients who were initially poor-grade. Among the poor-grade patients in whom ventriculostomy was done, there were 29 who recovered during CSF drainage and 21 cases who did not benefit from ventricular drainage.

Table 2. Frequency of rebleeding

Group	(*n*)	Rebleeding	Rebleeding after SAH (days[a])	VS after SAH (days[a])	H&H before rebleed[a]	H&H after rebleeding[a]	Survivors (%)
VS prior surgery, no preceding rebleeding	46	13[b]	9.2 ± 5	1.2 ± 2.5	3.9 ± 0.95	4.7 ± 0.8	15
Remaining cases	191	31	7.4 ± 8.3	–	2.8 ± 0.8	3.8 ± 1.0	45

[a] Mean ± standard deviation, VS; ventriculostomy; H&H; Hunt & Hess grade.
[b] Not significant (chi square, $p > 0.05$) in comparison to the rebleeding rate in patients without ventriculostomy prior surgery.

Risk of Rebleeding: Ventricular drainage was performed prior to aneurysmal surgery in 46 patients who had had no preceding rebleeding. In the remaining 191 patients, no ventriculostomy was performed prior to aneurysmal surgery or it was done *after* preceding rebleeding. In two groups we investigated the effect of ventricular drainage on the incidence of rebleeding. The rate of rebleeding during ventricular drainage prior to aneurysmal surgery was 28% in comparison to the 16% rate in the remaining patients. However, this was not statistically different (Table 2). The Kaplan-Meier [6] estimate of the probability of survival without rebleeding in the group of patients in whom ventricular drainage was performed before aneurysmal surgery and in whom rebleeding had not yet occurred ($n = 46$) was compared with the curve of the remaining cases ($n = 191$).

Within the first 10 days after the SAH no difference occurred between the probability curves of no rebleeding in these two groups. Thereafter patients in whom ventricular drainage was performed had an increased rate of rebleeding in comparison with those without ventricular drainage (Fig. 1).

Risk of Infection. Meningitis was found in 13% in those 91 cases in whom ventricular drainage had been performed. This complication was deleterious only in one

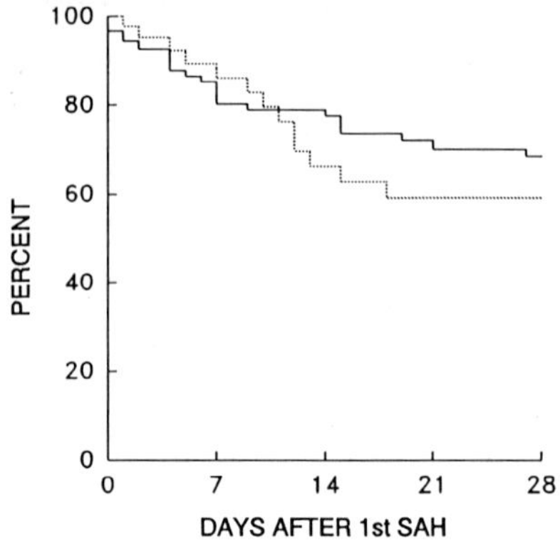

Fig. 1. The Kaplan-Meier estimated percentage of no rebleeding versus the time after the first SAH. *Solid line,* without ventricular drainage (*VD*) before aneurysmal surgery ($n = 191$). *Dotted line,* ventricular drainage was done before aneurysmal surgery ($n = 46$)

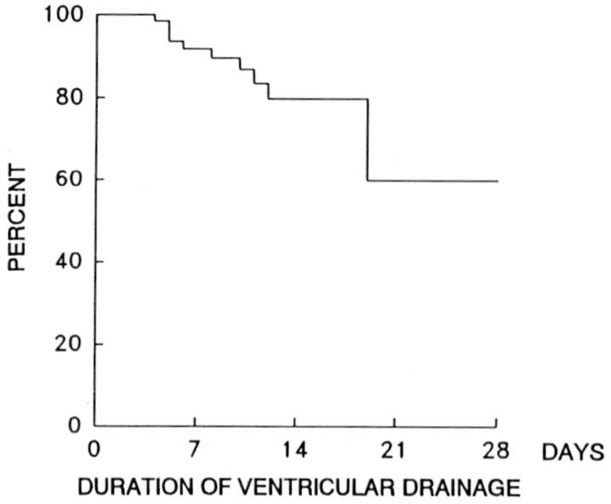

Fig. 2. The Kaplan-Meier estimated percentage of cases without infection versus the duration of ventricular drainage ($n = 91$)

patient. Closer analysis using a Kaplan-Meier estimate of the probability of survival without infection demonstrated that the incidence of infection depended strongly on the duration of ventricular drainage: after the 1st week an 8% infection rate was found, but after the 2nd week this increased to 21%, and after the 3rd week a 41% rate was found (Fig. 2).

Conclusion

In accordance with Bailes et al. [1], we suggest early ventricular drainage to be the decisive factor improving neurological condition of initially poor-grade patients. Our data show that after ventricular drainage definitive aneurysmal surgery may be delayed for several days. The preoperative neurological condition may thus be improved and the risk of immediate postoperative deficits after early surgery should be lowered.

References

1. Bailes JE, Spetzler RF, Hadley MN, Baldwin HZ (1990) Management morbidity and mortality of poor-grade aneurysm patients. J Neurosurg 72: 559–566
2. Gilsbach JM, Harders AG (1989) Morbidity and mortality after early aneurysm surgery – a prospective study with nimodipine prevention. Acta Neurochir (Wien) 96:1–7
3. Hasan D, Vermeulen M, Wijdicks EFM, Hijdra A, Van Gijn J (1989) Management problems in acute hydrocephalus after subarachnoid hemorrhage. Stroke 20:747–753
4. Heros RC (1989) Acute hydrocephalus after subarachnoid hemorrhage. Stroke 20:715–717
5. Hunt WE, Hess RM (1968) Surgical risk as related to time of intervention in the repair of intracranial aneurysms. J Neurosurg 28:14–20
6. Matthews DE, Farewell VT (1988) Using and understanding medical statistics. Karger, Basel, pp 67–78
7. Mayhall CG, Archer NH, Lamb A, Spadora AC, Baggett JW, Ward JD, Narayan RK (1984) Ventriculostomy related infections. A prospective epidemiologic study. N Engl J Med 310:553–559

8. Milhorat TH (1987) Acute hydrocephalus after aneurysmal subarachnoid hemorrhage. Neurosurgery 20:15–20
9. Nornes H (1973) The role of intracranial pressure in the arrest of hemorrhage in patients with ruptured intracranial aneurysm. J Neurosurg 39:226–234
10. Seifert V, Trost HA, Stolke D (1990) Management morbidity and mortality in grade IV and V patients with aneurysmal subarachnoid hemorrhage. Acta Neurochir (Wien) 103:5–10
11. Vassilouthis J, Richardson AE (1979) Ventricular dilatation and communicating hydrocephalus following spontaneous subarachnoid hemorrhage. J Neurosurg 51:341–351
12. Wyler AR, Kelly WA (1972) Use of antibiotics with external ventriculostomies. J Neurosurg 37:185–187

Complications and Clinical Course After Shunting of Normal Pressure Hydrocephalus

J. Meixensberger[1], M. Grimm[1], and M. Janka[1]

Introduction

The classical normal pressure hydrocephalus combines the clinical triad of dementia, gait disturbances, and urinary incontinence with ventricular dilatation on computed tomography (CT). Despite multiple diagnostic tools [e.g., continuous intracranial pressure (ICP) monitoring and cerebrospinal fluid (CSF) infusion tests, cerebral blood flow measurements, CSF tap tests and magnetic resonance imaging techniques] the therapeutic successes after shunting are obscured by shunt-related complications. Besides infection, overdrainage of implanted shunt systems is one of the problems caused by normal pressure hydrocephalus. Therefore in our present prospective study we evaluated a well-characterized group of shunted normal pressure hydrocephalus patients and were especially interested in the following issues:

1. How often are shunt-related complications after shunting of normal pressure hydrocephalus and what kind of complications occur?
2. Is there a benefit after shunting for these hydrocephalus patients in their follow-up?

Patients and Methods

Our series comprised 55 patients (29 males and 26 females). Their ages ranged from 22 to 78 years, with an average of 50.5 years. The clinical status was evaluated and we found unspecific symptoms such as headaches and dizziness in 64.2% and 43.4%, respectively. As classical clinical signs of normal pressure hydrocephalus we mentioned mental deficit in 74.5%, gait disturbances in 74.5%, and urinary incontinence in 50.9% of the cases. Presumed etiology of hydrocephalus was known in 29.1% of our patients (subarachnoid hemorrhage, trauma, meningitis) and unknown in 60.9%. All patients had a ventricular dilatation (Evans ratio > 0.35 [5]) on CT, additional signs of hydrocephalus such as periventricular lucencies, and no sign of intraventricular obstruction of CSF circulation. The indication for shunting was determined after continuous measurement of epidural ICP over a period of 2 nights and an additional lumbar bolus and infusion test. We

---

[1] Neurochirurgische Klinik und Poliklinik der Universität Würzburg,
Josef-Schneider-Straße 11, W-8700 Würzburg, FRG.

Advances in Neurosurgery, Vol. 21
R. Lorenz, M. Klinger, M. Brock (Eds.)

evaluated mean (ICP) (increased: > 10–15 mmHg), frequency of nightly B waves (pathological: > 20%), and calculated pressure volume index (decreased: < 25 ml) and resistance to outflow (pathological: > 12 mmHg · min · ml) [3, 6]. Ventriculoperitoneal CSF shunting was performed using a "Mishler" ($n = 42$) or a "Uni"- ($n = 13$) shunt with a medium ($n = 13$) or a high ($n = 42$) pressure valve. Additionally we implanted an "antisiphon device" ($n = 45$) to reduce the risk of overdrainage. Perioperative antibiotic therapy (cephalosporin, sulfonamide) was performed. Postoperatively we immobilized the patients for an average of 3 days. In the follow-up (mean: 22 months, range 12–48 months) we checked the neurological status, the CT scan, and the functional improvement of quality of life [2].

Results

Table 1 summarizes the evaluated complications after shunting. Three (5.5%) CSF infections (pathogen: *Staphylococcus aureus*) occurred in our hydrocephalus group. Removal of the shunt system and adequate antibiotic therapy guaranteed a recovery without permanent deficits. In total ten (18%) cases of overdrainage and hygroma could be verified on CT in the follow-up. In three (5.5%) patients an operation was once more necessary. One (1.8%) patient did not suffer from neurological deterioration. Analyzing the shunt systems we found an overdrainage in nine of ten patients in the Uni-shunt group without an antisiphon device. In the Mishler-shunt group with an antisiphon device only in one case could a small, clinically insignificant hygroma be detected (Fig. 1). Additionally, in three cases where we implanted a Uni-shunt with an antisiphon device no overdrainage could be found. One patient who first improved after shunting, deteriorated seriously af-

Table 1. Complications after shunting of normal pressure hydrocephalus

	Without permanent deficits		With permanent deficits	
	(*n*)	(%)	(*n*)	(%)
1. Infection				
Local	0		0	
Meningitis	3	5.5	0	
2. Overdrainage (hygroma)				
In total	10	18.1	0	
Operation necessary	2	3.6	1	1.8
3. Traumatic				
Subdural hematoma	0		1	1.8
4. Shunt dysfunction				
Obstruction	4	7.3	0	
Disconnection	3	5.5	0	
Valve dysfunction	1	1.8	0	

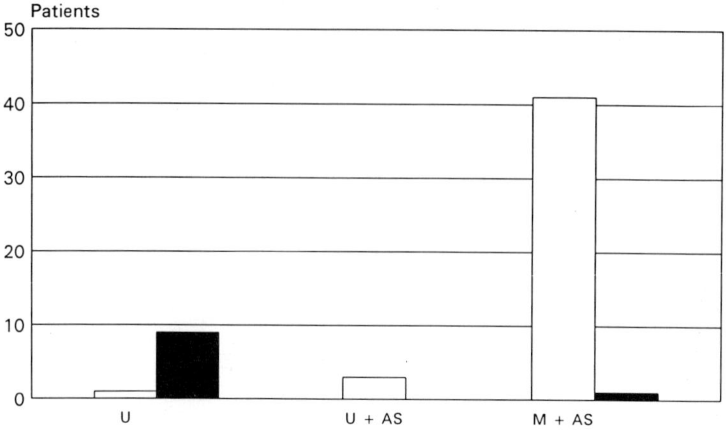

Fig. 1. Overdrainage after shunting of normal pressure hydrocephalus and the shunt valves used. *U*, Uni-shunt; *M*, Mishler shunt; with or without antisiphon device (AS). *Open columns*, no overdrainage; *solid columns*, overdrainage

ter a traumatic subdural hematoma. In the follow-up, shunt malfunction occurred in eight (14.6%) patients. After operative correction no permanent deficits were found.

In total 36 (65.4%) hydrocephalic patients improved after surgery. Despite normalizing ICP, 17 (31%) patients had no change in clinical condition. Only two (3.6%) patients got worse in the postoperative follow-up as we described above. Figure 2 summarizes the results of the analysis of the change in clinical signs during postoperative follow-up. Headaches and dizziness improved in nearly 90% of the patients. Additionally, our shunted patients suffered at different lower levels

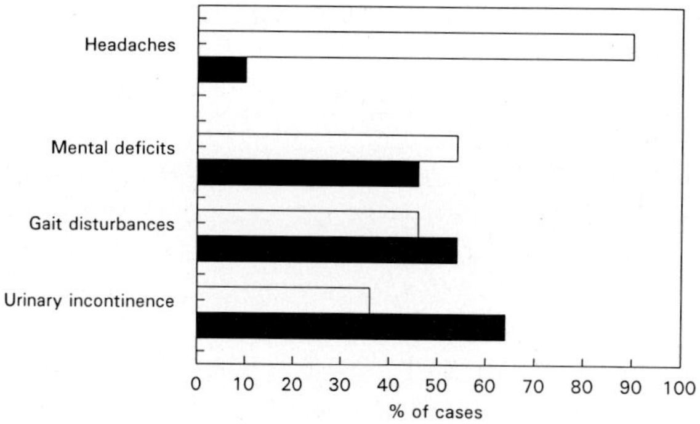

Fig. 2. Improvement of clinical symptoms after shunting of normal pressure hydrocephalus (mean follow-up 22 months, range 12–48 months). *Open columns*, improvement; *solid columns*, no improvement

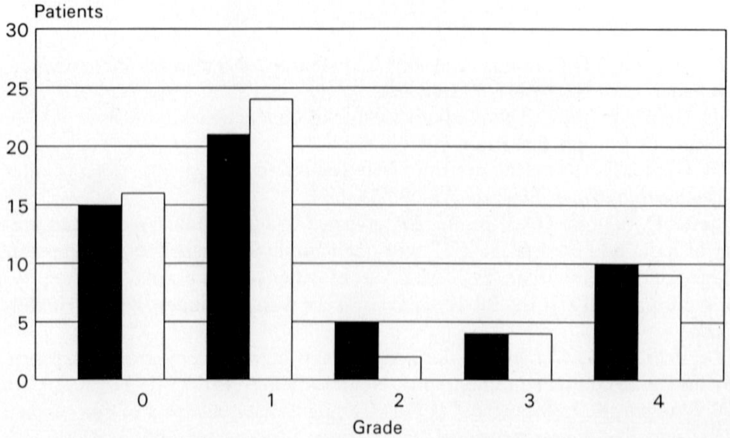

Fig. 3. Functional changes in daily life after shunting of normal pressure hydrocephalus. *0*, able to work, normal life; *1*, minor deficit, able to function independently at home; *2*, some supervision required at home; *3*, custodial care required despite considerable independent function; *4*, no practical capacity for independent function [2] (mean follow-up 22 months, range 12–48 months). *Solid columns*, preoperatively; *open columns*, postoperatively

from mental deficits, gait disturbances, and urinary incontinence. At least we could find a functional improvement of the shunted normal pressure hydrocephalus patients expressed by a lower number of patients who needed intensive care (Fig. 3).

Discussion

Risks of operation and benefit of therapy must be considered in the treatment of normal pressure hydrocephalus. Our series comprises no mortality and low morbidity with permanent deficits after shunting. Despite the fact that only patients with increased ICP and disturbances of ICP dynamics were treated, overdrainage exists. Here the siphon effect in the upright position could be almost prevented by the use of an antisiphon device [7] and immobilization for some days after the shunt operation. Additionally, in contrast to experimental evaluation of hydrodynamic quality of the Mishler valve [8], the clinical results are convincing.

In agreement with others, ventricular shunting leads to a substantial clinical improvement in about 65% of patients [1]. However, despite normalizing elevated ICP, nearly one third of our patients did not improve. Pathological ICP dynamics cannot be the only pathophysiological factor in normal pressure hydrocephalus. Disturbances of cerebral blood flow and brain metabolism must be considered as possible reasons [4]. These parameters might be more predictive and could improve our results in future.

References

1. Black P McL, Ojemann RG, Tzouras A (1985) CSF shunts for dementia, incontinence, and gait disturbance. Clin Neurosurg 32:632–651
2. Borgensen SE, Gjerris F (1982) The predictive value of conductance to outflow of CSF in normal pressure hydrocephalus. Brain 105:65–86
3. Borgensen SE, Gjerris F (1987) Relationships between intracranial pressure, ventricular size, and resistance to outflow. J Neurosurg 67:535–539
4. Delwel EJ, Hasan D, de Jong DA, Krening EP, Avezaat CJJ (1992) Diagnostic and predictive value of axial and coronal SPECT with technetium-99m labelled, D,L-hexamethyl-propylene amine oxime (99m TC HM-PAO) in patients with normal pressure hydrocephalus syndrome (NPH). In: Intracranial pressure VIII. Springer, Berlin Heidelberg New York
5. Gyldensted C (1977) Measurements of the normal ventricular system and hemispheric sulci of 100 adults with computed tomography. Neuroradiology 14:183–192
6. Marmarou A, Shulman K, LaMorgese J (1975) Compartmental analysis of compliance and outflow resistance of the cerebrospinal fluid system. J Neurosurg 43:523–524
7. Portnoy HD, Schulte RR, Fox JL et al. (1973) Anti-siphon and reversible occlusion valves for shunting in hydrocephalus and preventing post-shunt subdural hematomas. J Neurosurg 38:729–728
8. Trost HA, Claussen G, Heissler HE, Gaab MR (1992) Long term in vitro test results of various new and explanted hydrocephalus shunt valves. In: Intracranial pressure VIII. Springer, Berlin Heidelberg New York

Intrathecal Infusion Test: An Investigative Method to Treat Malresorptive Hydrocephalus by Shunt Operation

U. Meier[1], B. Reichmuth[1], W. Knopf[1], and A. Riederer[1]

The normal pressure hydrocephalus (NPH) is a clinical picture giving different results after a shunt operation [1, 2]. Because of these problems, we tried to form groups of patients on the basis of clinical symptoms and of the results of an intrathecal infusion test. Particularly the pictorial methods of representation in neuroradiology provide additional morphological information in difficult cases. Information regarding cerebral circulation is simultaneously received by xenon computed tomography (CT).

Materials and Methods

In the period from May 1982 to May 1992, 118 patients (148 examinations) were examined by means of an intrathecal infusion test. The average age of the 75 men and 43 women was 32.4 years (1 month–69 years). The mathematical basis, the normed conditions of examination, and the indications of the computer-aided infusion test are described in the literature [4, 5, 8]. The infusion test with constant flow and CT scan was performed simultaneously in 48 cases (53 examinations). Ventricular volume in cell media was verified by planimetry [6]. The size before and during the infusion test were compared. In 35 cases (37 examinations) a lumbar infusion test and the measurement of local cerebral circulation in the region of basal ganglia and circulatory area of the middle cerebral artery inside cell media were simultaneously performed by xenon CT.

Results

Hydrocephalus occlusus extraventricularis is characterized by the clinical triad dementia, gait ataxia, and urinary incontinence together with an intermittent increase of intracranial pressure with ascertainable impairment of absorption of the cerebrospinal fluid [1, 3]. Only in the case of gait ataxia was there a statistically significant difference ($p < 0.01$) between patients with normal pressure hydrocephalus and with cerebral atrophy. As a result of our liquor-dynamic examinations four groups were formed:

---

[1] Neurotraumatologische Klinik, Städtisches Krankenhaus im Friedrichshain, Landsberger Allee 49, O-1017 Berlin, FRG.

Advances in Neurosurgery, Vol. 21
R. Lorenz, M. Klinger, M. Brock (Eds.)

1. Normal pressure hydrocephalus in the early stages: resistance to outflow pathologically increased, compliance normal
2. Normal pressure hydrocephalus in the late stages: resistance to outflow pathologically increased, compliance very high
3. Hydrocephalic cerebral atrophy: resistance to outflow normal for ICP ≤ 25 Torr, pathological for ICP > 25 Torr, compliance high
4. Nonhydrocephalic cerebral atrophy: resistance to outflow normal, compliance very high

These groups were compared among themselves. There is a statistical difference for ventricular enlargement in CT scan during the infusion test between groups 1 and 2 and groups 1/2 and 3/4 (Fig. 1). The proportion of patients with periventricular lucencies in the CT scan decreases from group 1 to group 4, in contrast to those of coarse-structured sulci (Table 1). During xenon inhalation the intracranial pressure (ICP) increases by 3 Torr on average (Fig. 2). During the infusion test the proportion of patients with a decreased local cerebral circulation is greatest (100%) for patients with hydrocephalic atrophy, high (64%) for normal pressure hydrocephalus (NPH) in the late stage, and low (25%) for patients with nonhydrocephalic atrophy. One patient with NPH in the early stages was examined after shunt implantation, following slit ventricle syndrome, followed by shunt ligature. Only this patient (14%) had a decreased local circulation during the infusion test with xenon CT (Table 1). The self-assessment of the clinical course by the patients and their dependents shows significant differences with and without shunt (Fig. 3).

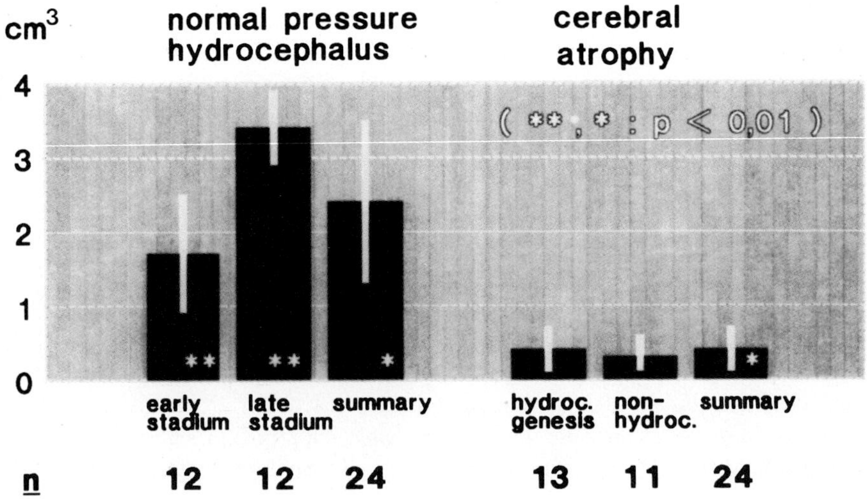

Fig. 1. Increase of ventricular volume during intrathecal infusion test in CT. Infusion rate, 1.5–2.0 ml/min; infusion volume, 10–30 ml; * ** p < 0.01

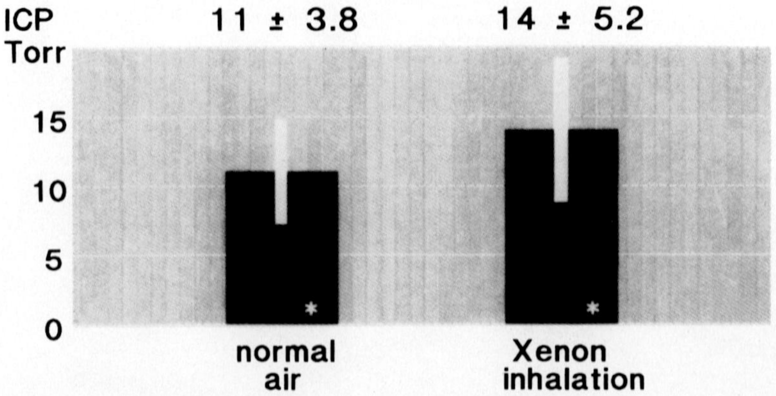

Fig. 2. ICP without volume-pressure load before and during xenon CT in 35 patients in bed position

Discussion

The computer-aided infusion test provides a 93% differentiation between patients with NPH and those with cerebro-atrophic processes. Functional checking of the valve systems is a further indication for the intrathecal infusion test. In patients with a classical pressure hydrocephalus or subdural hygromas, however, we do not see an indication for this invasive examination procedure [8]. Clinical findings are opposed to the results of liquor-dynamic investigations. The main syndrome in the case of NPH is gait ataxia. Forecast of the prognosis of disease is possible for patients with shunt by classifying according to clinical and liquor-dynamic results of investigation by differentiation of NPH in different stages just as hydrocephalic and nonhydrocephalic cerebral atrophy. Hydrocephalic cerebral atrophy could be regarded as a beginning senile or better arrested hydrocephalus. The postdiagnostic

Table 1. Results of CT and xenon CT

	Normal pressure hydrocephalus		Cerebral atrophy	
	Early stage	Late stage	Hydrocephalic genesis	Non-hydrocephalic
CT scan (*n*)	12	12	13	11
Periventricular luencies (%)	100	58	31	27
Cortical sulci to increase (%)	0	67	85	91
Xenon CT (*n*)	7	11	9	8
rCBF to decrease (%)	14	64	100	25

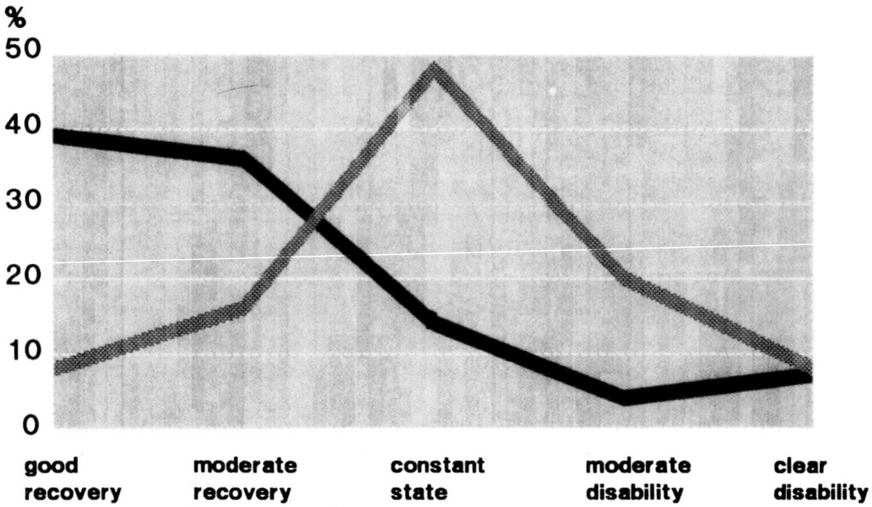

Fig. 3. Self-assessment of clinical course by patients and their dependents: outcome over a period longer than 1 year. *Solid line*, with shunt; *dotted line*, without shunt

results help to make a decision to treat by shunt operation and are critically estimated by self-assessment of the course of disease.

Exclusive CT examinations do not allow a differentiation of patients with NPH and patients with cerebral atrophy. In the simultaneous examinations the morphological substrate during the intrathecal infusion test is represented [7]. The results obtained indicate different reactions of the regional cerebral blood flow (rCBF) to increased ICP at different stages of NPH. On this basis, an assumption is made with regard to a disturbed cerebral autoregulation and the impact of ischemic processes on the pathogenesis of NPH in the late stage [9]. Without dynamic cerebrospinal fluid investigation it is not possible to exclude an NPH.

References

1. Dauch WA, Zimmermann R (1990) Der Normaldruck-Hydrozephalus. Eine Bilanz 25 Jahre nach der Erstbeschreibung Fortschr Neurol Psychiatr 58:178–190
2. Dommasch D, Mertens HG (1980) Cerebrospinalflüssigkeit – CSF. Thieme, Stuttgart, pp 212–272
3. Gjerris F, Borgesen SE, Sorensen PS (1989) Outflow of cerebrospinal fluid. Munksgaard, Copenhagen, pp 329–298
4. Künzel B, Klages G, Meier U (1987) Der intrathekale Infusionstest zur Untersuchung der kraniospinalen Liquordynamik. Ein neues Auswertverfahren. Zentralbl Neurochir 48:320–326
5. Meier U, Künzel B (1988) Rechnergestützte Modellversuche zur Liquordynamik des kraniospinalen Systems. Zentralbl Neurochir 49:233–237

6. Meier U, Michalik M, Planitzer J (1987) Computertomographische Untersuchungen zur Ventrikelgröße und Rinden-Mark-Relation des Gehirns bei einer Normalpopulation. Radiol Diagn 28:355–362
7. Meier U, Knopf W, Schmidt V, Prothmann KH, Ewert P, Reichmuth B, Michalik M, Planitzer J, Heinitz A, Lang G, Glawe H, Siedschlag WD, Gärtner F, Klötzer R, Huhnd T (1990) Typische CT-Befunde während des intrathekalen Infusionstestes bei posttraumatischen Störungen der Liquordynamik. Zentralbl Neurochir 51:102–106
8. Meier U, Knopf W, Gärtner F, Künzel B, Huhnd T (1990) Indikationen zum intrathekalen Infusionstest bei Störungen der Liquordynamik. Zentralbl Neurochir 51:107–111
9. Reichmuth B, Meier U (1991) Zerebrale Xenon-Computertomographie, Messung des regionalen zerebralen Blutflusses bei Patienten mit normal-pressure-hydrocephalus während lumbaler Druck-Volumen-Belastung (lumbaler Infusionstest). Radiol Diagn 32:42–45

Long-Term Follow-up and Computed Tomography Cisternography in the Evaluation of Normal-Pressure Hydrocephalus

C. Sprung[1], G. Gatzounis[1], and W. Lanksch[1]

Introduction

Patients with normal-pressure hydrocephalus (NPH) usually demonstrate significant early postoperative improvement, but significant clinical deterioration is observed in many cases. However, the majority of publications dealing with surgical results in NPH cover a rather short postoperative period of up to several months [1, 2, 11, 14, 19]. Only a few authors have reported longer follow-up periods [5, 15, 16, 23]. Therefore, we examined patients immediately after surgery and at long-term follow-up to determine the influence of a number of preoperative parameters on early and late results.

More than 25 years after the initial description of NPH by Hakim and Adams [7] no single diagnostic procedure offers sufficient accuracy to predict the outcome of shunt operations. Of the large number of diagnostic techniques employed in our Department [17, 18] we evaluated the results of computed tomography (CT) cisternography performed during the period 1982–1988 since this procedure has been endorsed by a number of authors as the diagnostic measure of choice in the preoperative evaluation of patients with NPH [6, 9, 10, 12, 20–22]. We reviewed long-term results in patients who had undergone metrizamide cisternography.

Patients and Methods

A total of 239 patients with clinical symptoms and CT findings characteristic of NPH were treated in our Department from 1980 to 1988. Patients with ventricular dilatation subsequent to trauma, subarachnoid hemorrhage, or meningitis, with cerebrospinal spinal fluid pressure below 18 cmH_2O at preoperative or intraoperative examination and with characteristic clinical signs of NPH were treated with a shunt procedure, without additional diagnostic measures in most cases. Patients with idiopathic NPH represent a major clinical challenge, since the diagnostic and therapeutic possibilities are still controversial in these cases. Therefore, the present study includes only two patients with meningitis and four with posttraumatic NPH.

Cisternography with metrizamide (Amipaque) was performed in 107 patients, who received 9.8 ml isotonic metrizamide solution (170 mg/ml = 1.7 g iodine) by

[1] Freie Universität Berlin, Universitätsklinikum Rudolf Virchow,
Abteilung für Neurochirurgie, Augustenburger Platz 1, W-1000 Berlin 65, FRG.

Advances in Neurosurgery, Vol. 21
R. Lorenz, M. Klinger, M. Brock (Eds.)

lumbar instillation. They were subsequently positioned with legs raised and head supported by a cushion, so that the contrast medium would collect at the craniocervical junction. In 80 cases CT studies were virtually free of motion artifacts and demonstrated passage of the contrast medium into the basal cisterns, the prerequisite for evaluation. The criteria of a negative or normal CT cisternogram were the presence of contrast medium in the basal cisterns and the 4th ventricle 3–6 h later and absence of reflux into the lateral ventricles at 12–24 h. The absence of contrast medium in the sulci and of enhancement of the cortex over the convexity (blush phenomenon) were additional criteria for a normal diagnosis. A positive (i.e., pathological) result was defined by the presence of reflux into the lateral ventricles lasting 12–24 h, stasis of the contrast medium at 24 h, absence of contrast medium in the sulci (so-called convexity block), and the absence of a blush phenomenon.

CT cisternograms were adequate for evaluation in 80 patients. There were 43 women and 37 men ranging in age from 21 to 80 years at diagnosis, with a mean age of 64.6 years. Clinical symptoms had been observed for less than 3 months in 12 patients, 3–12 months in 25, 1–2 years in 8, and more than 2 years in 17.

Preoperative symptoms were evaluated using a functional classification similar to that proposed by Stein and Langfitt [19]. Only 4 patients were in group I (indicating a mild disorder with the patient able to care for himself preoperatively), while 35 patients required some degree of assistance, and 23 patients were bedridden or hospitalized (group III). In addition, we ascertained whether dementia or motor dysfunction dominated the clinical presentation (Table 2).

On the basis of the clinical presentation, CT findings, and the results of CT cisternography, we established an indication for a drainage procedure in 63 patients, one of whom refused surgery. In the remaining 62 cases, 56 patients received a Holter valve, 5 a Sophy valve, and 1 a Hakim valve. A low-pressure valve was used in 6 cases, a medium-pressure valve in 47, and a high-pressure valve in 9.

We classified postoperative results as excellent (grade IV) when there was complete resolution of all preoperative symptoms. A good surgical result (grade III) was defined as incomplete resolution, while grade II results involved unchanged symptoms and grade I frank deterioration in comparison to the patient's preoperative condition. The initial evaluation was performed at an average of 4.3 months postoperatively and the second at a mean of 3.8 years (range 1–8 years) after surgery. Patients were evaluated using a number of psychometric tests and underwent clinical examination at least twice. In equivocal cases an additional opinion was sought from a relative or family physician.

Results

The results of the initial postoperative evaluation of the 62 surgically treated patients are presented in Table 1. In 17 patients (27.4%) there was an excellent initial result and in 34 (54.85%) a good outcome; there was no improvement in 9 (14.5%) and clinical deterioration in 2 (3.6%). At the second follow-up examination 15 of the 62 patients (24.2%) demonstrated an excellent result and 25 (40.3%) a good

Table 1. Preoperative clinical findings and outcome in patients with NPH

Preoperative condition	*n*	Outcome at 4.3 months				Outcome at 3.8 years			
		IV Excellent	III Good	II Unchanged	I Worse	IV Excellent	III Good	II Unchanged	I Worse
I (mild)	4	4	–	–	–	4	–	–	–
II (moderate)	35	7	24	3	1	7	19	9	–
III (severe)	23	6	10	6	1	4	6	8	5
Total (*n*)	62	17	34	9	2	15	25	17	5
Total (%)		27.4	54.85	15.5	3.6	24.2	40.3	27.4	8.1
Total (%)		82		18		64.5		35.5	

outcome; 17 patients (27.4%) were unchanged in comparison to their preoperative status, and deterioration was observed in 5 (8.1%). In summary, a good or excellent result was documented at the initial follow-up study in 82% of cases as compared to 64.5% of patients at 3.8 years. The proportion of unsatisfactory results increased from 18% at 4.3 months to 35.5% at 3.8 years (Table 1).

Postoperative results were superior and more stable in the six cases with defined etiologies than in the remaining patients with idiopathic NPH. Both the early and the late follow-up examinations documented good results in the four patients with posttraumatic NPH, and an excellent result was found in both patients with NPH secondary to meningitis.

There was no statistically significant relationship between treatment outcomes and duration of clinical symptoms or age at initial diagnosis.

In Table 1 early and late results are correlated with the severity of the preoperative presentation. The four patients with mild preoperative symptoms had excellent results at both early and late follow-up examinations, while less favorable long-term results were observed in cases with moderate to severe preoperative symptoms.

In Table 2 preoperative findings are classified in terms of the predominant disorder (dementia or motor dysfunction). The most favorable early outcomes were observed in patients with similar degrees of dementia and motor dysfunction. Early results were judged good or excellent in 73% of patients and satisfactory in patients with dementia as the dominant symptom. At long-term follow-up there was a slight reduction in the number of favorable outcomes among patients with predominantly motor disorders at their initial presentation, but only one patient with dementia demonstrated a good result.

Of the 80 metrizamide cisternograms suitable for evaluation, 55 demonstrated positive findings, and an operation was performed in all but one case, a patient who refused surgery. The results of 14 studies were classified as negative, but a drainage procedure was performed in three cases with pathognomonic CT scans and characteristic clinical symptoms. It was not possible to achieve an unequivocal diagnosis in 11 cases with technically adequate images (i.e., sufficient contrast in the basal cisterns and no motion artifacts). There was unilateral or partial filling of the lateral ventricle in three of these cases, defined reflux at 12 h, but incomplete resorption at 24 h in five patients and minimum contrast enhancement of the lateral ventricles at 24 or 48 h in three additional cases. Five of these patients underwent surgical treatment on the basis of clinical findings and other diagnostic measures. Table 3 presents a correlation of the results of CT cisternography with clinical findings at early and late follow-up examinations. Nine patients with unequivocally positive findings in the CT cisternogram demonstrated an unsatisfactory early postoperative result, and 14 patients had poor results at late follow-up. In contrast, two patients with negative cisternograms and four with equivocal results had good early postoperative clinical outcomes. However, at 3.8 years none of these patients demonstrated a satisfactory clinical result.

Postoperative complications were observed in 17 patients (27.4%). Surgical revision was required in one case with a large subcutaneous hematoma in the

Table 2. Symptoms and outcome in patients with NPH

Predominant symptom	Outcome at 4.3 months					Outcome at 3.8 years				
	IV Excellent		III Good	II Unchanged	I Worse	IV Excellent		III Good	II Unchanged	I Worse
Motor dysfunction	6		2	1	–	6		2	1	–
		82.1%					75%			
Motor dysfunction and mild dementia	3		12	4	–	3		10	4	2
Dementia and motor dysfunction of equal severity	5		12	1	1	4		8	4	1
		89.5%					70.6%			
Dementia and mild motor dysfunction	2		7	2	1	–		1	6	2
		73.3%					9%			
Dementia	1		1	1	–	–		–	2	–
Total (*n*)	17		34	9	2	13		21	17	5
Total (%)	27.4		54.8	14.5	3.3	23.2		37.5	30.4	8.9

Table 3. CT cisternography and postoperative outcome

Result	Outcome at 4.3 months				Outcome at 3.8 years			
	IV Excellent	III Good	II Unchanged	I Worse	IV Excellent	III Good	II Unchanged	I Worse
Positive	15	28	[illegible]	2	14	26	11	3
Negative	–	2	[illegible]	–	–	–	2	1
Equivocal	–	4	[illegible]	–	–	–	4	1
Total	17	34	9	2	14	26	17	5

abdominal wall and in two patients with shunt infection. Seven patients required additional interventions for correction of partial or complete malfunction of the shunt. A clinically symptomatic hygroma developed in seven patients, although adjustment of the Sophy valve was sufficient to obviate revision in four of these.

Discussion

After initial reports of successful drainage operations in NPH there have been descriptions of less favorable outcomes, especially in idiopathic hydrocephalus [3, 14, 15, 19, 23]. Evaluation of surgical results in patients with NPH is difficult since a wide variety of criteria have been employed. Some authors have considered improved clinical findings at 3 months a success, while others have required clinical improvement of several years duration. In addition, it is impossible to determine whether patients who were not treated surgically might have benefited from a shunt procedure. Hughes et al. [11] analyzed outcomes in this group of patients, and their findings have raised questions about the value of surgical treatment. Our series confirms the results of other authors [2, 5, 15, 19, 23] who performed repeated follow-up examinations and found less favorable outcomes at subsequent examinations (Table 4). The reduction in the number of positive results at long-term follow-up in our series is comparable to the deterioration in clinical status described in the series published by Borgesen and Petersen [2, 15]. We did not find a correlation between the clinical outcomes following surgery and duration of the preoperative symptoms or age at diagnosis, and our findings concur with those published by the majority of authors [1, 5, 11, 19], although two groups have reported contrary results [2, 15]. There was an apparent relationship between the degree of preoperative disability and outcome. We observed better postoperative results in patients with motor dysfunction than in those with dementia, but this difference became apparent only at late follow-up. Several other groups have reported similar findings [1, 5, 14].

The results in our series, most of which cases were of idiopathic NPH, indicate significantly better postoperative findings than those recently reported by Vanneste et al. [23], who found improvement in only 15% of cases with idiopathic NPH.

Several authors have reported equivalent findings with CT cisternography and isotope cisternography [6, 9, 10], and others have emphasized the advantages of superior spatial resolution and reduced radiation exposure with CT cisternography [4, 12, 20–22]. Radionuclide cisternography has achieved improved spatial resolution with single photon emission CT and three-dimensional techniques [8]. Several reports provide correlations between the results of isotope cisternography and clinical outcome [2, 13, 24]. However, the present study constitutes the first systematic evaluation of the predictive value of metrizamide cisternography in terms of surgical outcome in patients with NPH, although case reports [20] have been published, and the method has been recommended as a diagnostic technique in recent review articles [1, 16].

Table 4. Results of shunting in NPH

Authors	Year	*n*	Percentage clinical improvement (2nd evaluation)	Length of follow-up
Stein and Langfitt [19]	1974	43	67 (37)	6–30 months (mean 18 months)
Laws and Mokri [14]	1976	56	50	21.5 months
Greenberg et al. [5]	1977	73	45 (37)	9.5 months/3 years
Hughes et al. [11]	1978	27	33	18 months
Börgensen [2]	1984	64	76 (58)	3 months/12 months
Petersen et al. [15]	1985	45	75.5 (42)	10–157 months
Spanu et al. [16]	1986	54	72	3–12 months + yearly
Vanneste et al. [24]	1992	152	36	2 months–8 years (mean 3.1 years)
Present series		62	82 (64.5)	4.3 months/3.8 years

It should be noted that only 80 of 107 CT cisternograms were technically adequate. Exclusion of the studies with equivocal findings reduced this number to 57 cases. Correct prediction of the early postoperative result was possible in 81% of these patients (45 cases with correct positive CT cisternograms and 1 correct negative study). There were 9 false positive and 2 false negative results. The preoperative cisternogram predicted late outcome in 75% of cases (40 correct positive and 3 correct negative studies), while there were 40 false positive but no false negative results.

When the specificity of the diagnostic technique was calculated as suggested by Borgesen [2] the result (0.83) was slightly lower than that reported by the authors when using the constant pressure infusion test. In terms of late outcome, specificity was significantly worse at 0.74. A possible cause of the failure of CT cisternography to predict outcome may be the lack of international standardization for patient position and amount of contrast medium [18]. Even moderate degrees of aqueduct stenosis, which would not be detected by CT, would result in negative cisternograms. In addition, we are convinced that CSF circulation may be affected by movement of these patients, many of whom suffer from dementia and are very restless.

Although CT cisternography offers advantages over isotope cisternography in terms of superior spatial resolution and lower radiation exposure, we concur with Vanneste et al. [24] that CT cisternography – like isotope cisternography – "has no advantage over selecting patients for a shunt on the basis of combined clinical and CT data alone."

In contrast to other reported series [2, 16], there were no deaths during the follow-up period in our 62 surgically treated patients. The surgical complication rate was 27.4%, comparable to results reported by other authors [2, 14, 19, 23].

Conclusions

Patients with defined etiologies have better and more stable postoperative outcomes than do patients with idiopathic NPH. Outcome is also better in cases with motor disorders rather than dementia, especially in terms of long-term results. Our series confirms the fact that postoperative results vary with the interval between treatment and follow-up examination. This underscores the necessity of late follow-up examinations for evaluation of surgical treatment.

Twenty-five examinations were technically inadequate. Of 62 surgically treated patients 57 had unequivocal findings in the CT cisternogram. These correctly predicted outcome at early follow-up examination in 81% of cases, while 18% of results were incorrect in terms of predictive accuracy; 75% of studies correctly predicted late outcome, while 25% were inaccurate. On the basis of these findings we believe that this diagnostic procedure is no longer indicated for the preoperative evaluation of this group of patients. Examination of CSF pulsation and circulation by means of MRI and measurements of cerebral blood flow may provide improved accuracy in terms of surgical outcomes.

References

1. Black PM, Ojemann RG, Izouras A (1985) CSF shunts for dementia, incontinence, and gait disturbance. Clin Neurosurg 32:632–656
2. Borgesen SE (1984) Conductance to outflow of CSF in normal pressure hydrocephalus. Acta Neurochir (Wien) 71:1–45
3. Clarfield AM (1989) Normal-pressure hydrocephalus: saga or swamp? (editorial) JAMA 262:2592–2593
4. Drayer BP, Rosenbaum AE, Higman HB (1977) Cerebrospinal fluid imaging using serial metrizamide. CT cisternography. Neuroradiology 13:7–17
5. Greenberg JO, Shenkin HA, Adam R (1977) Idiopathic normal pressure hydrocephalus: a report of 73 patients. J Neurol Neurosurg Psychiatry 40:336–341
6. Greitz T, Hindmarsh T (1974) Computer assisted tomography of intracranial CSF circulation using a watersoluble contrast medium. Acta Radiol 15:497–507
7. Hakim S, Adams RD (1965) The special clinical problem of symptomatic hydrocephalus with normal cerebrospinal fluid pressure: observations on cerebrospinal fluid hydrodynamics. J Neurol Sci 2:307–327
8. Henkes H, Huber G, Hierholzer J, Cordes M, Kujat C, Piepgras M (1991) Radionuklidzisternographie: SPECT- und 3D-Technik. Radiologie 31:489–495
9. Hindmarsh T, Greitz T (1975) Computer cisternography in the diagnosis of communicating hydrocephalus. Acta Radiol Suppl (Stockh) 346:91–97
10. Hindmarsh T, Greitz T (1977) Hydrocephalus, atrophy and their differential diagnosis: CSF dynamics investigated by computer cisternography. In: du Boulay GH, Moseley IF (eds) Computerized axial tomography in clinical practice. Springer, Berlin Heidelberg New York, pp 205–212
11. Hughes CP, Siegel BA, Coxe WS et al. (1978) Adult idiopathic communicating hydrocephalus with and without shunting. J Neurol Neurosurg Psychiatry 41:961–971
12. Inaba Y, Hiratsuka H, Tsuyumu M, Suganuma Y, Okada K, Fujiwara K, Takasato Y (1978) Diagnostic value of CT cisternography with intrathecal metrizamide enhancement, comparison with isotope cisternography. Neuroradiology 16:214–215
13. Larsson A, Moonen M, Bergh AC, Lindberg S, Wikkelsö C (1990) Predictive value of quantitative cisternography in normal pressure hydrocephalus. Acta Neurol Scand 81:327–332
14. Laws ER Jr, Mokri B (1977) Occult hydrocephalus: results of shunting correlated with diagnostic tests. In: Keener EB (ed) Clinical neurosurgery. Williams & Wilkins, Baltimore, 316–333
15. Petersen RC, Mokri B, Laws ER Jr (1985) Surgical treatment of idiopathic hydrocephalus in elderly patients. Neurology 35:307–311
16. Spanu G, Sangiovanni G, Locatelli D (1986) Normal-pressure hydrocephalus: twelve years experience. Neurochirurgia 29:15–19
17. Sprung C, Collmann H, Fuchs EC, Suwito S, Duisberg R (1977) Pre- and postoperative evaluation of hydrocephalus using the infusion test. In: Wüllenweber R, Brock M, Hamer J, Klinger M, Spoerri O (eds) Advances in Neurosurgery 4. Springer, Berlin Heidelberg New York, pp 161–167
18. Sprung C, Grumme T (1979) Use of CT cisternography, RISA cisternography, and the infusion test for predicting shunting results in normal pressure hydrocephalus (NPH). In: Marguth F, Brock M, Kazner E, Klinger M, Schmiedek P (eds) Advances in Neurosurgery 7. Springer, Berlin Heidelberg New York, pp 350–360
19. Stein SC, Langfitt TW (1974) Normal pressure hydrocephalus. Predicting the results of cerebrospinal fluid shunting. J Neurosurg 41:463–470
20. Takahashi M, Arii H, Tamakawa Y (1978) Comparison of metrizamide CT cisternography with radionuclide cisternography in abnormal cerebrospinal fluid dynamics. Neuroradiology 16:199–202

21. Tamaki N, Kanazawa Y, Asada M, Kusunoki T, Matsumoto S (1978) Comparison of cerebrospinal fluid dynamics studied by computed tomography (CT) and radioisotope (RI) cisternography. Neuroradiology 16:193–198
22. Tamaki N, Kanazawa Y, Asada M, Kusunoki T, Matsumoto S (1979) Dynamics of cerebrospinal fluid circulation evaluated by metrizamide CT cisternography. Compt Assist Tomogr 3 (2):209–216
23. Vanneste J, Augustijn P, Dirven C, Tan WF, Goedhart ZD (1992) Shunting normal-pressure hydrocephalus: do the benefits outweigh the risks? A multicenter study and literature review. Neurology 42:54–59
24. Vanneste J, Augustijn P, Davies, Gareth AG, Dirven C, Tan WF (1992) Normal-pressure hydrocephalus: is cisternography still useful in selecting patients for a shunt? Arch Neurol 49:366–370

Narrow Sulci at the Medial Brain Surface: A Feature of Normal-Pressure Hydrocephalus in Computerized Tomography ?

D. Van Roost[1], L. Solymosi[1], and P. M. Wallenfels[1]

Introduction

In computerized tomography (CT), obliterated cerebral sulci represent a common sign of raised intracranial pressure, which is found in obstructive hydrocephalus; the sign more or less fails in malresorptive hydrocephalus and is totally missing in ex vacuo hydrocephalus. Whereas it is hardly possible to distinguish between a malresorptive and an ex vacuo hydrocephalus on the basis of the sulci of the convexity, the sulci of the medial brain surface seem to present themselves as a differentiating feature. Figure 1 shows a malresorptive hydrocephalus with open sulci at the convexity, but not at the medial brain surface. Figure 2 shows an ex vacuo hydrocephalus with wide sulci both at the medial brain surface and at the convexity.

Method

We retrospectively assessed 12 patients with a mean age of 64 (± 14) years, who were treated for malresorptive hydrocephalus with a cerebrospinal fluid (CSF) shunt. Preoperatively, these patients showed the clinical signs of a normal-pressure hydrocephalus except for a dilatation of the inner CSF spaces and preserved convexity sulci: five out of 12 patients showed the entire triad with dementia gait, and micturition disorders, four patients showed dementia with or without a gait disorder, but without a micturition disorder. Three patients did not present with dementia, one of them without either gait or micturition disorders, but only with a vague headache and intermittent vertigo. In all 12 patients the diagnosis was confirmed by a CT study of CSF dynamics, disclosing a protracted enhancement of the intraventricular CSF after lumbar intrathecal application of contrast medium. In three patients the intraventricular pressure was monitored over 48 h. After CSF shunt placement, a clear improvement of clinical signs was seen in eight, a partial improvement in one and a questionable improvement in two out of the 12 patients.

On the pre- and postoperative CT scans we measured the volume of the inner and outer CSF spaces. The outer CSF spaces were divided in convexity and medial brain surface. For the volumetric measurement we used a stereologic method based

[1] Neurochirurgische Klinik, Universität Bonn, Sigmund-Freud-Straße 25, W-5300 Bonn 1, FRG.

Advances in Neurosurgery, Vol. 21
R. Lorenz, M. Klinger, M. Brock (Eds.)

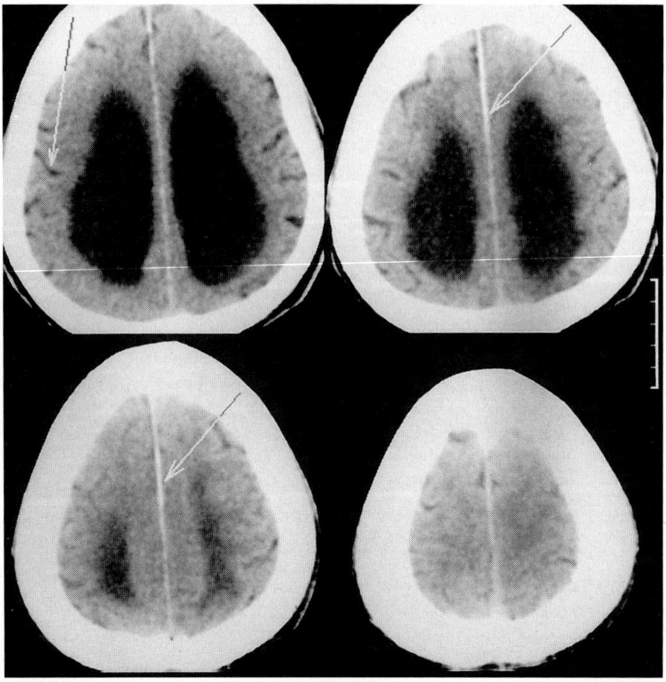

Fig. 1. Malresorptive hydrocephalus: open sulci at the convexity, obliterated sulci at the medial brain surface

on the Cavalieri theorem of systematic sampling [1, 2]. For this purpose a transparent counting grid is superimposed on the CT film. For every CT slice, the grid points that hit the area of interest are counted and multiplied by the slice thickness. We chose a 5 x 5-mm point spacing of the grid to measure the intracranial space and the ventricles, and a 1 x 1-mm point spacing to measure the sulci. Finally, the cumulative value for all the slices can be translated into an absolute volumetric quantity by taking the CT scale into account. In order to make an easier comparison of the figures, however, we calculated relative CSF volumes with the respective intracranial space as a reference.

Results

One patient showed a ratio of 0.2448 of ventricular to intracranial space before the shunt and a ratio of 0.1796 after the shunt, i.e., a change of – 27%. In the same patient, the part of the convexity sulci in the skull content preoperatively amounted to 0.0243, postoperatively to 0.0354, i.e., a change of + 45%. The sulci of the medial brain surface participate in the skull content preoperatively to 0.0061 and postoperatively to 0.0108, which is a change of + 78%. These changes are the product of

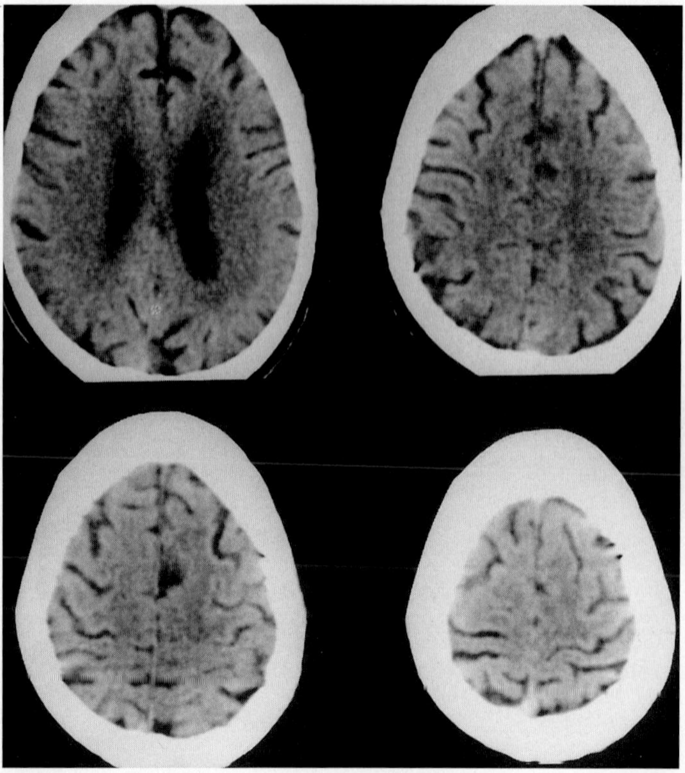

Fig. 2. Ex vacuo hydrocephalus: wide sulci both at the medial brain surface and at the convexity

measurements and not very conspicuous at first glance on the CT slices. Only by turning one's attention to the sulci of the medial brain surface can one visually recognize the increase in size.

Averaging these measurements for all 12 patients, we find, after shunting, a volume reduction of the lateral ventricles of 19% ± 16% and a volume increase of the convexity sulci of 13% ± 17%. The volume increase of the sulci of the medial brain surface, however, amounts to 59% ± 21%. A histogram (Fig. 3) displays even better the relative percentual changes of the inner and outer CSF spaces after shunting.

Conclusion

In malresorptive hydrocephalus, the regularization of the CSF pressure by a shunt obviously produces a proportionally well-balanced decrease of the inner and increase of the outer CSF spaces, whereas the sulci of the medial brain surface

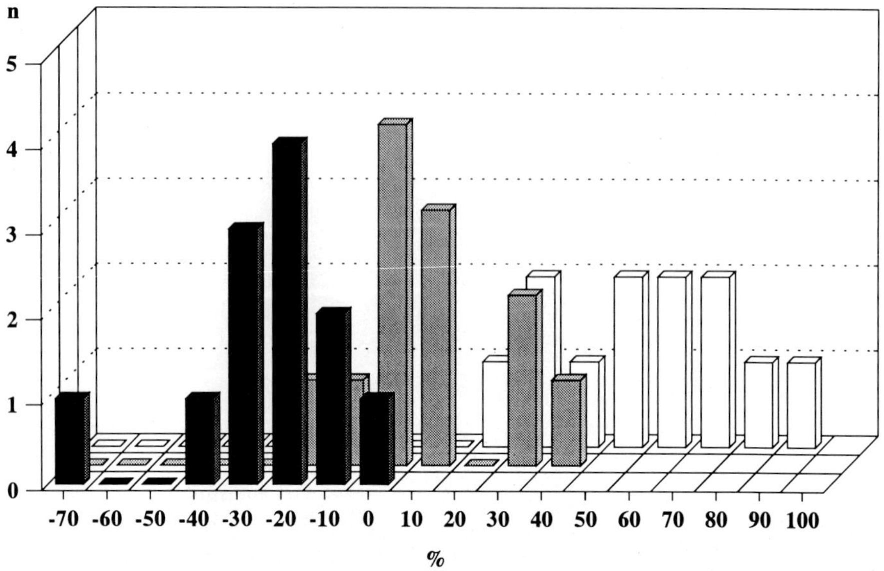

Fig. 3. Histogram displaying the percentual changes of the inner and outer CSF spaces after shunting in malresorptive hydrocephalus. The lateral ventricles (*solid columns*) decrease by 20% on average, the sulci of the convexity (*shaded columns*) increase by 10% on average, and the sulci of the medial brain surface (*open columns*) show a broad scattering around the 50%–60% mark

increase in an unproportional manner. Inversely, the sulci of the medial brain surface in untreated malresorptive hydrocephalus are distinctly narrower than the sulci of the convexity, and even in a nonenhanced CT scan they represent a characteristic feature. The value of this feature lies in the availability of a sign on routine CT scan that helps to distinguish a malresorptive from an ex vacuo hydrocephalus and, in consequence, to indicate a shunt for treatment.

References

1. Cavalieri B (1966) Geometria degli indivisibili. Unione Tipographico, Torino
2. Pakkenberg B, Boesen J, Albeck M, Gjerris F (1989) Unbiased and efficient estimation of total ventricular volume of the brain obtained from CT-scans by a stereological method. Neuroradiology 31:413–417

Aqueductal Cerebrospinal Fluid Flow Phenomena on Magnetic Resonance Imaging: Comparison with Intracranial Pressure and Cerebrospinal Fluid Dynamics

E. Hofmann[1], J. Meixensberger[1], M. Warmuth-Metz[1], T. Becker[1], K. Pfister[1], and M. Jackel[1]

Introduction

Magnetic resonance imaging (MRI), in contrast to computed tomography (CT), yields not only a description of static anatomy, but can also be used to assess certain functional aspects, e.g., cerebrospinal fluid (CSF) flow. Aqueductal stenosis and conditions with excessive CSF flow can easily be distinguished using proper MRI pulse sequences [1, 5]. Cardiac-gated gradient-echo sequences, among others, have proved useful in evaluating CSF pulsations [8]. CSF flow presents as a rhythmic change in signal intensity which can be visualized on a fast closed-loop display ("cine" or "movie" mode).

It has been stated that MRI techniques need clinical verification before being recognized as valid diagnostic tools [3]. The present study aimed to correlate results of invasive clinical tests with findings at MRI.

Material and Methods

We used a cardiac-gated fast field echo (FFE) sequence, a gradient-echo sequence installed on our Philips Gyroscan S15 scanner. A low flip angle (10°) and long echo time (35 ms) resulted in T2*-weighted images with CSF appearing bright. Per heartbeat interval, eight individual images representing the corresponding heart phases were obtained. On midsagittal images, pulsatile CSF flow through the mesencepahalic aqueduct resulted in oscillating signal void (Fig. 1) which could be measured and calculated. The resulting signal vs. time graph was evaluated.

Mean signal value over all eight heart phases was regarded as a measure for pulsatility of aqueductal CSF flow. Fast flow corresponded with strong signal loss. A total of 26 hydrocephalic patients (14 males and 12 females aged 18–73 years, mean age 47 years) were evaluated. Their main clinical symptoms were headache (16/26), gait disturbance (16/26), dementia (14/26), and urinary incontinence (5/26). All patients underwent continuous epidural pressure monitoring for at least 24 h. In all cases additional dynamic CSF studies were performed using the bolus injection method.

---

[1] Abteilung Neuroradiologie, Universität Würzburg, Josef-Schneider-Straße 11, W-8700 Würzburg, FRG.

Advances in Neurosurgery, Vol. 21
R. Lorenz, M. Klinger, M. Brock (Eds.)

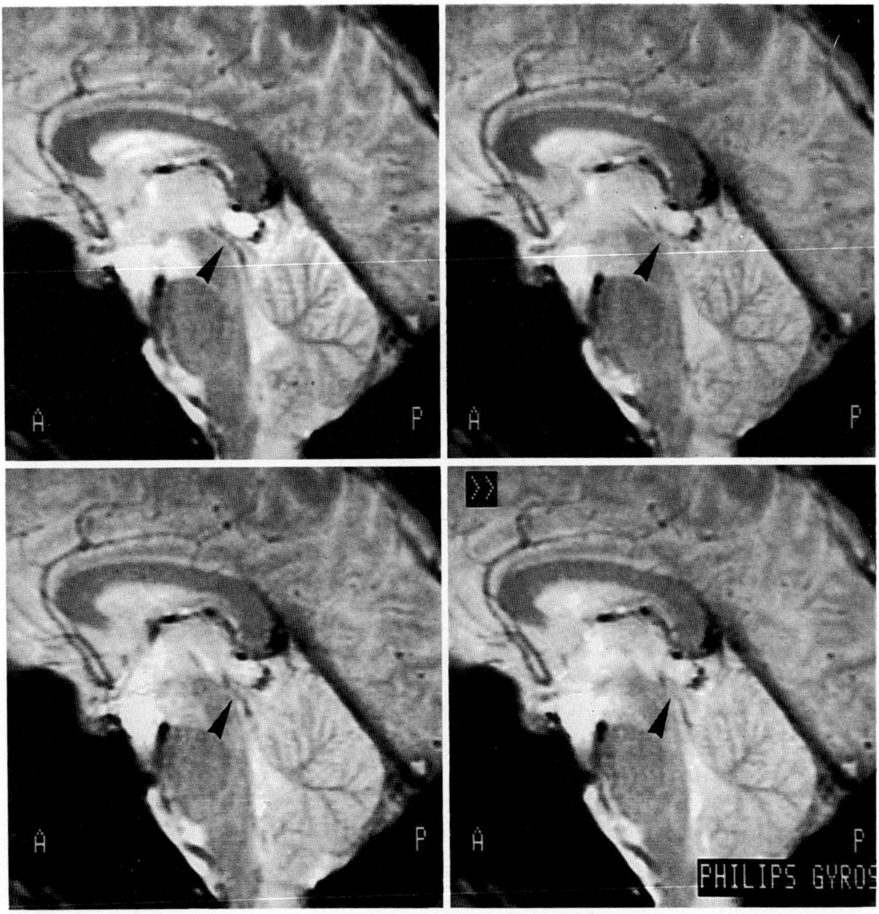

Fig. 1. Representative sagittal images of a healthy volunteer. *Top left* to *bottom right*, heart phases 8, 138, 268, and 398 ms after R wave. Initial signal loss due to retrograde aqueductal flow, subsequent hyperintensity represents stagnant CSF during flow reversal. Second signal void due to antegrade flow. *Arrowheads*, aqueduct

Magnetic resonance findings in our patients could be compared with a control group of 21 healthy volunteers (eight males and 13 females aged 22–92 years, mean age 45 years). Pathology of aqueductal CSF pulsation was assumed either when there was no detectable flow or when the calculated value was beyond the normal value plus or minus the double standard deviation range.

Implantation of a shunt was indicated when B wave activity exceeded 40% or outflow resistance was above 12 Torr/ml per minute ($n = 14$). In one additional patient with only a moderate increase of outflow resistance and B wave activity, clinical deterioration made shunting necessary.

Results

A summary of findings is given in Table 1. Of those patients in whom a shunt had to be implanted ($n = 15$), only one had an MRI study within the normal range. This patient had typical signs and symptoms of idiopathic intracranial hypertension (pseudotumor cerebri) in spite of a massive dilatation of ventricles as well as of external CSF spaces. Among the remaining 14 patients, aqueductal CSF pulsations were absent ("aqueductal stenosis") in eight (Fig. 2), reduced in one, and intensified in five (Fig. 3).

Among 11 patients in whom shunting was not warranted, ten abnormal MRI studies were noted. Four individuals had aqueductal stenosis, six showed increased CSF pulsations.

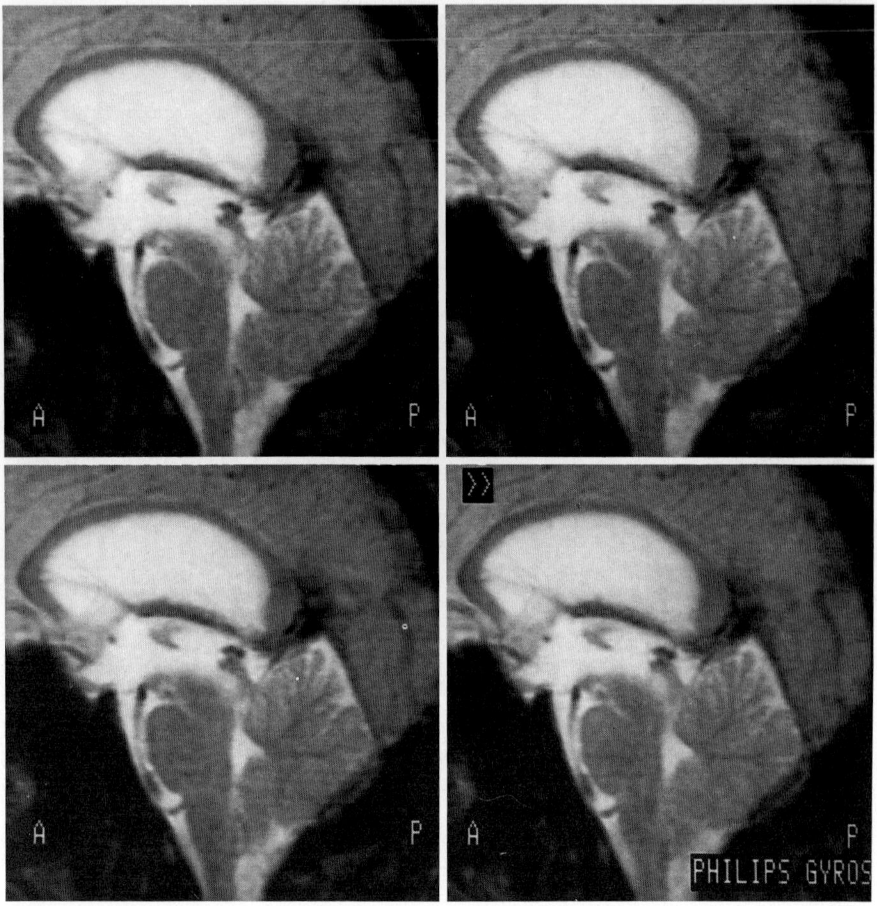

Fig. 2. A 31-year-old male with gait disturbances, increased outflow resistance, and B wave activity. No detectable aqueductal CSF flow on MRI 102, 289, 477, and 664 ms after R wave (aqueductal stenosis)

Table 1. MR findings in patients with and without indication for shunting

	MR normal	MR pathologic
Shunting indicated	1[a]	14
Shunting not indicated	1	10[b]

[a] Patient with idiopathic intracranial hypertension (pseudotumor cerebri) and dilatation of internal and external CSF spaces.
[b] One patient with clearly pathologic findings at MRI and invasive measurement was not shunted as she had only minor complaints.

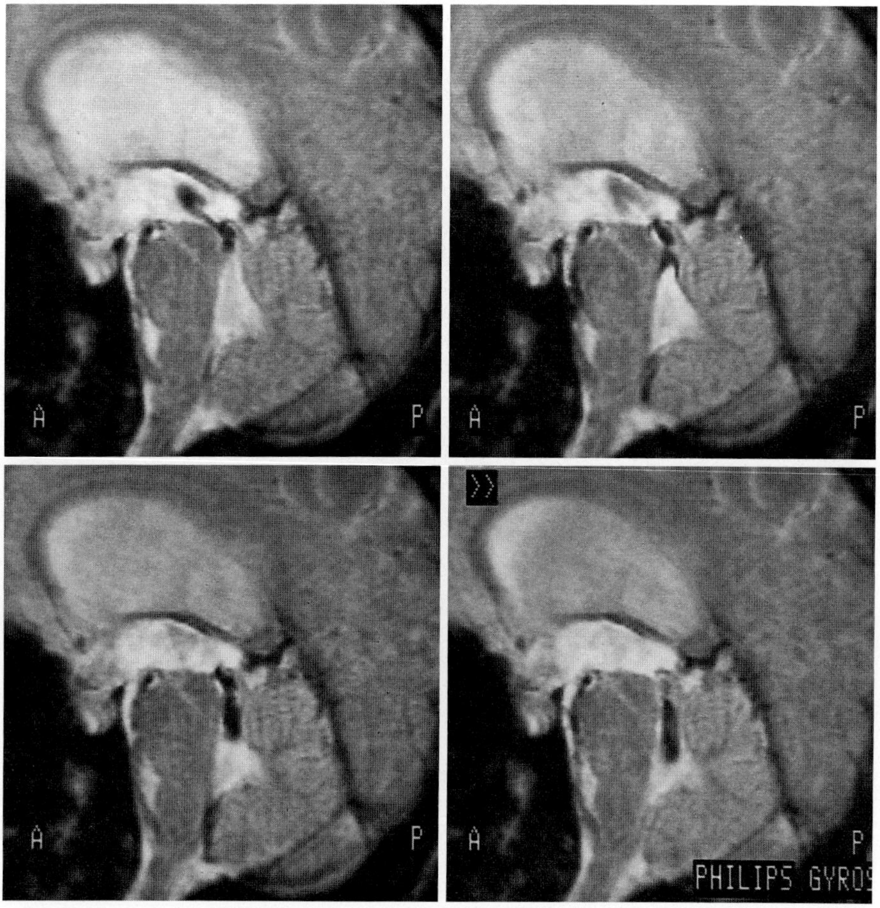

Fig. 3. A 59-year-old female with gait disturbances, increased outflow resistance, and B wave activity. Pronounced aqueductal signal loss 70, 195, 320, and 445 ms after R wave. Note synchronous flow void in foramen of Magendie

Discussion

Before the advent of MRI, the pulsatile nature of CSF flow was a familiar observation on fluoroscopic studies. DuBoulay et al. [4] gave a detailed description of pulsatile movements in the CSF pathways. His finding of rhythmic to-and-fro pulsations through the aqueduct is fully confirmed by our results and those of others [6, 8].

Magnetic resonance imaging has attracted new interest to the study of CSF dynamics. On conventional "static" MRI, the presence of marked aqueductal CSF flow void has been associated with normal-pressure hydrocephalus [2]. This sign, however, is of limited diagnostic value as it is subject to technical and patient-associated factors. Special imaging techniques can overcome these shortcomings. Gradient-echo sequences do not give a quantitative analysis of flow, but they are widely used and can permit a semiquantitative assessment of CSF flow. Protons moving in-plane lead to a loss of signal due to phase shift, phase dispersion, and turbulence. The method outlined above is unable to detect slow bulk flow of CSF. With cardiac gating, however, we can visualize rhythmic CSF pulsations by assessing flow-dependent signal void.

Few communications have described correlations of CSF flow on MRI with intracranial pressure [7]. Our preliminary results indicate that the technique is a simple, noninvasive, and sensitive method of detecting pathologic aqueductal flow. A normal CSF flow pattern established by the above-mentioned method suggests caution before proceeding to invasive pressure monitoring. However, we are unable, so far, to predict which patients might benefit from shunting. This decision must be based on clinical findings, course, and invasive testing.

References

1. Atlas SW, Mark AS, Fram EK (1988) Aqueductal stenosis: evaluation with gradient-echo rapid MR imaging. Radiology 169:449–453
2. Bradley WG, Whittemore AR, Kortman KE, Watanabe AS, Homyak M, Teresi LM, Davis SJ (1991) Marked cerebrospinal fluid void: indicator of successful shunt in patients with suspected normal-pressure hydrocepahus. Radiology 178:459–466
3. Clark WC, Muhlbauer MS (1992) Disorders of cerebrospinal fluid circulation and edema. Curr Opin Neurol Neurosurg 5:22–24
4. Du Boulay G, O'Connell J, Currie J, Bostick T, Verity P (1972) Further investigations on pulsatile movements in the cerebrospinal fluid pathways. Acta Radiol [Diagn] 13:496–523
5. Jack CR, Mokri B, Laws ER, Houser OW, Baker HL, Petersen RC (1987) MR findings in normal-pressure hydrocephalus: significance and comparison with other forms of dementia. J Comput Assist Tomogr 11:923–931
6. Mark AS, Feinberg DA, Brant-Zawadzki MN (1987) Changes in size and magnetic resonance signal intensity of the cerebral CSF spaces during the cardiac cycle as studied by gated, high-resolution magnetic resonance imaging. Invest Radiology 22:290–297
7. Ohara S, Nagai H, Ueda Y (1989) CSF pulsatile flow on MRI and its relation to intracranial pressure. In: Hoff JT, Betz AL (eds) Intracranial pressure, vol 7. Springer, Berlin Heidelberg New York, pp 410–415

8. Quencer RM, Donovan Post MJ, Hinks RS (1990) Cine MR in the evaluation of normal and abnormal CSF flow: intracranial and intraspinal studies. Neuroradiology 32:371–391

Clinical Experience with a New Flow-Regulating Hydrocephalus Shunt System

H. Wiedemayer[1] and S. Sackers[1]

Introduction

To date, most shunt systems for surgical treatment of hydrocephalus are differential pressure valves with fairly constant resistance. The amount of cerebrospinal fluid (CSF) drained by these systems varies widely following variations of differential pressure. Particularly when the patient is in an upright position, differential pressure increases extremely, leading to considerable overdrainage of CSF (siphon effect). Overdrainage of CSF may cause clinical manifestations such as slit ventricles and subdural effusions.

To overcome these complications related to overdrainage, a new shunt system was introduced [7], which is now commercially available (Orbis-Sigma Valve, Cordis). This shunt system maintains constant CSF drainage by means of a variable resistance between certain differential pressure limits. Complications of overdrainage of CSF should be reduced using this shunt device. This open study was performed to evaluate the significance of these advantages in clinical practice.

Patients and Methods

Between 1988 and 1990 52 patients with hydrocephalus of differing origins were treated by insertion of an Orbis-Sigma Valve (group 1) and another 52 patients (group 2) received a conventional differential pressure valve, which had been used routinely in our unit up to that date (Pudenz-Schulte Valve, PS-medical, medium pressure).

Age, sex distribution, and diagnosis of both groups are listed in Table 1. Thirty-five patients in group 1 and 37 patients in group 2 received their first shunt system. The other patients underwent operative revisions of previously implanted devices. In these patients, a complete new shunt system was implanted including ventricular catheter, valve, and distal catheter. Details of operative procedures are listed in Table 2.

All the patients in both groups 1 and 2 were followed by means of clinical controls for a mean of 410 and 333 days, respectively. At least one computed

[1] Universitätsklinikum Essen, Neurochirurgische Klinik und Poliklinik, Hufelandstraße 55, W-4300 Essen 1, FRG.

Advances in Neurosurgery, Vol. 21
R. Lorenz, M. Klinger, M. Brock (Eds.)

Table 1. Patients and diagnosis

	Group 1 ($n = 52$)	Group 2 ($n = 52$)
Mean age (years)	32.2	25.6
Newborns (*n*)	12	11
Female (*n*)	23	31
Male (*n*)	29	21
Congenital hydrocephalus (*n*)	6	4
Hydrocephalus and myelocele (*n*)	8	7
Occlusive hydrocephalus (*n*)	15	14
Normal-pressure hydrocephalus (*n*)	15	14
Others (*n*)	8	13

Table 2. Operative procedures

	Group 1 (*n*)	Group 2 (*n*)
First operation	35	37
Revision	17	15
Biventricular shunt	1	4
Peritoneal shunt	46	34
Atrial shunt	6	18

tomographic (CT) scan was performed in all patients 3 months or later following operation.

The postoperative complications are listed in Table 3. The rate of shunt infections was about 6% overall: five patients in group 2 and one patient in group 1. Dysfunction of the shunt system with consecutive underdrainage of CSF occurred in five patients in each group. In two of these patients of each group, occlusion of the ventricular catheter was detected intraoperatively.

Table 3. Postoperative complications

	Group 1	Group 2
Mean follow-up (days)	410	333
Complications		
Infection (*n*)	1	5
Dysfunction (*n*)	5	5
Ventricular catheter (*n*)	2	2
Others (*n*)	8	5
Subdural effusion (*n*)	4	3
Slit ventricle (*n*)	0	1

Table 4. Patients with overdrainage: age and diagnosis

Group 1			Group 2		
Patient no.	Age	Diagnosis	Patient no.	Age	Diagnosis
1.	3 days	Occlusive hydrocephalus	5.	69 years	Normal-pressure hydrocephalus
2.	68 years	Normal-pressure hydrocephalus	6.	39 years	Occlusive hydrocephalus
3.	69 years	Normal-pressure hydrocephalus	7.	54 years	Normal-pressure hydrocephalus[a]
4.	76 years	Normal-pressure hydrocephalus[a]	8.	20 years	Hydrocephalus following meningitis

[a] Patients 1–7 had subdural effusions and patient 8 slit ventride. Patients remained completely free of clinical symptoms.

Other minor complications such as local hematomas or subcutaneous CSF accumulations were observed in eight patients in group 1 and five patients in group 2. These minor complications resolved spontaneously without further operative intervention.

Finally, subdural effusions were observed in four patients in group 1 and in three patients in group 2. Two of these patients with subdural effusions – one of each group – remained completely free of clinical symptoms (Table 4). Subdural effusions were detected on routine CT scan only. These two patients were followed clinically and subdural effusions resolved spontaneously. In the other patients, operative treatment including subdural drainage and temporary occlusion of the shunt system was necessary.

Those patients with complications related to overdrainage are listed separately in Table 4. Particularly older patients with normal-pressure hydrocephalus were at risk. Symptomatic slit ventricles were observed in one patient only. This patient, suffering from hydrocephalus following meningitis, belonged to group 2.

Discussion

Treatment of hydrocephalus with conventional differential pressure valves leads to considerable overdrainage of CSF when the patient is in the upright position. In vivo studies in shunt-treated patients demonstrated a lowering of intracranial pressure down to –370 mm H_20 in the upright position [3, 4]. Clinical complications following overdrainage of CSF are slit ventricles and subdural effusions [1, 2, 5].

To overcome this problem, modifications of the shunt systems have been developed, e.g., antisiphon devices [3, 6, 8] and programmable valves.

Antisiphon devices change the opening pressure and the resistance of the valve [4] and in this way can cause underdrainage of CSF. Shunt systems with programmable resistance are, in our opinion, inadequate because they do not respond to the postural changes of differential pressure.

The Orbis-Sigma Valve is an interesting approach to this problem because of its variable resistance that maintains a fairly constant flow of between 20 and 30 ml/h, near the ranges of normal CSF secretion, at differential pressures of 80–360 mm H_2O [7]. Within these ranges of differential pressure, overdrainge should be avoided or reduced.

Nevertheless, our clinical experience using this shunt system is in contrast to these theoretical advantages. Subdural effusions – considered as a typical consequence of overdrainage – occurred in four of 52 patients (group 1) who were fitted with the Orbis-Sigma Valve. Using a conventional differential pressure valve in another 52 patients (group 2), subdural effusions were encountered in three patients. One additional patient of this group suffered from slit ventricles. Overall complications of overdrainage were equal in both groups.

The antisiphon effect of the Orbis-Sigma Valve is apparently not sufficient to overcome the clinical complications due to overdrainage.

Considering the hydrodynamic characteristics of this valve one can state that, at differential pressures greater than 350 mm H_2O, CSF flow rates rapidly increase. In adult patients, differential pressure reaches values of up to 400 mm H_2O or higher in the upright position causing remarkable overdrainage in this shunt system too.

Finally, complications of underdrainage were equal in both patient groups. Underdrainage was related to dysfunction of the peripheral catheter in three patients and to occlusion of the ventricular catheter in two patients in each group. Overall, the new shunt system is, in our experience, as reliable as the conventional device which had been used in our unit up until then.

Conclusions

1. The Orbis-Sigma Valve is as reliable as a conventional differential pressure valve with regard to the incidence of shunt dysfunctions.
2. Overdrainage of CSF with clinical manifestation of subdural effusions is not prevented or significantly reduced using this valve.

References

1. Faulhauer K, Schmitz P (1978) Overdrainage phenomena in shunt treated hydrocephalus. Acta Neurochir (Wien) 45:98–101
2. Forrest DM, Cooper DGW (1968) Complications of ventriculoatrial shunts. A review of 455 cases. J Neurosurg 29:506–512
3. Fox JL, Portnoy HD, Shulte RR (1973) Cerebrospinal fluid shunts: an experimental evaluation of flow rates and pressure values in the anti-siphon valve. Surg Neurol 1:299–302
4. Fox JL, McCullough DC, Green RC (1973) Effect of cerebrospinal fluid shunts on intracranial pressure and on cerebrospinal fluid dynamics. II. A new technique of pressure

measurements: results and concepts. III. A concept of hydrocephalus. J Neurol Neurosurg Psychiatry 36:302–312

5. Liesegang J, Strahl EW, Streicher HR (1980) Complications following shunt operations in children. In: Grote W, Brock M, Clar HE, Klinger M, Nau HE (eds) Advances in Neurosurgery, vol 8. Springer, Berlin Heidelberg New York, pp 222–226
6. Portnoy HD, Tripp L, Croissant PD (1976) Hydrodynamics of shunt valves. Childs Brain 2:242–256
7. Sainte-Rose C, Hooven MD, Hirsch JF (1987) A new approach in the treatment of hydrocephalus. J Neurosurg 66:213–226
8. Yamada H (1982) A flow-regulating device to control differential pressure in CSF shunt systems. J Neurosurg 57:570–573

Management of Hydrocephalus in Craniosynostosis

H. Collmann[1], N. Sörensen[1], J. Krauß[1], C. Michel[2], and J. Mühling[2]

Introduction

Ventricular dilation in patients with primary craniosynostosis raises several questions concerning etiology and pathogenesis, clinical significance, and indication for shunt treatment. In a few previous reports hydrocephalus in these patients has been attributed to either coincidental cerebral malformations [5], constriction of the subarachnoid space [4, 8] or venous obstruction [11]. Golabi found that some 4% of patients with craniosynostosis develop shunt-dependent hydrostatic hydrocephalus. More often, however, ventricular dilation represents only a kind of dysmorphic ventriculomegaly (hydrocephalus ex vacuo), as stated by Noetzel et al. [9] and confirmed in our own previous study [3].

Since intracranial hypertension may be due to both craniostenosis and CSF accumulation, hydrostatic hydrocephalus may not easily be recognized in these patients. The objective of the present study was to obtain more information about the characteristics of hydrostatic hydrocephalus in craniosynostosis.

Methods

During the last 9 years routine examination of patients operated on for craniosynostosis at our institution included examination of the CSF spaces. Most patients underwent computed tomography and some magnetic resonance imaging. Only in simple scaphocephaly was information based predominantly on pre- or early postoperative ultrasound examination. Most patients with enlarged ventricles had follow-up studies. Classification of syndromic craniosynostosis followed published criteria [1]. Intracranial hypertension was confirmed either by epidural or fontanometric pressure monitoring [10] or by papilledema or marked dural tension during operation. Decompressive surgery consisted of large craniectomies or enlargement of skull capacity using various techniques of cranial vault reshapement including fronto-orbital advancement.

[1] Abteilung Pädiatrische Neurochirurgie, Neurochirurgische Universitätsklinik, Josef-Schneider-Straße 11, W-8700 Würzburg, FRG.
[2] Universitätsklinik für Mund-Kiefer-Gesichtschirurgie, Pleicherwall 2, W-8700 Würzburg, FRG.

Advances in Neurosurgery, Vol. 21
R. Lorenz, M. Klinger, M. Brock (Eds.)

Table 1. Frequency and degree of ventricular dilation in various types of craniosynostosis, including number of patients with hydrostatic hydrocephalus

	n	Ventricular Dilation Mild	Moderate	Severe	Total	Shunt dependent
Isolated Synostosis	349	4	2	4	10	5
Frontal	59	–	–	1	1	1
Sagittal	181	1	–	–	1	–
Unicoronary	47	1	–	2	3	2
Bicoronary	25	–	1	1	2	2
Multiple sutures	37	2	1	–	3	0
Syndromes	159	36	18	7	61	14
Crouzon	38	9	6	1	16	3
Pfeiffer	10	3	3	3	9	5
Apert	41	16	5	–	21	2
Chotzen	39	4	1	–	5	1
Others	31	4	3	3	10	3
Total	508	40	20	11	71	19

Results

Prevalence of Ventricular Dilation. From a total of 508 patients – most of them children – 71 presented with some degree of ventricular dilation (Table 1). There was a striking difference between isolated and syndromic synostosis, the prevalence being 3% in the former and 38% in the latter. Additional differences were noted in the group of genetic syndromes (Table 1; Figs. 1–3).

In 19 patients the hydrocephalus turned out to be shunt dependent. Again, prevalence differed considerably for various types of isolated synostosis and syndromes, most strikingly between Pfeiffer's and Apert's syndrome (Table 1; Figs. 1, 2).

Associated Disorders. Analysis disclosed seven patients in whom hydrocephalus was caused by a coincidental disorder unrelated to synostosis: perinatal hemorrhage (three), amniotic band syndrome (one), and myelomeningocele (three patients with isolated synostosis of coronary suture); five of these needed a shunt. Excluding these seven patients, there were only three hydrocephalics left in the group of isolated synostosis; none had proven hydrostatic hydrocephalus. Therefore the following analysis is confined to the group with syndromic synostosis.

Morphologic Features. Ventricular dilation was marked in seven patients; each needed a shunt. Of 18 patients presenting with moderately enlarged ventricles six were shunt dependent. Even in one case of mild enlargement, shunting turned out to be the only way for effective control of intracranial hypertension. A dilated third ventricle was noted in all but two shunt-dependent patients, but in three shunt-

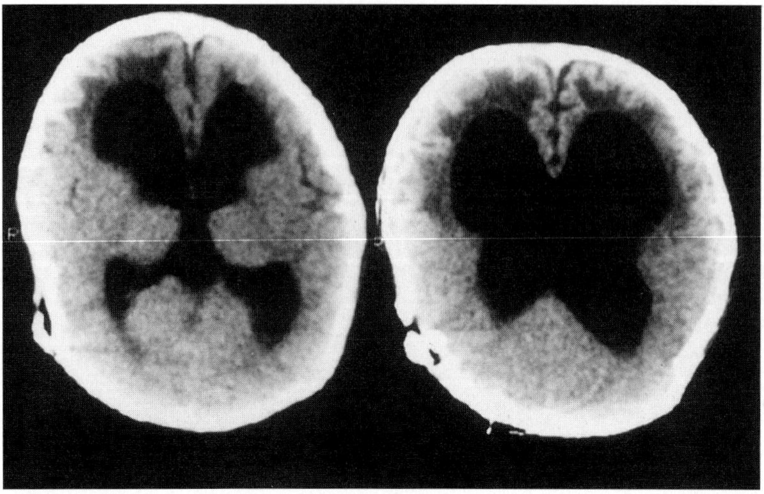

Fig. 1. Severe ventricular enlargement in hydrostatic hydrocephalus, 3 months after decompressive surgery; at that time normal ventricular size (6 month-old boy, Pfeiffer's syndrome)

independent patients as well (Figs. 2, 3). All shunt-dependent patients had compromised CSF spaces within the posterior fossa, but this was also found in many non-hydrocephalic patients with craniostenosis. No case of hydrostatic hydrocephalus could be attributed to a particular associated malformation of the brain.

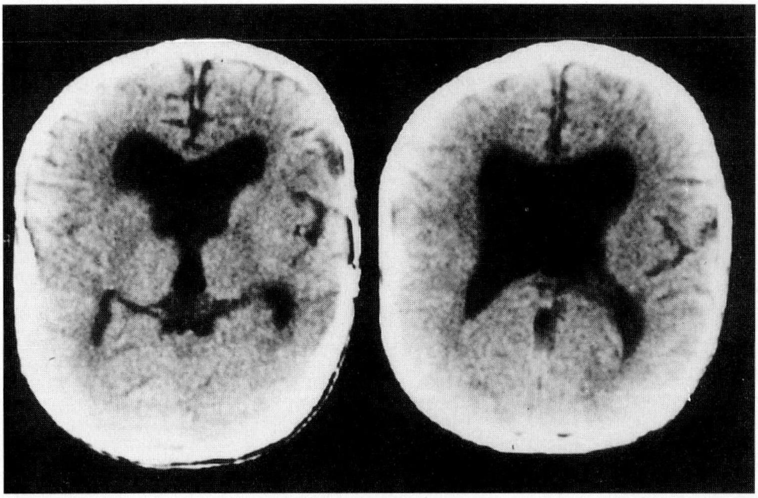

Fig. 2. Moderate shunt-independent ventriculomegaly (5-year-old boy, Apert's syndrome)

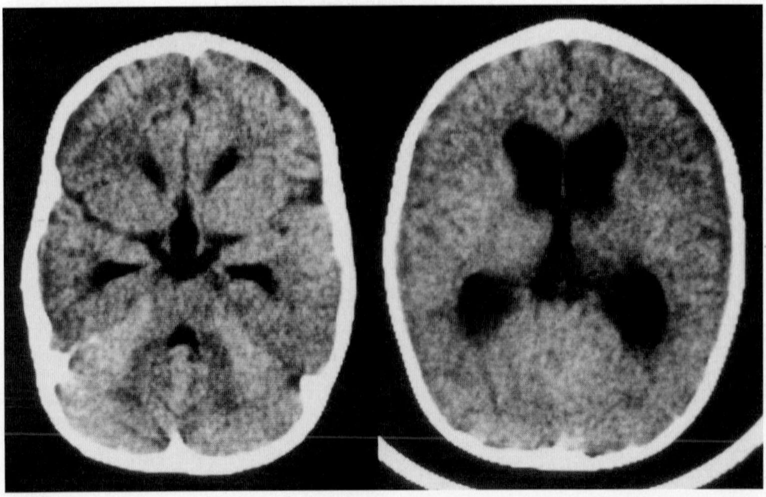

Fig. 3. Moderately enlarged ventricles in hydrostatic hydrocephalus, normal ventricles at birth, rapidly developing intracranial hypertension (14 month-old girl, Crouzon's syndrome)

Evolution of Hydrocephalus. At birth only two patients had severely enlarged ventricles. Spontaneous progression was noted in all cases of hydrostatic hydrocephalus. On the other hand, some increment of ventricular size was also documented in two-thirds of patients with ventriculomegaly. Following surgery for craniostenosis local enlargement of the ventricles was frequently observed, but this did not confirm hydrostatic hydrocephalus. The effect was most evident after surgery of severely distorted skulls such as those with clover leaf skull syndrome.

Response to Treatment. Prior to any treatment intracranial hypertension was confirmed in 38 of the 61 hydrocephalic patients with syndromous synostosis. Twenty of these received a shunt. Regarding the response to treatment three groups were identified. In seven patients intracranial pressure was effectively controlled by inserting a shunt first (group A). Age at shunting was 2–14 months (median, 6 months). Four of these needed decompressive surgery for recurrent intracranial hypertension due to craniostenosis after an interval of 5–20 months. In one case of extreme ventricular dilation pressure remained normal for at least 5 years. Two patients died soon after shunting because of severe associated anomalies. In six other patients shunting was not followed by resolution of intracranial hypertension (group B). All but one had only mildly enlarged ventricles. All were finally treated successfully by decompressive surgery. Finally, seven patients received a shunt as second procedure (group C) after an interval of 2 months–4 years following surgery for synostosis. Shunting was chosen either because of persistent or early recurrent intracranial hypertension despite adequate treatment of craniostenosis, or because of conspicuous progression of ventricular dilation. Patients' ages at shunting ranged from 3 months to 6 years (median, 20 months). Treatment was successful in all cases. In an effort to avoid shunt insertion suboccipital craniectomy was performed in two hydrocephalic patients, but failed in both.

Discussion

The concurrence of hydrostatic hydrocephalus and primary craniosynostosis is a unique condition, in that opposite forces are acting upon the brain. Accumulating CSF tends to blow up the brain and its coverings, but at the same time the deficient skull growth restrains it from expanding. Intracranial pressure may be elevated by both mechanisms. Hence, classical signs of childhood hydrocephalus such as accelerated head growth and bulging fontanelle are not available for identification of shunt-dependent CSF circulation disorder. Moreover, adding to the diagnostic problem, only a minority of patients with dilated ventricles have hydrostatic hydrocephalus. Intracranial hypertension by craniostenosis and ventriculomegaly may coincide, but in these cases successful treatment cannot be expected from shunting.

Our own observations as well as the data of other authors [2, 5, 6, 9] suggest that ventricular enlargement in primary craniosynostosis may reflect quite different pathological conditions: primary cerebral dysplasia, for instance, in Apert's syndrome [2], secondary brain atrophy as a consequence of long-standing craniostenosis, or CSF circulation disorder. High-pressure hydrocephalus must be considered as well as normal pressure hydrocephalus and even arrested hydrocephalus. Finally, various etiologic factors may be involved at the same time.

For these reasons there are as yet no reliable criteria for differentiation between shunt-dependent hydrostatic hydrocephalus and shunt-independent ventriculomegaly. Studies of CSF dynamics may be expected to overcome this problem, but no exact data are available now [12].

Our study provides some practical guidelines. Patients with severe or rapidly progressing ventricular enlargement should be shunted without delay. In these patients surgery for synostosis should be postponed for at least several months to avoid the risk of persistent epidural dead space following cranial vault reshapement. In mild or moderate ventricular dilation with slow progression a dilated 3rd ventricle or a constricted posterior fossa may provide additional arguments. In doubtful cases it seems advisable to operate on the synostosis first and to wait for the resolution of intracranial hypertension. If necessary, a shunt may be added in a second procedure. The remodeled skull will not collapse if the bone fragments are securely fixed [7].

References

1. Cohen MM (1986) Syndromes with craniosynostosis. In: Cohen MM (ed) Craniosynostosis: diagnosis, evaluation, and management. Raven, New York, pp 413–590
2. Cohen MM, Kreiborg S (1990) The central nervous system in the Apert syndrome. Am J Med Genet, 35:36–45
3. Collmann H, Sörensen N, Krauß J, Mühling J (1988) Hydrocephalus in craniosynostosis. Childs Nerv Syst 4:279–285
4. David DJ, Poswillo D, Simpson D (1982) The craniosynostoses. Causes, natural history, and management. Springer, Berlin Heidelberg New York
5. Fishman MA, Hogen GR, Dodge PR (1971) The concurrence of hydrocephalus and craniosynostosis. J Neurosurg 34:621–629
6. Golabi H (1957) Zur Kenntnis der Beziehungen zwischen Gehirn und Schädelkapsel bei den turricephalen craniostenostischen Dysostosen. Virchows Arch [A] 33:365–383
7. Mühling J, Collmann H, Reuther J, Sörensen N (1989) Functional and anatomic aspects of the osteotomy in craniofacial surgery. Neurosurg Rev 12:21–23
8. Müller PJ, Hoffmann HJ (1975) Cloverleaf skull syndrome. J Neurosurg 43:86–91
9. Noetzel MJ, Marsh JL, Palkes H, Gado M (1985) Hydrocephalus and mental retardation in craniosynostosis. J Pediatr 107:885–892
10. Renier D, Sainte-Rose CH, Marchac D, Hirsch J-F (1982) Intracranial pressure in craniostenosis. J Neurosurg 57:370–377
11. Sainte-Rose CH, LaCombe J, Pierre-Kahn A, Renier D, Hirsch J-F (1984) Intracranial venous sinus hypertension: cause or consequence of hydrocephalus in infants? J Neurosurg 60:727–736
12. Scarfo GB, Tomaccini D, Gambacorta D, Piane R (1981) Disturbance of cerebrospinal flow in craniostenosis. Z Kinderchir 34:193–197

Intensive Care

Effect of Head Elevation on Intracranial Pressure, Cerebral Perfusion Pressure, and Cerebrovenous Oxygen Saturation

G.-H. Schneider[1], R. Franke[1], A. von Helden[1], A. Unterberg[1], and W. Lanksch[1]

Introduction

Treatment of elevated intracranial pressure (ICP) has been shown to decrease mortality and to improve neurological outcome in severe head injury [4, 8].

Up to now head elevation has been the first of a series of standard procedures to control raised ICP. Though there is general agreement that this maneuver significantly reduces ICP [1–3, 6], this practice has been increasingly challenged recently [6, 7]. Elevating the head not only lowers ICP, it may also significantly reduce cerebral perfusion pressure (CPP) [1, 2, 6].

It still remains uncertain which body position is the most beneficial for patients with compromised intracranial compliance. Recently, it has been shown that cerebrovenous oxygen saturation can be used as an estimate of cerebral blood flow [5]. Furthermore, continuous monitoring of cerebrovenous oxygen saturation has become feasible.

The aim of this study was to determine the effect of head elevation on cerebrovenous oxygen saturation (CVOS), as an indicator for cerebral perfusion, as well as ICP and CPP in comatose patients with intracranial hypertension.

Material and Methods

Twenty-one comatose patients were included in the study. Table 1 describes the study group.

Treatment of patients was done in accordance with international standards which included prompt evacuation of intracranial masses, if necessary, and aggressive management of ICP [moderate hyperventilation, sedation, cerebrospinal fluid (CSF) drainage, mannitol, and finally barbiturates].

Mean arterial pressure (MAP) was measured in the radial artery and care was taken to keep the transducer at the level of the external auditory canal. CPP was calculated as the difference of MAP and ICP.

To monitor CVOS a fiberoptic catheter (Abbott Laboratories, Illinois, USA) was placed in the jugular bulb on the side of the main lesion where its position was checked by X-ray.

[1] Neurochirurgische Forschung Universitätsklinikum Rudolf Virchow,
Freie Universität Berlin, Spanndauer Damm 130, W-1000 Berlin 19, FRG

Advances in Neurosurgery, Vol. 21
R. Lorenz, M. Klinger, M. Brock (Eds.)

Table 1. Characteristics of study group

Sex ratio (M:F)	14:7
Mean age (years)	47 (range 20–79)
Diagnosis	
Severe head injury (*n*)	14
Subarachnoid hemorrhage (Hunt and Hess grade IV) (*n*)	4
Intracerebral hemorrhage (*n*)	3
GCS on admittance	4–8 (mean: 6)
Initial ICP (15° head elevation) (mmHg)	22.2 ± 2.8 (range 9–60)

Study measurements were performed within 72 h after admittance. The head was lowered from 45° by three 15° steps (each for 20 min) to the horizontal position. At each position ICP, MAP, and CVOS were recorded. Arterial and jugular venous blood samples were obtained for determination of blood gases, pH, oxygen saturation, as well as lactate concentration.

For statistical evaluation the Friedman test for paired values was used.

Results and Discussion

The effect of head elevation on ICP, CPP, and CVOS is given in Fig. 1. Table 2 is a survey of mean values (± SEM) of all pertinent parameters measured.

Intracranial pressure was significantly lower at 45° (10.6 ± 1.3 mmHg), 30° (11.6 ± 1.3 mmHg), and 15° (14.9 ± 1.6 mmHg) compared to the supine position at 0° (20.7 ± 1.4 mmHg). At 15° of head elevation 57%, at 30° even 90% of the total reduction of ICP was achieved. This clearly demonstrates that, for the purposes of controlling acute intracranial hypertension, it is not necessary to elevate the head above 30°.

Mean arterial pressure, recorded at head level as an estimate of mean carotid pressure [6], gradually rose from 70.6 ± 2.3 mmHg at 45° to 81.0 ± 2.5 mmHg with the patient lying flat ($p < 0.001$). As the change in MAP and ICP grossly equalled each other, head position had no effect on CPP, which remained constant. Also, CVOS remained unaffected by the degree of head elevation with an average reading of 65%.

As parameters indicative of cerebral metabolism, such as cerebral arteriovenous difference of oxygen saturation ($AVDO_2$), $PaCO_2$ and cerebral arteriovenous difference of lactate (AVDL), showed no significant change either, it seems justified to use jugular venous saturation to evaluate the quality of cerebral blood flow. Obviously the supine position has no negative influence on cerebral perfusion even though ICP is above 20 mmHg.

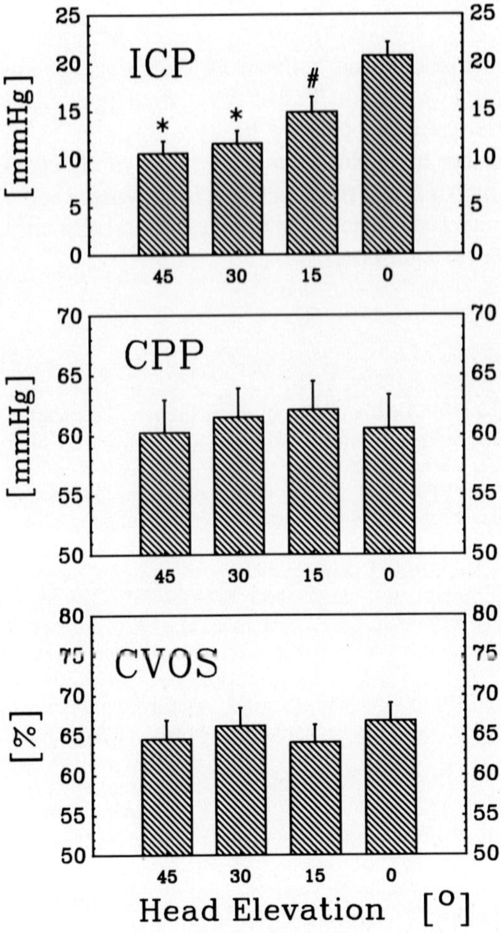

Fig. 1. Effect of body position on intracranial pressure (*ICP*), cerebral perfusion pressure (*CPP*), and cerebrovenous oxygen saturation (*CVOS*). While ICP significantly decreased, CPP and CVOS, as an estimate for cerebral blood flow, remained unchanged

Table 2. Effect of head elevation on cerebral and systemic parameters

Parameter	Head elevation 45°	30°	15°	0°
MAP (mmHg)	70.6 ± 2.3	72.9 ± 2.3	76.5 ± 2.4	81.0 ± 2.5*
ICP (mmHg)	10.6 ± 1.3*	11.6 ± 1.3*	14.9 ± 1.6***	20.7 ± 1.4
CPP (mmHg)	60.3 ± 2.7	61.5 ± 2.4	62.1 ± 2.4	60.6 ± 2.8
CVOS (%)	64.6 ± 2.4	66.2 ± 2.3	64.1 ± 2.2	66.8 ± 2.2
$AVDO_2$ (Δ%)	31.2 ± 2.3	30.6 ± 2.3	32.1 ± 2.2	29.6 ± 2.3
$PaCO_2$ (mmHg)	33.8 ± 0.8	33.6 ± 0.9	33.7 ± 0.8	33.4 ± 0.8
AVDL (mg/dl)	–0.4 ± 0.2	–0.4 ± 0.2	–0.3 ± 0.2	–0.4 ± 0.1

* $p < 0.001$, ** $p < 0.05$, *** $p < 0.01$

Summary and Conclusions

This study demonstrates that head position does not influence CVOS, i.e., cerebral perfusion, even in patients with moderately raised ICP. In order to treat intracranial hypertension, it is not necessary to elevate the head above 30°.

It still remains to be studied whether head elevation has a negative effect on cerebral blood flow in patients with higher levels of intracranial hypertension and a more significantly reduced intracranial compliance. Continuous jugular oximetry seems to be an apt new tool to answer this question.

References

1. Davenport A, Will EJ, Davidson AM (1990) Effect of posture on intracranial pressure and cerebral perfusion pressure in patients with fulminant hepatic and renal failure after acetaminophen self-poisoning. Crit Care Med 18:286–289
2. Durward QJ, Amacher AL, Del Maestro RF et al. (1983) Cerebral and cardiovascular responses to changes in head elevation in patients with intracranial hypertension. J Neurosurg 59:938–944
3. Kenning JA, Toutnant SM, Saunders RL (1981) Upright patient positioning in the management of intracranial hypertension. Surg Neurol 15:148–152
4. Mararou A, Eisenberg HM, Foulkes MA, Marshall LF, Jane JA et al. (1991) Impact of ICP instability and hypotension on outcome in patients with severe head trauma. J Neurosurg 75:S59–S66
5. Robertson CS, Narayan RK, Gokaslan ZL et al. (1989) Cerebral arteriovenous oxygen difference as an estimate of cerebral blood flow in comatose patients. J Neurosurg 70:222–230
6. Rosner MJ, Coley IB (1986) Cerebral perfusion pressure, intracranial pressure and head elevation. J Neurosurgery 65:636–641
7. Rosner MJ, Daughton S (1990) Cerebral perfusion pressure management in head injury. J Trauma 30:933–941
8. Saul TG, Ducker TB (1982) Effect of intracranial pressure monitoring and aggressive treatment on mortality in severe head injury. J Neurosurg 56:498–503

Interhemispheric Gradients in Head-Injured Patients: Their Evidence in Epidural Intracranial Pressure Measurement

D. Woischneck[1], M.R. Gaab[1], and T. Barner[1]

Introduction

Intracranial pressure (ICP) in clinical use is monitored by epidural sensors. From subarachnoidal measurement, pressure gradients between different intracranial compartments are known, mainly transtentorially and on both sides of the falx cerebri. While the transtentorial differences are well known, the interhemispheric gradients in brain-injured patients so far have not sufficiently been quantified, especially for epidural evaluation.

Material and Methods

In 15 patients ICP was monitored by epidural, frontal measurements on the right and left sides, in reference to the foramen of Monro. We used the sensor of the Geltec company. For calculation of the cerebral perfusion pressure (CPP), we cannulate the radial artery for continuous blood pressure recording by a Statham transducer. Measurement started 22 h after the accident and was performed on average of 79 h. It was performed until ICP was in a normal range (12 patients) or brain death occurred (3 patients). For analysis we divided the total time of measurement for each patient into 3-h intervals. The average ICP and CPP values of these intervals were used as our main criteria for evaluating study results.

Results

Of our 15 patients 12 showed an ICP gradient between the right and left hemispheres: in 7 cases the gradient was noticed once in the clinical course and in 5 cases twice. The gradient in these 12 patients averaged 15 mmHg, with a maximum of 30 mmHg maximally, due to 3-h intervals. When it occurred, we always noticed significant differences for longer than 24 h – a maximum of 3 days in one course.

In cases of an cerebral contusion, the side of the high or low ICP corresponded to CT criteria. Figure 1 shows the ICP course of a 37-year-old patient with

[1] Neurochirurgische Klinik, Medizinische Hochschule Hannover, Konstanty-Gutschow-Straße 8, W-3000 Hannover 61, FRG.

Advances in Neurosurgery, Vol. 21
R. Lorenz, M. Klinger, M. Brock (Eds.)

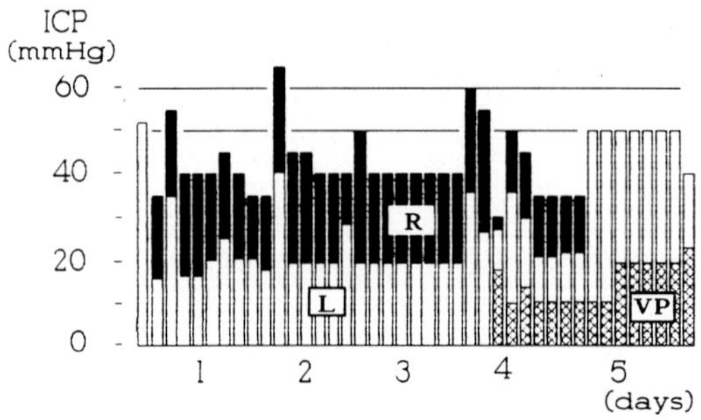

Fig. 1. ICP course after bifrontal contusion (37-year-old man, measurement starting 6 h after the accident). Each column is the average ICP for 3 h. *R*, Right side; *L*, left side; *VP*, intraventricular pressure

bifrontal contusion areas. The ICP on the right side is up to 30 mmHg higher than on the left. This gradient occurred twice during the measurement period. In the case of this patient, we temporarily also measured the intraventricular pressure, which was lower than ICP on both sides and led to completely different evaluations of the patient's situation. On the other hand, the CPP in cases of mainly a traumatic brain swelling showed significant gradients up to 20 mmHg, although computed tomography revealed no differences concerning formation of the right/left edema.

When an acute ICP rise was induced (for example, upon coughing against the respirator; Fig. 2), we observed a characteristic pressure curve in all patients. The side of the primarily higher ICP showed a proportionally higher mounting, and the plateau was reached earlier on this side. In the phase of the final ICP fall, the higher side showed a delay in reaching the basic pressure again.

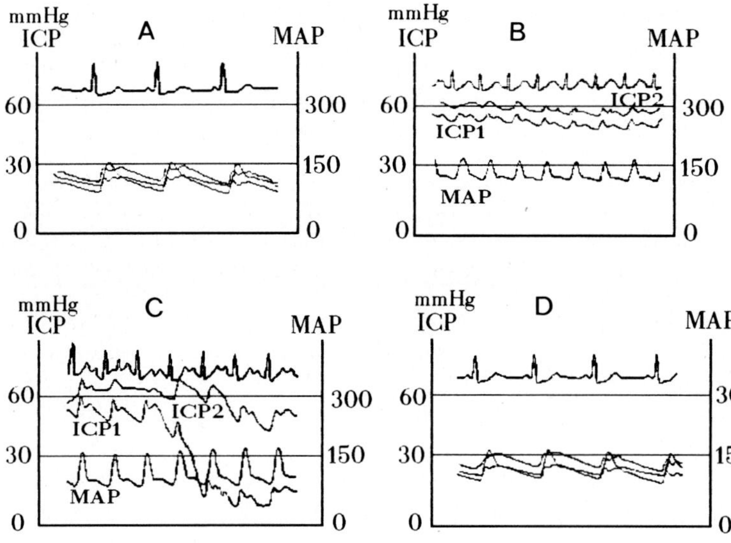

Fig. 2 A–D. ICP course in acute crisis in case of a traumatic brain swelling. **A** Before coughing against the respirator. **B** 1 min after coughing. **C** 5 min after coughing. **D** normalization

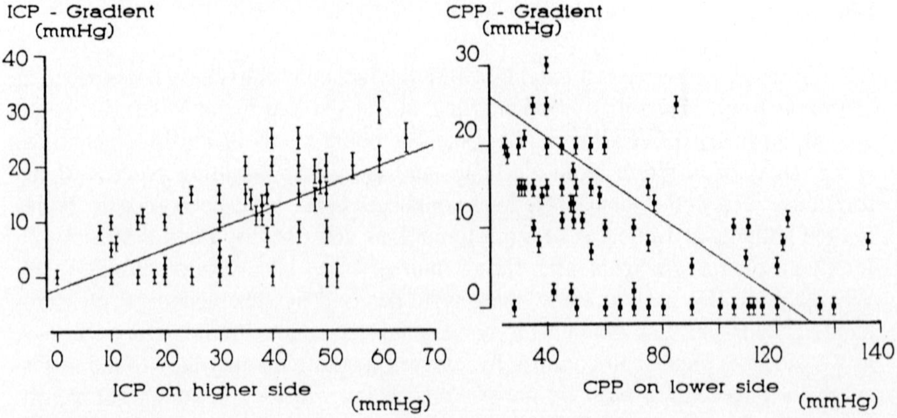

Fig. 3. Correlation of the ICP (*left*) and CPP (*right*) with the grade of intracranial hypertension (defined by the ICP on the side of the maximal swelling or contusion)

Figure 3 summarizes values in all the patients when a gradient was seen. We related this gradient to the ICP of the side of the higher pressure, and ICP differences between right and left showed a positive correlation with the amount of the intracranial hypertension.

As noted above, in three cases a gradient was not observed. In two cases these were patients with maximal brain swelling in a state of supratentorial herniation; one was a patient with a contusion of the midbrain without significant swelling.

Table 1 summarizes the ICP and CPP values of all patients with a significant gradient. As one can see here, for therapeutic intervention (mannitol administration, decompressive operation) this would have meant an astonishing difference in a number of decisions whether we measured right or left.

In summary, we found right/left gradients in ICP and CPP due to the side of the brain where computed tomography had suggested differences in ICP. On the other hand, we describe patients in whom the results of computed tomography were differences of edema generation, although epidural measurement revealed significant ICP differences. In cases of such gradient, it was always longer than 24 h. Sometimes it occurred twice in the clinical course. It showed a positive correlation to the degree of intracranial hypertension.

Table 1. Interhemispheric gradient and average ICP over 3 h

Side of	ICP > 20	ICP > 40	CPP < 50	*n*
High ICP	99	53	57	195
Low ICP	65	9	18	195

Discussion

ICP differences between right and left from the falx cerebri have been described in laboratory animals especially by Langfitt et al. [1] and Leech and Miller [2]. These are explained by different principles, such as obliterations of the subarachnoidal space, areas of different brain elasticity, and the time-consuming process of the formation of a brain edema [4]. Intracranial gradients have been seen in brain-injured patients and in cases of brain tumors, as described by Pick and Bock [3]. Interhemispheric gradients after head injuries have been explored mainly by Weaver et al. [5]. In their study, these were detected by subarachnoidal measurement. They found such gradients to correspond to computed tomography findings, as we did in our study. In contrast, by subarachnoidal recording they found differences for only 24 h at most. In our patients, 1 day was the minimum that we observed. Furthermore, neither Weaver et al. [5] nor, as far as we know, any other author has reported intracranial gradients between right and left which vanish in the clinical course and return secondarily. This may of course be explained by the secondary typical brain swelling 2–4 days after the trauma.

The positive correlation of the gradient with the intracranial hypertension (Table 1) is a result known from subarachnoidal measurement [5]. The behavior of right and left ICP during acute crisis (Fig. 3) has not been described until now.

References

1. Langfitt TW, Weinstein JD, Kassell NF (1964) Transmission of increased intracranial pressure. II. Within the supratentorial space. J Neurosurg 21:998–1005
2. Leech PJ, Miller JD (1974) Intracranial pressure-volume relationships during experimental brain compression in primates. J Neurol Neurosurg Psychiatry 37:1093–1098
3. Piek J, Bock WJ (1988) Intrahemispheric gradients of brain tissue pressure in patients with brain tumors. Acta Neurochir 93:129–132
4. Reulen HJ, Kreysch HG (1973) Measurement of brain tissue pressure in cold induced cerebral edema. Acta Neurochir 29:29–40
5. Weaver D, Winn HR, Jane JA (1982) Differential intracranial pressure with mass lesions. J Neurosurg 56:660–665

Improved Outcome from Traumatic Coma Using Only Ventricular Cerebrospinal Fluid Drainage for Intracranial Pressure Control

J. B. G. Ghajar[1], R. J. Hariri[1], and R. H. Patterson[1]

Treatment of intracranial hypertension is essential in the management of patients with traumatic brain injuries. Patients with persistently high intracranial hypertension are likely to die [1], and treatments to reduce intracranial hypertension are performed with the aim of improving cerebral perfusion. While mortality from severe head injury has been reduced from 50% to 35% over the past 15 years [2], the contribution of the treatment of elevated intracranial pressure (ICP) has never been isolated from the contributions of advances in surgical management, diagnostic radiology and general intensive unit (ICU) care. It is at least theoretically possible that the prognosis of severely head-injured patients is no better with treatment of elevated ICP than without treatment, given adequate surgical and ICU care. Similarly, the question of whether or not treatment of elevated ICP simply increases the number of vegetative survivors has never been answered directly. Commonly employed therapeutic measures to reduce ICP are hyperventilation, mannitol, barbiturates, and ventricular cerebrospinal fluid (CSF) drainage. We hypothesized that CSF drainage alone would decrease morbidity and mortality to a greater extent than other treatments because it has the potential to improve cerebral perfusion as well as decrease intracranial pressure [3]. Hyperventilation, in contrast, can potentially reduce cerebral perfusion below ischemic thresholds by vasoconstriction [4]. Osmotic diuretics [5] and barbiturates [6] can also theoretically reduce cerebral perfusion to a deleterious extent by systemic hypotension. These factors are crucial in the consideration of a traumatized brain with an already marginal blood flow, especially during the early stages of treatment [7]. However, studies of patients with severe head injury in the past 15 years have used a combination of therapies and not ventricular CSF drainage alone as the principal method of reducing increased intracranial pressure.

We initiated a prospective study to evaluate and compare the outcome of two groups of patients with severe head injury, one managed with ventricular intracranial pressure monitoring and therapeutic drainage and a second group of patients treated without ICP monitoring or therapeutic drainage of ventricular CSF.

[1] The Aitken Neurosurgery Laboratory, 1300 York Avenue, Room LC-807, New York, NY 10021, USA.

Advances in Neurosurgery, Vol. 21
R. Lorenz, M. Klinger, M. Brock (Eds.)

Patient Population

The patient population for this study consisted of patients between the ages of 16 and 70 admitted to the New York Hospital Cornell Medical Center or to the Jamaica Hospital Cornell Trauma Center with a nonpenetrating severe head injury during the 3-year period from January 1989 through December 1991. Severe head injury was defined as Glasgow Coma Score (GCS) ≤ 7 for at least 24 h following initial resuscitation. Patients who met brain death criteria within 24 h of admission were excluded.

Clinical Management

Patients were assigned to one of two groups depending on the neurosurgeon on call for the day. Group 1 patients had placement of ventricular catheters for ICP monitoring and were treated by CSF drainage when ICP exceeded 15 mmHg. Group 2 patients had no ICP monitoring device placed and were not treated for intracranial hypertension.

All patients were managed by a neurotrauma protocol that included intubation and ventilation to a PaO_2 of 100 mmHg and a $PaCO_2$ of 35 mmHg, CT scans, and prompt evacuation of significant subdural hematomas. The head of the bed was elevated to 30° from horizontal. Fluid resuscitation in the emergency room was performed according to Advanced Trauma Life Support Program (ATLS) guidelines. Patients were maintained normovolemic and monitored for blood pressure and arterial PaO_2, $PaCO_2$, and pH with an indwelling arterial line and, if hypotensive on admission, with Swan-Ganz monitoring. Some patients were given 1 g/kg mannitol on admission if they showed signs of impending cerebral herniation, but thereafter mannitol was not administered for ICP management.

In group 1 patients a right frontal ventriculostomy was performed using the right-angle technique [8] within 4 h of their arrival to the emergency room. The ventriculostomy catheter was placed on the contralateral side in the presence of a subdural hematoma or significant cerebral contusion that produced a midline shift. The catheter was connected by a three-way valve to a pressure transducer which displayed the ICP pressure on a monitor and to a drainage system which was set to drain CSF at 15 mmHg pressure to an ideal endpoint of 10 mmHg. Ventricular CSF pressure was measured every hour and was averaged over an 8 h shift. Ventricular CSF was cultured and analyzed for protein, glucose, and cell count in patients who became febrile with ventriculostomy catheters in place. Catheters were removed if the CSF culture was positive and a contralateral catheter was placed if ICP was elevated. Ventricular catheters were removed if the ICP remained on average less than 15 mmHg without drainage over a 24–48 h period.

Forty-nine consecutive patients were entered into the study: 34 in group 1 and 15 in group 2. The larger number of patients in group 1 compared to group 2 reflects the larger proportion of on-call days by neurosurgeons admitting patients for group 1 protocol (ICP monitoring and treatment).

Table 1. Demographics and clinical features

Factor	Group 1	Group 2
Patients (*n*)	34	15
Average age (years)	33	41
Motor vehicle accident (%)	76	53
Evacuated acute subdural hematoma (%)	29	27
Average GCS post resuscitation	5	6

Results

Table 1 shows the demographic data and some clinical features for both groups. The average GCS in group 1 (GCS = 5) was significantly ($p < .05$) lower than in group 2 (GCS = 6). In both groups there was a similar percentage of patients who had craniotomies for acute subdural hematomas.

Table 2 shows that ventricular ICP was monitored on average for 4.3 days. ICP averaged 13.3 mmHg in all patients, which demonstrated that CSF drainage was successful in maintaining average ICP below 15 mmHg. The incidence of intracranial hypertension (ICP > 20 mmHg) was low (10%), as was the rate of CSF infection (6%). Three patients out of 15 in group 2 received either steroids or mannitol during their course of ICU care; none of the patients in group 1 received mannitol or steroids during their ICU stays. The average $PaCO_2$ during ICP monitoring was not different between the two groups (group 1, 33 mmHg; group 2, 34 mmHg).

Table 3 shows the Glasgow Outcome Score (GOS) for both groups at 6 months to 3 years following discharge. A 100% follow-up review was obtained. Mortality in group 1 patients was approximately four times less than mortality in group 2 patients, and the percentage of group 1 patients living independently was approximately three times greater than the percentage of group 2 patients living independently. The percentage of patients who were vegetative or dependent was not significantly different between the two groups.

Table 2. Ventricular ICP and $PaCO_2$ parameters

Factor	Group 1	Group 2
Average duration of ICP monitoring (days)	4.3	N/A
Average ICP during treatment (mmHg)	13	N/A
Incidence of intracranial hypertension (%)	10	N/A
Ventricular CSF infection rate (%)	6	N/A
Average $PaCO_2$ during ICP monitoring (mmHg)	33	34

Table 3. Discharge outcome

Status	GOS	Group 1 (%)	Group 2 (%)
Dead	1	12	53
Vegetative	2	9	7
Dependent	3	20	20
Living independently	4/5	59	20

Conclusion

This study indicates that ventricular ICP monitoring and CSF drainage for intracranial hypertension in severely head-injured patients significantly decreases mortality without significantly increasing the percentage of vegetative or dependent patients compared to a control group that was neither monitored nor treated for intracranial hypertension.

We believe that the favorable outcomes demonstrated with our treated group of severely head-injured patients are attributable to our stepwise approach to ICP management, with CSF drainage as the first step. Our current protocol is shown in Fig. 1. The efficacy of CSF drainage alone prevents us from having to resort to further methods of treatment in most patients. In addition, our protocol uses

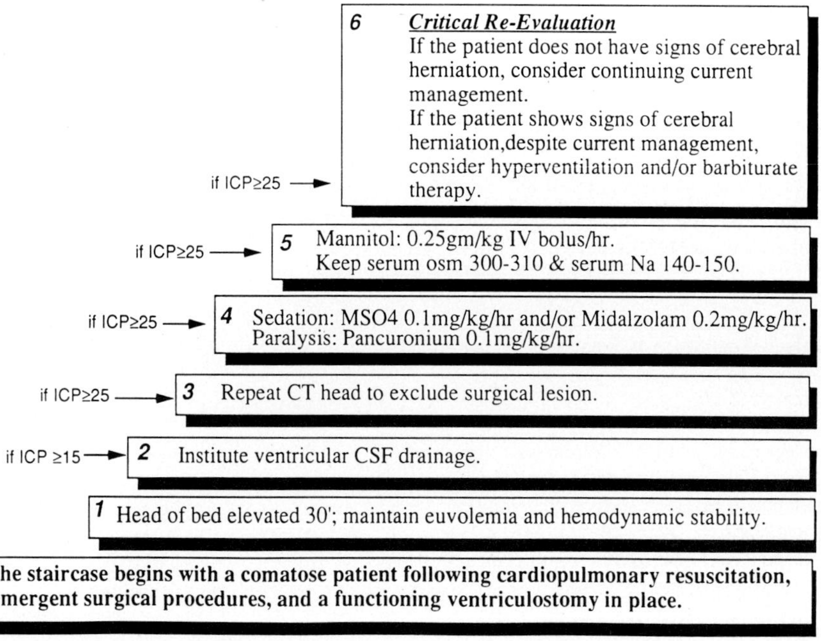

Fig. 1. The ICP management climb. ICP is measured in mmHG. ICP ≥ 25 is defined as the average ICP over an 8-h period

ICP > 15 mmHg as the indication for treatment, in contrast to many other protocols that use ICP > 20 or 25 mmHg as the indication for treatment.

References

1. Miller JD, Becker DP, Ward JD et al. (1977) Significance of intracranial hypertension in severe head injury. J Neurosurg 47:503–516
2. Miller JD (1991) Changing patterns in acute management of head injury. J Neurol Sci 103:S33–S37
3. Goh D, Minns R, Pye SD et al. (1991) Cerebral blood flow velocity changes after ventricular taps and ventriculoperitoneal shunting. Childs Nerv Syst 7:452–457
4. Muizelaar JP, Marmarou A, Ward JD et al. (1991) Adverse effects of prolonged hyperventilation in patients with severe head injury: a randomized clinical trial. J Neurosurg 75:731–739
5. Cote CJ, Greenhow DE, Marshall BE (1979) The hypotensive response to rapid intravenous administration of hypertonic solution in man and in the rabbit. Anesthesiology 50:30–35
6. Etsten B, Li TH (1955) Hemodynamic changes during thiopental anesthesia in humans: cardiac output, stroke volume, total peripheral resistance and intrathoracic blood volume. J Clin Invest 34:500–510
7. Bouma GJ, Muizelaar JP, Choi SC et al. (1991) Cerebral circulation and metabolism after severe traumatic brain injury. The elusive role of ischemia. J Neurosurg 75:685–693
8. Ghajar JBG (1985) A guide for ventricular catheter placement. A technical note. J Neurosurg 63:985–986

Barbiturate Coma in Patients with Severe Head Injuries: Long-Term Outcome in 79 Patients

J. Piek[1]

Introduction

Barbiturates have been used in the treatment of raised intracranial pressure (ICP) for more than 15 years [3, 4, 6]. Recently Eisenberg et al. [1] reported the results of a multicenter, randomized study on the efficacy of using barbiturates in severe head-injured patients. They concluded that high-dose barbiturates are an effective additional therapy in decreasing ICP in selected patients. In the present study we report the clinical results of thiopentone therapy in 79 patients with severe head injuries.

Material and Methods

A total of 79 patients (Table 1) with severe head injuries (initial Glasgow Coma Score, GCS [7], ≤ 8 or during the next 48 h were treated. Barbiturate coma with thiopentone was installed when ICP rose above 25 mmHg and did not respond to conventional methods (algorithm for therapy in Fig. 1). Initially repeated doses of 100 mg were injected until ICP fell below 25 mmHg. This loading dose was followed by continuous drug infusion calculated by weight, pharmacological data, and effect on ICP. Barbiturate infusion was reduced when EEG suppression periods reached a length of 10 s.

Results

Immediate Effects

In 72 patients barbiturate therapy was initiated during the first 72 h following trauma as conventional methods failed to maintain ICP below 25 mmHg. The length of barbiturate therapy varied from 2 to 12 days with a mean duration of 6.7 days. The average daily dose administered varied from 2354 to 3506 mg. Initially 43 patients responded to therapy (i.e., ICP fell more than 15 mmHg following the

[1] Neurochirurgische Klinik, Heinrich-Heine-Universität, Moorenstr. 5, W-4000 Düsseldorf, FRG.

Advances in Neurosurgery, Vol. 21
R. Lorenz, M. Klinger, M. Brock (Eds.)

Table 1. Patient data

Age	
Range (years)	3–71
Mean (years)	29.32
Median (years)	27
Sex	
Mal (*n*)	53
Femal (*n*)	26
GCS (at admission)	
Range	3–13
Mean	6
Maximum ICP	
Range (mmHg)	25–180
Mean (mmHg)	49.90
Median (mmHg)	45
Minimum ICP	
Range (mmHg)	2–30
Mean (mmHg)	11.87
Median (mmHg)	10
Type of intracranial lesion	
Epidural hematoma (*n*)	3
Subdural hematoma (*n*)	10
Intracerebral hematoma (*n*)	8
Two hematomas (*n*)	4
Three hematomas (*n*)	2
No hematoma (*n*)	52
Associated injuries	
Thorax (*n*)	7
Abdomen (*n*)	7
Thorax and Abdomen (*n*)	26
Spinal column (*n*)	9
Extremities (*n*)	15
None (*n*)	15

initial "loading dose"). In 21 patients ICP was reduced by less than 15 mmHg, in another 15 patients ICP remained unchanged (36 nonresponders).

Outcome

Tables 2–4 give details of the outcome. A total of 46 patients died – 38 within the first two posttraumatic weeks – mainly because of their primary brain injury or due to uncontrollable ICP. Five patients died from day 14 to 28 post injury; the

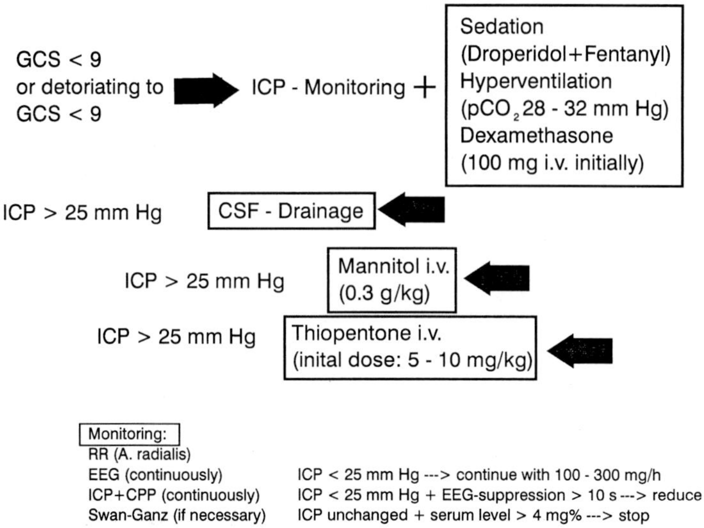

Fig. 1. Algorithm for treatment of raised ICP in the study group

remaining three patients were either severely disabled or vegetative at discharge and died due to infectious complications in other hospitals.

Thirty-three patients had a follow-up examination with a minimal follow-up time of 370 days (mean: 663 days). At this time 11 patients were severely disabled, ten had a moderate outcome, and 12 patients survived in a good condition.

Severe neurological deficits (paresis, aphasia) often combined with severe neuropsychological alterations were the main causes for a bad outcome, whereas incomplete cranial nerve palsies (especially cranial nerves I, II, VII, and VIII), mild aphasia and hemipareses were present in the better-outcome groups. A better outcome was predominantly observed in patients with initially low GCS scores (4–6), whereas patients with initial GCS scores of > 8 and secondary deterioration to lower scores exclusively had a Glasgow outcome score of 3. A good or moderate outcome was observed in 20 of 43 patients (46.51%) who initially responded to thiopentone injection, whereas in the nonresponder group only two of 36 patients showed a moderate or a good outcome. Patients with a good or moderate outcome in a remarkable percentage (45%) complained of severe psychological problems in spite of their minor neurological handicaps; some of them still stayed in psychological therapy. Three of these 22 patients had thought of committing suicide; another two had been divorced in the meantime. Family problems were most common in patients with severe disabilities (25%). Of 22 patients with a good or a moderate outcome, 17 (77%) had finally reached their pretraumatic socioeconomic status, whereas only five of 11 patients with a Glasgow Outcome Scale (GOS) [2] score of 3 were in same job following their trauma.

Table 2. Outcome in 33 surviving patients following high-dose barbiturate therapy for raised ICP

	Responders[a]	Nonresponders[b]	Total
Dead	12	34	46
Vegetative	–	–	–
Severe	11	0	11
Moderate	10	0	10
Good	10	2	12
	43	36	79

[a] ICP falls more than 15 mmHg after loading dose.
[b] ICP falls less than 15 mmHg after loading dose of barbiturates.

Table 3. Results of follow-up examination in 33 surviving patients: cranial nerve deficits

Cranial nerve	Incomplete, one/both (*n*)	Complete, one (*n*)	Complete, both (*n*)	Total (*n*)
I	2	1	5	8
II	10	4	1	15
III	4	4	0	8
IV	4	2	0	6
V	3	3	0	6
VI	3	3	0	6
VII	5	4	0	9
VIII	15	1	1	17
IX	1	3	0	4
X	0	3	0	3
XI	6	3	0	9
XII	0	1	0	1

Table 4. Results of follow-up examination in 33 surviving patients: other findings

	None (*n*)	Mild/moderate (*n*)	Severe/complete (*n*)
Hemiparesis	25	5	3
Aphasia	17	11	5
Akalkulia	17	7	9
Agraphia	19	9	5
Neuropsychological handicaps	16	11	6

Discussion

Following the pioneering work of the San Diego Group from 1975 to 1979 [3, 4, 6], barbiturate coma has been widely used for ICP control in severely head-injured patients. In numerous studies it has been shown that barbiturates are effective in controlling elevated levels of ICP. Concerning long-term outcome, however, its use compared to conventional therapy has been doubted [5, 8].

In three controlled, randomized trials by the Richmond [8] group, in Toronto [5], and recently in Galveston [1], only Eisenberg et al. [1] could show a beneficial effect of barbiturate coma on ICP control and short-term outcome in head-injured patients. In the Richmond study a patient group was defined which was believed at risk for developing elevated ICP; in Toronto the effect of barbiturates versus mannitol was studied. Therefore high-dose barbiturates were given as an initial therapy. Only Eisenberg et al. [1] could demonstrate a beneficial effect of high-dose barbiturates when they were administered after conventional therapy failed. In their study approximately one third of the patients in whom conventional therapy failed reacted to additional doses of barbiturates, which is fewer compared to our study. In their study only one patient whose ICP responded to barbiturates died, whereas in nonresponders only three of 22 patients survived 1 month. In the present study the percentage of deaths (27.9%) and severe outcome (25.6%) is higher compared to Eisenberg et al.'s patients but is mainly due to a longer follow-up time.

From our results and the literature, we conclude that high-dose barbiturate therapy in patients with severe head injuries should be initiated whenever conventional therapy fails to control ICP, but should not be used as a primary therapeutical instrument. In this situation approximately 30% – 50% of the patients will respond to a "loading dose" of barbiturates with an ICP reduction of more than 15 mmHg. About half of the responders to barbiturate therapy will have a moderate or good outcome, whereas a favorable outcome is very unlikely if a reduction of ICP is not observed following an initial loading dose of thiopentone.

References

1. Eisenberg HM, Frankowski RF, Contant CF et al. (1988) High-dose barbiturate control of elevated intracranial pressure in patients with severe head injury. J Neurosurg 69:15–23
2. Jennett B., Bond M (1975) Assessment of outcome after severe brain damage. A practical scale. Lancet 1:480–484
3. Marshall LF, Smith RW, Shapiro HM (1979) The outcome with aggressive treatment in severe head injuries. Part II. J Neurosurg 50:25–30
4. Rockoff MA, Marshall LF, Shapiro HM (1979) High-dose barbiturate therapy in humans: clinical review of 60 patients. Ann Neurol 6:194–199
5. Schwartz ML, Tator CH, Rowed DW et al. (1984) The University of Toronto Head Injury Treatment Study: a prospective, randomized comparison of pentobarbital and mannitol. Can J Neurol Sci 11:434–440

6. Shapiro HM (1975) Intracranial hypertension. Therapeutic and anesthetic considerations. Anesthesiology 43:445–471
7. Teasdale G, Jennett B (1974) Assessment of coma and impaired consciousness. A practical scale. Lancet 2:81–84
8. Ward JD, Becker DP, Miller JD et al. (1985) Failure of prophylactic barbiturate coma in the treatment of severe head injury. J Neurosurg 62:383–388

Pre-hospital Airway Care and Control of Ventilation in Patients with Head Injuries: A Retrospective Analysis in 1623 Head Trauma Victims

E. J. Wahjoepramono[1], J. Piek[2], and W. J. Bock[2]

Introduction

Emergency care of a head-injured patient is based on the principles of rapid diagnosis and treatment of the primary injury and early and aggressive management in order to prevent secondary insults to the injured brain. Frost [4] and Frost et al. [5] showed that even patients who seem to ventilate adequately are often hypoxic with PaO_2 values of 65 mmHg or even less. Experiences from the Traumatic Coma Data Bank (TCDB) [2] and from previous studies [3, 7] have shown that hypoxemia as well as hypotension and hypercapnia significantly worsen the prognosis of a patient with a severe head injury. In San Diego County, Klauber et al. [6] have shown that improved pre-hospital care improves the outcome of patients with severe head injuries.

To evaluate the quality of pre-hospital ventilatory care of patients with head injuries, we retrospectively analyzed the admission data of 1623 head trauma victims admitted to our department from 1981 to 1989.

Patient Group and Methods

Admission data [arterial blood gas analysis, admission Glasgow Coma Score (GCS), pre-hospital care data] of 1623 head trauma victims admitted to our department from 1981 to 1989 were retrospectively analyzed. Hypoxemia was defined as an arterial $PO_2 < 80$ mmHg, hypercapnia as an arterial $PCO_2 > 50$ mmHg.

Of these 1623 patients, 1136 (69.99%) had a severe head injury (GCS < 9). In 148 patients (9.12%) the severity of head injury was moderate (GCS 9–12) and in 339 patients (20.89%) only minor. A total of 28.65% of the patients had multiple trauma to chest, abdomen, spinal column, or multiple fractures of the extremities; whereas 71.35% of the patients had isolated head injuries or head injuries with fracture of only one extremity.

A total of 35.3% of the patients had been transported directly from the scene of accident to our hospital, either by helicopter or by ambulance, whereas 22.36% had

---

[1] Department of Neurosurgery, University Padjadjaran, Hasan Sadihin Hospital, Bandung, Indonesia.
[2] Neurochirurgische Klinik, Heinrich-Heine-Universität, Moorenstr. 5, W-4000 Düsseldorf, FRG.

Advances in Neurosurgery, Vol. 21
R. Lorenz, M. Klinger, M. Brock (Eds.)

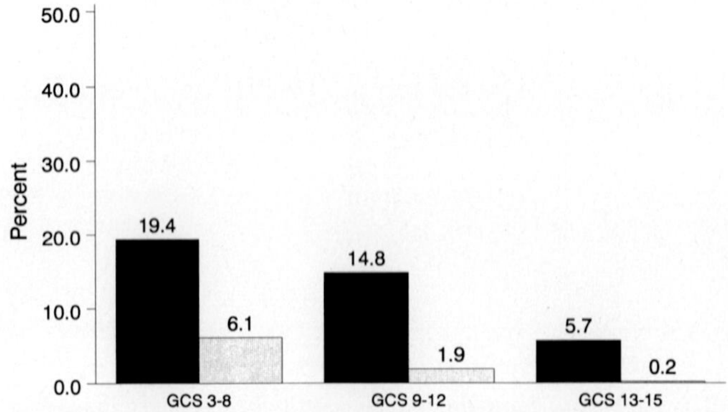

Fig. 1. Admission blood gas analysis of 1623 patients with head injuries. Hypoxemia (*solid columns*) = $PaO_2 < 80$ mmHg; hypercapnia (*shaded columns*) = $PaCO_2 > 50$ mmHg

been transferred from other hospitals in Düsseldorf, and 42.20% from hospitals outside town.

Results

A total of 19.4% of all patients with severe head injuries were hypoxic on arrival to our unit; 6.1% were hypercapnic. The corresponding figures for moderate head injuries were hypoxemia in 14.8% of the patients and hypercapnia in 1.9%. The corresponding figures in patients with minor head injuries were 5.7% for hypoxemia and 0.2% for hypercapnia, respectively (Fig. 1).

Further analysis of the admission data explained this high rate of hypoxemic patients: whereas 78.10% of all patients with severe head injuries had been intubated at the scene or for transport to our hospital, controlled ventilation was performed in only half of them (Fig. 2). Therefore median values of PaO_2 were

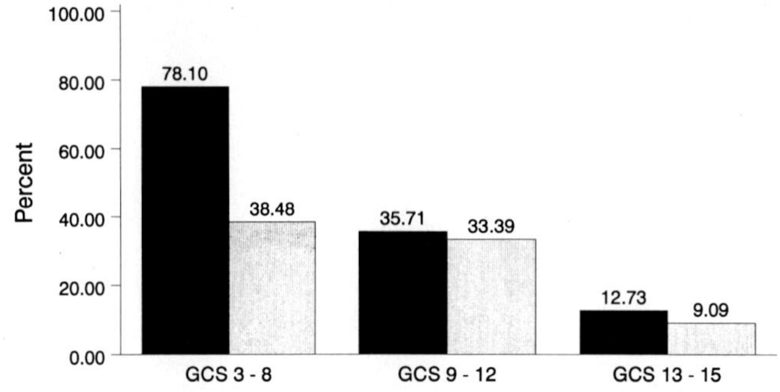

Fig. 2. Ventilatory care depending on the severity of head injury in 1623 patients with head injuries. *Solid columns*, total intubation; *shaded columns*, intubation and spontaneous ventilation

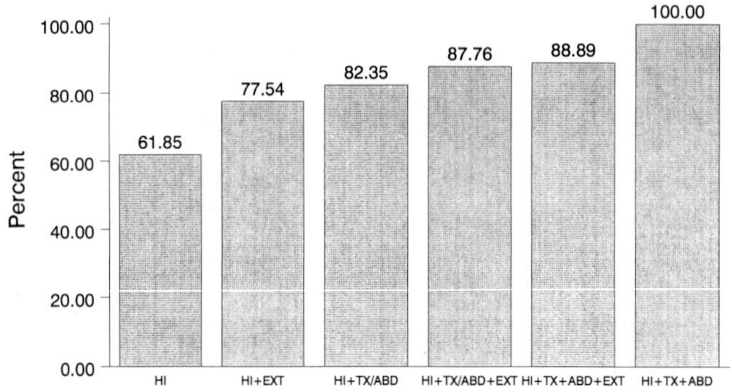

Fig. 3. Ventilatory care (i.e., intubation) depending on the severity of associated injuries in 1623 head-injured patients. *HI*, head injury; *TX*, chest trauma; *ABD*, abdominal trauma; *EXT*, fracture(s) of the extremities

significantly lower in patients who were breathing spontaneously on admission (median PaO_2 128 mmHg), but did not differ significantly between patients who were intubated with spontaneous ventilation (median PaO_2 158.4 mmHg) and patients who were under controlled ventilation (median PaO_2 161 mmHg). There was also no difference in the rate of hypoxic patients who were intubated and breathing spontaneously (22.35%) and patients who were intubated but breathing spontaneously (21%). Only controlled ventilation in intubated patients resulted in a lower rate of hypoxemia (16.3%). Further analysis was done to evaluate the reasons and indications for intubation of patients with head injuries. It was found that the rate of intubated patients was influenced by the type of transport, the expected transport time, and the type of injury, respectively.

The more severe the associated injuries were, the higher was the rate of intubated patients. Whereas only 68% of patients with isolated head injuries were intubated at the scene of the accident, the number rose when associated injuries were present and was 100% for patients with head injuries plus thoracic plus abdominal trauma (Fig. 3).

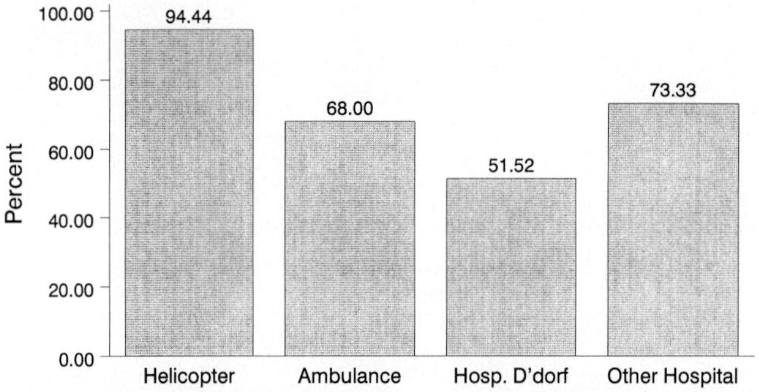

Fig. 4. Ventilatory care (i.e., intubation) depending on the type of transport in 1623 patients with head injuries. *Hosp. D'dorf*, hospital in Düsseldorf

Patients brought directly to our hospital by helicopter were more often intubated than patients for whom an ambulance had been chosen as transport.

Patients who were transferred from another hospital were less often intubated if the distance between our department and the referring hospital was short (Fig. 4).

Discussion

It is widely known that severe head injuries may be followed by numerous extracranial complications. Previous studies by Eisenberg et al. [3], Miller et al. [7], and Bowers and Marshall [1] clearly indicated that hypotension and hypoxemia adversely influenced outcome. Recent information from the TCDB [2] demonstrated that hypoxemia alone has only a small effect, but the combination of hypoxemia and hypotension has a dramatic impact on the outcome of severely head-injured patients. The present study clearly shows that, in spite of advanced care in pre-hospital treatment, hypoxemia and hypercapnia still play an important role as secondary insults to the injured brain. In the present series, airway protection by intubation was only performed in 68% of the severely injured patients with isolated head injuries. Adequate ventilation was assured in only part of the patients who had been intubated. It seems that the indication to intubate and ventilate a patient is based more on external factors (e.g., presence of associated injuries, length and type of transport) than on the severity of the head injury itself.

Therefore intensified training of all physicians involved in pre-hospital care of head trauma victims is urgently required for the initial assessment and early management of these patients.

References

1. Bowers SA, Marshall LF (1980) Outcome of 200 consecutive cases of severe head injury treated in San Diego County:a prospective analysis. Neurosurgery 6:237–242
2. Chesnut RM, Marshall LF (1989) The role of secondary brain injury in determining outcome from severe head injury. Paper presented in receipt of the Volvo Neurotrauma Award from the Neurotraumatology Section of the World Federation of Neurosurgical Societies, New Delhi
3. Eisenberg HM, Cayard CA, Papanicolaou RL et al. (1983) The effects of three potentially preventable complications on outcome after severe closed head injury. In: Ishii S, Nugui H, Brock M (eds) Intracranial pressure V. Springer, Berlin Heidelberg New York
4. Frost EAM (1979) The physiopathology of respirations in neurosurgical patients. J Neurosurg 50:699–714
5. Frost EAM, Arancibia CU, Shulman K (1979) Pulmonary shunt as a prognostic indicator in head injury. J Neurosurg 50:768–772
6. Klauber MR, Marshall LF, Toole BM (1985) Cause of decline in head-injury mortality rate in San Diego County. J Neurosurg 62:528–531
7. Miller JD, Sweet RC, Narayan R et al. (1978) Early insults to the injured brain. JAMA 240:439–442
8. Teasdale G, Jennett B (1974) Assessment of coma and impaired consciousness. A practical scale. Lancet 2:81–84

Influence of Volume- and Pressure-Controlled Ventilation on the Intracranial Pressure with Continuous Propofol Sedation in Neurosurgical Patients

J. Nadstawek[1], C. Cedzich[2], R. Priem[2], S. Albrecht[1] and K. Müller[2]

Introduction

Patients with craniocerebral trauma endangered by an increase of intracranial pressure (ICP) must be sedated and artificially ventilated. At the same time, the neurosurgeon must have the possibility of establishing the patient's neurological status at any time, or at least after discontinuing sedation. Pressure-controlled ventilation has numerous advantages in preventing pulmonary complications in multiple trauma patients [1].

This study was designed to evaluate the influence of pressure- and volume-controlled ventilation on ICP of neurotraumatized patients. The effects of the short-acting anesthetic propofol, used for continuous sedation, on ICP and cerebral perfusion pressure were also analyzed.

Patients and Methods

Fifteen patients, 17–50 years old, with craniocerebral trauma and a score of between 4 and 8 on the Glagow Coma Scale (GCS), were included in this study. ICP was measured using an intraventricular catheter. Volume-controlled ventilation (Siemens Servo 900 C) was used for the first 24 h after the patient's admission to the intensive care unit, followed by pressure-controlled ventilation with a maximal inspiratory pressure of 30 mmHg for the next 24 h period. ICP was measured continuously; PCO_2 was kept at 30 mmHg. All patients were sedated with propofol 5–8 mg/kg body weight per minute intravenously, starting 2 h after the beginning of the respiratory therapy. Before switching to pressure-controlled ventilation, propofol infusion was again interrupted for 2 h. Mean arterial pressure (MAP) and cerebral perfusion pressure (CPP) were also evaluated during the whole observation period of 48 h.

We compared the effects of volume-controlled and pressure-controlled ventilation with and without propofol sedation on ICP values, CPP, and MAP. Owing to the oily solution of propofol, serum triglycerides and cholesterol were analyzed before, during (every 48 h), and after discontinuing the propofol infusion. The time

[1] Institut für Anästhesiologie, Universität Bonn, Sigmund-Freud-Str. 25, W-5300 Bonn 1, FRG.
[2] Neurochirurgische Klinik, Universität Bonn, Sigmund-Freud-Str. 25, W-5300 Bonn 1, FRG.

Advances in Neurosurgery, Vol. 21
R. Lorenz, M. Klinger, M. Brock (Eds.)

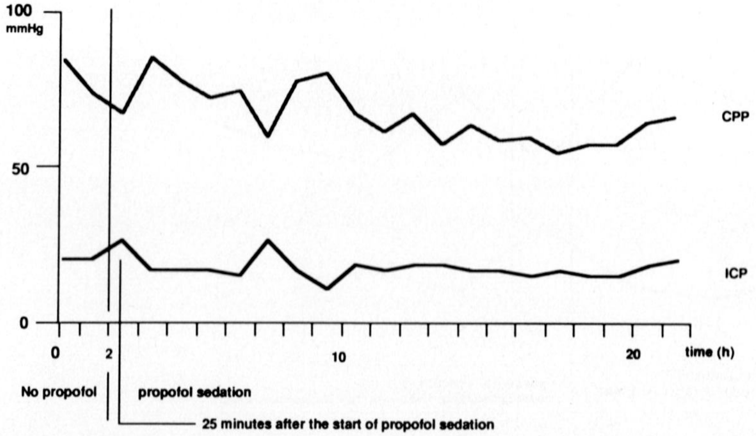

Fig. 1. Mean ICP and CPP during volume-controlled ventilation

between interrupting the propofol administration and the first possible neurological examination was also evaluated.

Data were analyzed using Mann-Whitney's U test; $p < 0.05$ was considered significant.

Results

Initial ICP under volume-controlled hyperventilation was 24 ± 4.1 mmHg. No significant changes in ICP and CPP could be observed during the whole time of volume-controlled hyperventilation without propofol sedation (Fig. 1). A slight and short decrease of ICP and an insignificant increase of CPP were observed 25 min after starting the propofol infuser. Slightly lower CPPs were noted during the whole time course of propofol administration (Fig. 2). Similar results were found by Van-Hemelrijk et al. [3] using a bolus technique.

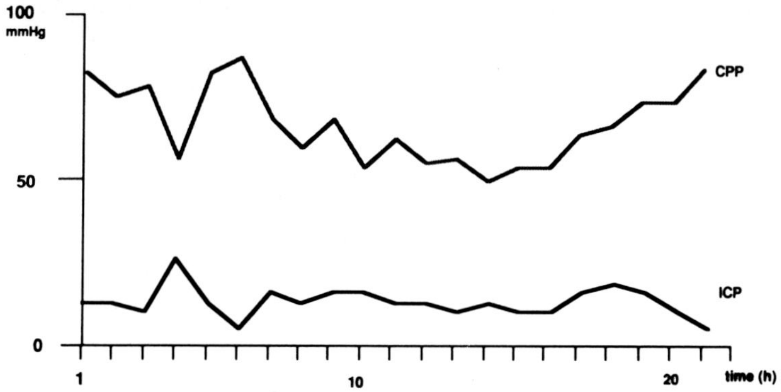

Fig. 2. Mean ICP and CPP during continuous infusion of propofol (average levels for volume- and pressure-controlled ventilation)

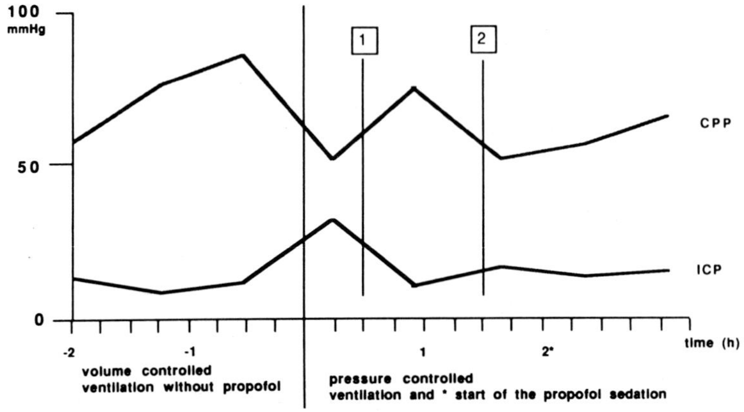

Fig. 3. Mean ICP and CCP during pressure-controlled ventilation (*1*, reversal of ICP change; *2*, reversal of CPP change)

After switching the artificial ventilation to a pressure-controlled mode without propofol sedation, a short period of ICP increase and a drop in CPP were registered. These alterations reversed after 30 min (ICP) and 90 min (CPP) (Fig. 3). Insignificant changes in ICP, CPP, and MAP were found after starting the propofol sedation (Figs. 2, 3).

Although there were initial changes in ICP and CPP during pressure-controlled ventilation, no significant differences regarding ICP, CPP, and MAP were seen for either ventilation modes with or without propofol sedation.

Neurological examination was possible 30–60 min after discontinuing propofol administration regardless which artificial ventilation mode was applied.

Triglyceride and cholesterol serum levels were increased during propofol infusion, but dropped to normal values within 24 h after discontinuing infusion (Fig. 4).

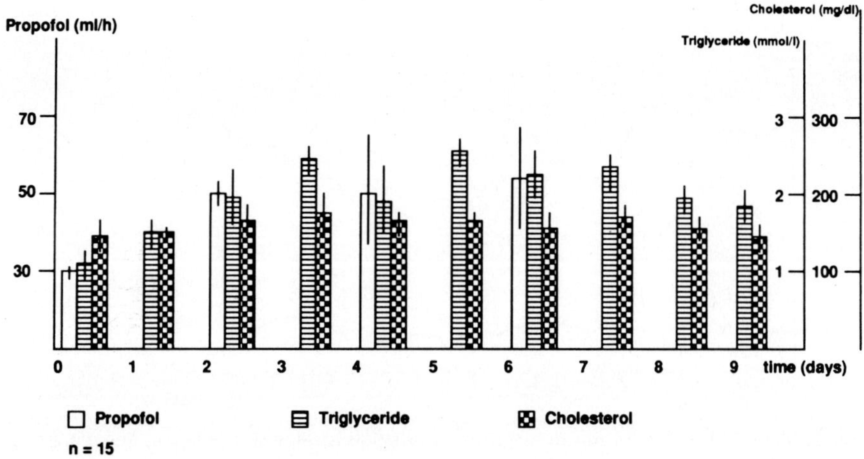

Fig. 4. Triglyceride and cholesterol serum values during continuous propofol infusion

Conclusion

Pressure-controlled ventilation does not lead to an increase of ICP. Continuous administration of propofol in patients with moderately increased ICP seems to be a superior alternative to barbiturate therapy, especially if the problem of neurological examination and adverse effects has to be considered. One of the major side effects of propofol (besides seizures and extrapyramidal disorders [2]), namely, higher levels of serum cholesterol and triglycerides, was reversible within 24 h after interrupting administration.

References

1. Neuhaus R, Lips U, Zenz M (1981) Kritische Bewertung des Atemtrainings mit intermittierendem Überdruck bei akuten pulmonalen Störungen. Anasth Intensivther Notfallmed 16:203–210
2. Rogers EM (1991) Diprivan intensive care sedation in children. Br J Anaesth 67:505
3. Van-Hemelrijk J, Van-Aken H, Plets C, Goffin J, Vermaut G (1989) The effects of propofol on intracranial pressure and cerebral perfusion pressure in patients with brain tumors. Acta Anaesthesiol Belg 40 (2):95–100

The Influence of Nosocomial Pneumonia on Outcome of Severely Head-Injured Patients

J. Piek[1], R. M. Chesnut[2], L. F. Marshall[2], M. van Berkum-Clark[2], M. R. Klauber[3], B. A. Blunt[3], H. Eisenberg[4], J. A. Jane[5], A. Marmarou[6], and M. Foulkes[7]

Introduction

As the outcome of most patients suffering from severe head injury is determined by the primary brain lesion itself, numerous studies have focussed on the type and severity of this lesion as predictors of outcome in this patient group. On the other hand, it is widely known that severe head injury may be followed by many extracranial complications [1, 2]. However, little attention has been paid to the question of how these complications influence outcome, and what patient groups are at particular risk [12]. To answer these questions, we studied a subgroup of patients from the Traumatic Coma Data Bank (TCDB) [9] with special regard to the role of nosocomial pneumonia.

Material and Methods

Between April 1983 and April 1988 data on prehospital and hospital acute care and on the rehabilitation period were collected prospectively on 1030 patients with severe head injuries (Glasgow Coma Scale, GCS, [14] score of 8 or less on admission or during the ensuing 2 days) admitted to four major trauma centers (Medical College of Virginia at Richmond, University of California at San Diego, University of Virginia at Charlottesville, University of Texas Medical Branch). Of these, 613 were available for logistic regression analysis; the others included 284 brain death on arrival from gunshot wounds, 82 missing preresuscitation GCS scores, 39 missing data on hypoxia or hypotension, and 23 missing complication forms (some patients fulfilled more than one of these criteria).

The evolution and development of various extra- and intracranial complications were recorded daily from 1 to day 14 following injury.

---

[1] Neurochirurgische Klinik, Heinrich-Heine-Universität Düsseldorf, Moorenstr. 5, W-4000 Düsseldorf, FRG.
[2] Division of Neurological Surgery, UCSD Medical Center, San Diego, California, USA.
[3] Department of Community and Family Medicine, UCSD Medical Center, San Diego, California, USA.
[4] University of Texas Medical Branch, Galveston, Texas, USA.
[5] University of Virginia School of Medicine, Charlottesville, Virginia, USA
[6] Medical College of Virginia, Richmond, Virginia, USA.
[7] National Institute of Neurological Disorders and Stroke, Bethesda, Maryland, USA.

Advances in Neurosurgery, Vol. 21
R. Lorenz, M. Klinger, M. Brock (Eds.)

Intracranial complications included: intracranial hemorrhage, intraventricular hemorrhage, subdural hematoma, epidural hematoma, cerebral fluid leak, intracranial pressure trace loss, postsurgical ventriculitits/meningitis, abscess, and wound infection.

Extracranial complications were: pulmonary (adult respiratory distress syndrome, atelectasis, pleural effusion, pulmonary embolus, respiratory failure), cardiovascular (arrhythmias, congestive heart failure, myocardial ischemia, hypotension < 90 mmHg, hypertension > 160 mmHg), peripheral vascular (deep vein thrombosis), gastrointestinal (gastrointestinal hemorrhage, pancreatitis, gastric perforation), renal (acute renal failure), hepatic (liver failure, cholangitis, hepatic renal syndrome), electrolyte imbalance, coagulopathy, *SIADH*, diabetes insipidus, nonsurgical meningitis/ventriculitis, septicemia.

The diagnosis of pneumonia was made by the presence of infiltration on the chest X-ray and positive sputum for organism on the Gram stain specimen or culture. Lung empyemas were coded considered as pulmonary complications. Although patients may have suffered a particular complication more than once, it was counted only once during their stay.

All definitions are available in the TCDB Manual of Operations and data forms, National Technical Information Service (NITS), United States Department of Commerce, 5285 Port Royal Road, Springfield, VA 22161 (NITS Accession No. 228060/AS).

Outcome was dichotomized for statistical analysis. favorable (follow-up Glasgow Outcome Scale [8] score "good" or "moderate") or unfavorable (follow-up Glasgow Outcome Scale score "severe," "vegetative," or "dead"). A backward elimination, stepwise logistic regression model [6] was used to model the dependent variable, i.e., the log odds of unfavorable outcome. The Hosmer-Lemeshow approach was used to test the goodness of fit of the logistic model. This model included the following variables: (a) age on admission, divides at age 40 years, (b) maximum preresuscitation GCS motor score, (c) hypoxia upon arrival at TCDB hospital emergency room, (d) hypotension upon arrival at TCDB hospital emergency room, (e) multiple trauma to any extracranial system with an abbreviated injury score of 3 or greater, (f) presence or absence of any intracranial complication (see above).

Age, maximum preresuscitation GCS motor score, hypoxia, and hypotension were included in the model because previous TCDB research has shown these factors to be closely correlated to outcome [3, 10]. The 5% level was used for statistical significance.

Results

There were 1709 individual extracranial complications, ranging in severity from mild to life threatening. Among the patients 27.1% had a good outcome, 16.5% moderate, 15.5% severe, 5% vegetative, and 35.8% of the patients died (i.e., 43.6% "favorable" versus 56.4% "unfavorable" outcome). As can be seen in Fig. 1,

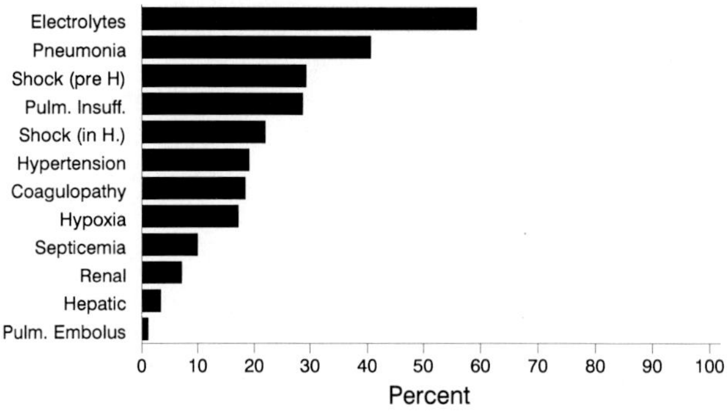

Fig. 1. Frequency of extracranial complications in 613 patients with severe head injury

disturbance of electrolytes was the most common complication, followed by pneumonia with a frequency of 40.6%. Shock of at least 30-min duration (29.3%), disturbances of blood coagulation (18.4%), and septicemia (10%) were the next most common, whereas complications of the digestive tract, liver, or kidneys occurred rarely.

Age ($p < 0.001$), maximun preresuscitation GCS motor score ($p = < 0.001$), shock upon arrival ($p = 0.0077$), shock during the hospital course ($p < 0.001$), coagulopathy ($p = 0.0036$), septicemia ($p = 0.0036$), and septicemia ... ($p = 0.047$) were found to be significant predictors of an unfavorable outcome. The significance level for pneumonia was $p = 0.037$. All other complications (including presence of any intracranial complication) could not be identified as being significantly responsible for an overall unfavorable outcome in patients with severe head injuries.

The model used had an acceptable sensitivity (75.4%) and specificity (75.8%). Further analysis showed that about one-fifth of the patients had an estimated 40%–60% probability of unfavorable outcome. This indicates a large subgroup of patients with an uncertain prognosis at the time of injury whose outcome may be influenced by minimizing or eliminating complications.

Looking at the time course of pneumonia as an extracranial complication that influences outcome in severely head-injured patients, we found that it reached its peak occurrence from day 5 through day 11. By removing the complications using the backward elimination, stepwise logistic regression model described above, we found that the estimated reduction in unfavorable outcome for pneumonia was 2.9% in the patient group. It should be noted that in the statistical model each complication is removed separately, holding the others constant.

Discussion

Extracranial complications occur frequently in head-injured patients. Although the outcome of an individual patient may be adversely affected by numerous complications, pneumonia was identified to have an independent influence on outcome in severe head injury. It was further shown that this occurs late in the hospital course (from days 5 through 11) and therefore may be preventable. This would reduce the number of patients with unfavorable outcome since, for eliminating pneumonia as a single complication, the estimated statistical reduction in unfavorable outcome in the present patient group was 2.9%. As severe pneumonia is often associated with other factors such as hypotension, hypoxia, septicemia, and coagulation disorders, from a clinical point of view the estimated reduction in unfavorable outcome may be much greater. Improved strategies for the prevention or effective treatment of pulmonary infections should therefore have a major positive effect on the outcome of severe head injuries.

The risk of pneumonia in an intensive care unit increases with impairment of airway reflexes, a history of aspiration, and more than 24 h of artificial ventilation [4, 13], all common situations in severely head-injured patients. Barbiturate therapy also may increase the rate of pneumonia [11]. Therefore, a certain proportion of pneumonias will be not preventable, but their effects should be minimized by rapid diagnosis and prompt identification and treatment of the causing organism. The neutralization of gastric pH by antacids [5], H_2 receptor blockers [5], or enteral nutrition [7] has been found to be associated with a higher incidence of pneumonia. The use of sucralfate, which is equally protective against gastric ulcers but may not raise gastric pH to the same extent, may be useful in reducing gram-negative colonization of [5, 7] the oropharynx, thus preventing pneumonia. Intravenous antibiotics, combined with selective decontamination of the digestive tract, may also be effective in decreasing nosocomial pneumonia in general [13].

From the results of this study we conclude that these concepts should be rigorously investigated in severely head-injured patients.

Acknowledgements. This work was supported by the Traumatic Coma Data Bank (TCDB) under Contracts N01-NS-3-2339, N01-NS-3-2341, N01-NS-3-2342, N01-NS-6-2305 from the National Institute of Neurological Disorders and Stroke (NINDS) and the Wilhelm Tönnis Foundation of the German Society for Neurosurgery. The TCDB Manual of Operations, which includes the TCDB data forms, is available from the National Technical Information Service (NITS), United States Department of Commerce, 5285 Port Royal Road, Springfield, VA 22161 (NITS Accession No. 228060/AS).

References

1. Baigelman W, O'Brien JC (1981) Pulmonary effects of head trauma. Neurosurgery 9:729–740
2. Bloomfield EL (1989) Extracerebral complications of head injury. Crit Care Clin 5:881–892
3. Chesnut RM, Marshall LF (1989) The role of secondary brain injury in determining outcome from severe head injury. Paper presented in receipt of the Volvo Neurotrauma Award from the Neurotraumatology Section of the WFNS, New Delhi, India
4. Craven DE, Kunches LM, Kilinsky V et al. (1986) Risk factors for pneumonia and fatality in patients receiving continuous mechanical ventilation. Am Rev Respir Dis 133:792–796

5. Driks MR, Craven DE, Celli BR et al. (1987) Nosocomial pneumonia in intubated patients given sucralfate as compared with antacids or histamine type 2 blockers. The role of gastric colonization. N Engl J Med 317:1376–1382
6. Hosmer DW, Lameshow S (1989) Applied logistic regression. Wiley, New York
7. Jacobs S, Chang RW, Lee B et al. (1990) Continuous enteral feeding: a major cause of pneumonia among ventilated intensive care unit patients. JPEN J Parenter Enteral Nutr 14:353–356
8. Jennett B, Bond M (1975) Assessment of outcome after severe brain damage: a practical scale. Lancet I:1031–1034
9. Marshall LF, Becker DP, Bowers SA et al. (1983) The National Traumatic Coma Data Bank. I. Design, purpose, goals, and results. J Neurosurg 59:276–284
10. Marshall LF, Gautille TH, Klauber MR et al. (1991) The outcome of severe closed head injury. J Neurosurg [Suppl]:S28–S38
11. Nadstawek J, Moskopp D, Fischer M et al. (1991) Susceptibility to infection during continuous thiopentone therapy. In: Bock WJ, Lumenta C, Brock M, Klinger M (eds) Advances in neurosurgery 19. Springer, Berlin Heidelberg New York pp 217–221
12. Price JE, Murray A (1972) The influence of hypoxia and hypotension on recovery from head injury. Br J Acc Surg 3:218–224
13. Stoutenbeck CP, van Saene HK, Miranda DR et al. (1987) The effect of oropharyngeal decontamination using topical nonabsorbable antibiotics on the incidence of nosocomial respiratory tract infections in multiple trauma patients. J Trauma 27:357–364
14. Teasdale G, Jennett B (1974) Assessment of coma and impaired consciousness: practical scale. Lancet II:81–84
15. Torres A, Aznar R, Gatell JM et al. (1990) Incidence, risk, and prognostic factors of nosocomial pneumonia in mechanically ventilated patients. Am Rev Respir Dis 142:523–528

Peripheral Nerves

Treatment of Peripheral Nerve Lesions

G. Penkert[1]

Classification of Nerve Lesions

Depending on the amount of compressing and destroying forces, Seddon, in 1943 [4], created the well-known idea of neurapraxia – functional blockade of the electrical nerve conductivity due to myelin degeneration, axonotmesis – interruption of continuity of the axons, and neurotmesis – complete interruption of nerve continuity. In comparison, Sunderland [5] distinguished five degrees of nerve lesion in 1951. We consider this division to be much more helpful in understanding the different disturbing events which occur within the nerves:

Grade I

Sunderland's grade I lesion is identical with Seddon's neurapraxia. The myelin sheath is the most sensitive part of the nerve fiber; thus focal demyelination occurs first. The rearrangement of the myelin sheath will last 3–4 weeks. After this short period, the nerve regains its function.

Grade II

Owing to further compressing forces, the axons undergo wallerian degeneration. Nevertheless, each axon remains enclosed by its basal membrane and endoneurium so that it can reach its former muscle end plate. This process of axon sprouting will last some months, but the end result is nearly a complete return to health.

Grade III

At this stage of lesion we find the endoneural structures being destroyed to a greater degree so that motor axons may sprout into a sensory pathway or vice versa.

This leads to a certain amount of "missprouting" with simultaneous functional defects.

---

[1] Neurochirurgische Klinik, Krankenhaus Nordstadt, Haltenhoffstr. 41,
W-3000 Hannover 1, FRG.

Advances in Neurosurgery, Vol. 21
R. Lorenz, M. Klinger, M. Brock (Eds.)

Table 1. Nerve lesions according to Seddon [4] and Sunderland [5]

Seddon 1943	Sunderland 1951		
Neurapraxia	Grade I:	Focal demyelinization	
Axonotmesis	Grade II: Grade III: Grade IV:	Continuity of axons interrupted Architecture of perineurium destroyed Architecture of endoneurium destroyed	Wallerian degeneration of the nerve fiber
Neurotmesis	Grade V:	Continuity of all nerve structures interrupted	

Grade IV

Because of the disarranged perineurial structures found here, the degree of missprouting improves rapidly on one side, but, on the other hand, the surrounding connective tissue of each fascicle and fascicle group becomes fibrotic and compresses the outgrowth of the axons in a circular manner. The amount of missprouting occurs so much that, for example, antagonistic muscles will be innervated simultaneously. From a certain degree of compressing fibrosis, the axon sprouts are blocked completely, and there will be a "neuroma in continuity" without any nerve function. This is now comparable to a nerve interruption.

Thus the idea of axonotmesis contains a wide field of different types of nerve lesion; we are now able to explain the possible unexpected by poor results after a neurolysis.

Grade V

A grade V lesion is again identical with Seddon's neurotmesis, i.e., a complete interruption of the whole nerve (Table 1).

Tinel Sign

The time span between a nerve lesion and possible regeneration will often be several months. During this period we can test the behavior of the axon sprouts only by provoking the "Tinel sign". The palpation of the nerve and where sprouting occurs triggers an "electric" pain which is experienced in the sensitive area previously belonging to the injured nerve. If the trigger point moves downwards over this period of several months, an outgrowth of axons is taking place. This would signify a positive prognostic factor.

Operative Procedures

Lesions Without Loss of Continuity

These are lesions which can be overcome by axon sprouting without any surgical reconstruction, the so-called pseudoneuromas. The first step is to open the outer epineurium in a longitudinal direction from proximal and distal towards the level of the lesion. If there is a persisting compression, it will be necessary to peel and remove the surrounding epineurium. In the case of an interfascicular fibrosis, it will be necessary to dissect between the fascicle groups.

The numerous fascicles of each nerve are arranged into groups of fascicles, but their arrangement changes from the central levels to the periphery: nerve roots consists of fewer but thicker fascicles which can be divided into sectors. Whereas more peripherally the nerve has its typical group arrangement – three to five groups of fascicles – between these groups there is only loose connective tissue with longitudinally oriented vessels. At the peripheral end these groups also divide into many small fascicles so that the nerve structure acquires a multifascicular nature. In summary, the nerve begins in a mono- or oligo-fascicular fashion, in the middle it contains a typical group arrangement, and at the end this grouping is again lost in favor of multiple small, no longer distinguishable fascicle groups. The surgeon has to be aware of this changing arrangement. An interfascicular microsurgical neurolysis is only possible in the case of a group arrangement, whereas at root level a dissection of fascicles would damage their continuity!

Lesions with Loss of Continuity

These are lesions which cannot be overcome by axon sprouts, i.e., completely interrupted nerves (grade V lesion) and also cases with real neuroma formation in continuity. The treatment of choice is to restore the nerve continuity. For the last 30 years, free autologous nerve grafts have been used for interposition between the nerve stumps. In the case of nerve segments with the typical, previously mentioned group arrangement, each fascicle group can be coaptated to one nerve graft (Figs. 1–4). This method ensures control on the individual coaptation and avoids any disturbing tension which induces tissue fibrosis in the area of the coaptation [1–3]. One suture through the epineurium of the sural nerve graft and through the epineurium of each fascicle group is sufficient to avoid foreign body granulomas.

If the nerve is unifascicular or multifascicular, the grafts have to be coaptated over the whole cross-section of the nerve stump. The question of increased scar tissue formation by gluing or stitching is often discussed controversially, but it has not been completely answered yet. In introducing laser techniques to maintain the coaptation, one should always consider the costs of this method. It is important to remember that the patient's own fibrin will maintain the coaptation after perhaps 10–20 min [1]! However, despite several coaptation methods, postoperative immobilization of the area is advisable.

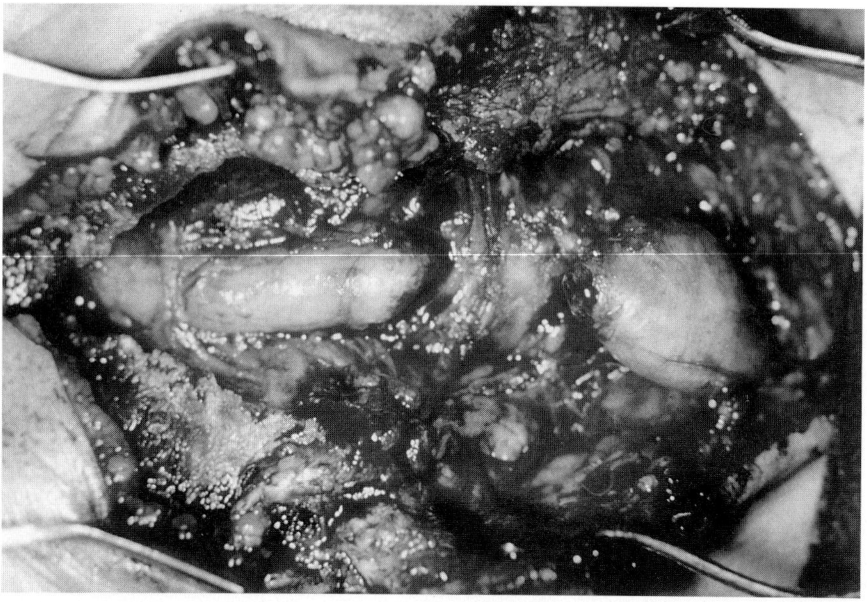

Fig. 1. Transected median nerve with neuroma at the proximal stump

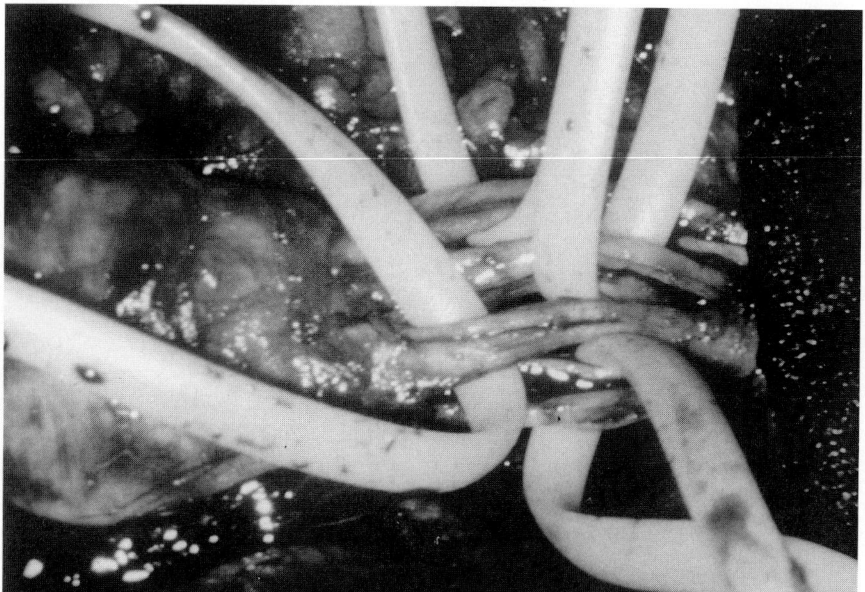

Fig. 2. Separation of the fascicle groups

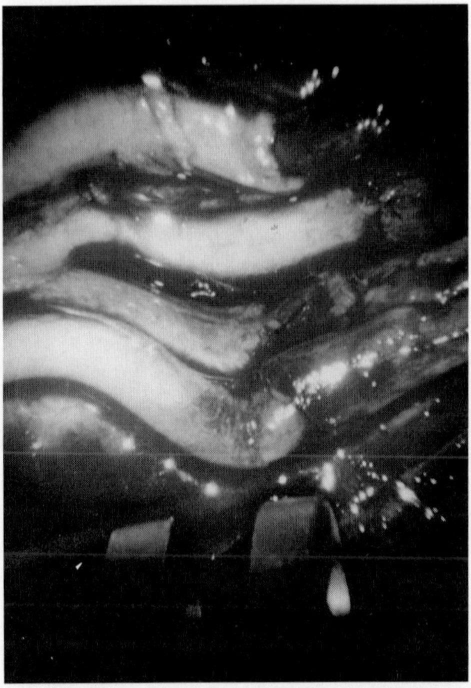

Fig. 3. Coaptation of sural grafts (proximal suture line)

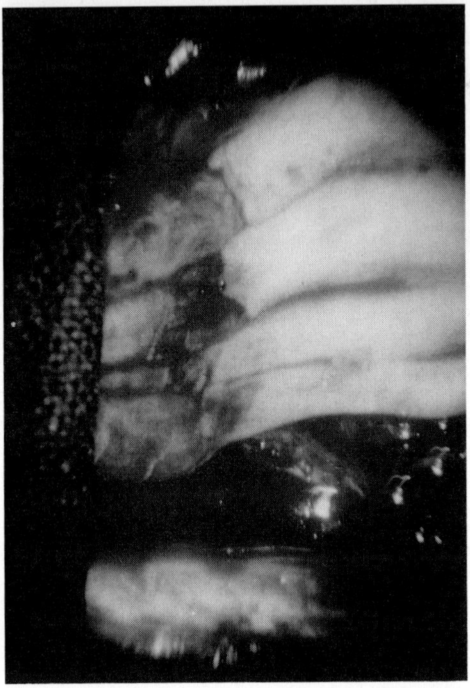

Fig. 4. Distal suture line

References

1. Millesi H (1983) Microsurgery of peripheral nerves. In: Kibbin B Mc (ed) Recent advances in orthopaedics. Churchill Livingstone, Edinburgh, pp 1–22
2. Samii M, Penkert G (1988) Verletzungen der peripheren Nerven. In: Koslowski L, Bushe K-A, Junginger T, Schwemmle K (eds) Lehrbuch Chirurgie. Schattauer, Stuttgart, pp 439–446
3. Samii M, Penkert G (1988) Chirurgie bei peripheren Nervenverletzungen. In: Berchtold R, Hamelmann H, Peiper H (eds). Lehrbuch der Chirurgie. Urban and Schwarzenberg, Munich, pp 819–841
4. Seddon H-J (1943) Three types of nerve injury. Brain 66:237–288
5. Sunderland S (1951) A classification of peripheral nerve injuries producing loss of function. Brain 74:491–516

What Is Special About Traumatic Brachial Plexus Lesions ?*

A. C. J. Slooff[1]

Diversity of the Pathological Condition

Our experience (Table 1) covers a period from 1976 to May 1992 but the series is not representative of the real incidence of brachial plexus lesions. Minor lesions are not presented to us nor are many of the severe lesions. They are masked by the multitrauma or are considered as inoperable – an expression of incredible defeatism. Iatrogenic lesions are increasing and obstetrical lesions have been our special interest for the last 5 years.

Traffic accidents, especially motorcycle accidents, still count as the most frequent cause of brachial plexus lesions. Gunshot lesions and stab wounds will undoubtedly increase and the same is true for lesions caused by sport.

Traumatic lesions are often associated with other injuries such as craniocerebral lesions, fractures of the clavicula, scapula, humerus, cervical spine, with spinal cord and thoracic lesions, and vascular injuries.

Table 1. Etiology of brachial plexus lesions

	Total cases (*n*)	Operated cases (*n*)
Traumatic lesions	507	227
Traction/crush lesions Lacerations	295	
Gunshot wounds	186	70
Obstetric lesions		
Iatrogenic lesions	26	
Tumors	30	19
Entrapment syndromes	12	8
Lesions due to irradiation	9	
Others	21	
	579	254

* Dedicated to Algir Narakas.

[1] Neurosurgical Department, De Wever Hospital, Postbus 4446, 6401 Cy Heerlen, The Netherlands.

Advances in Neurosurgery, Vol. 21
R. Lorenz, M. Klinger, M. Brock (Eds.)

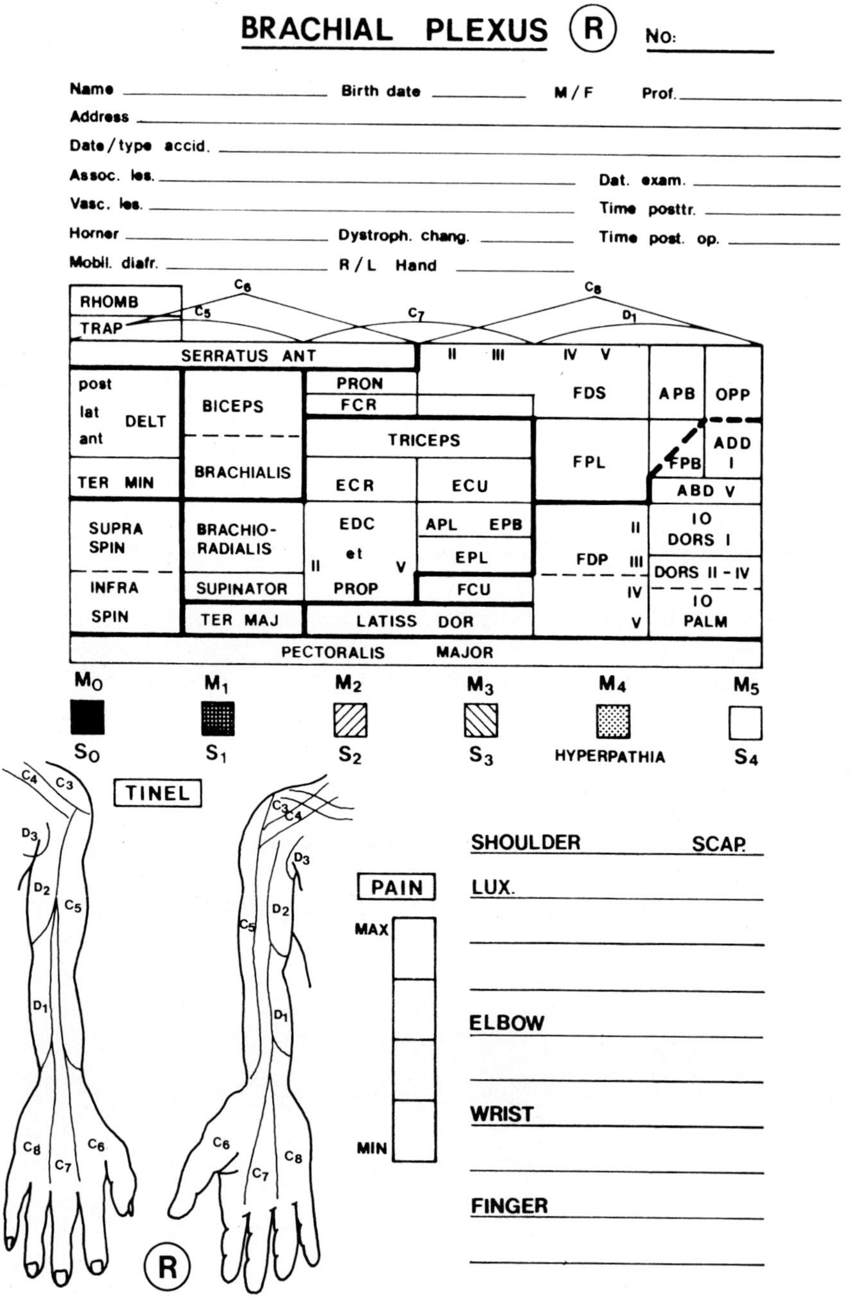

Fig. 1. Chart recording traumatic brachial plexus lesions

Multitrauma is found in 50% of cases and in 70% of the patients operated on. This association is an indication of the severity of the lesion, pointing to the site of the trauma, and serves as a reference point for a possible second level lesion, e.g., radial, axillary, suprascapular or musculocutaneous nerves. Vascular lesions are noted in 10%–15% of patients and are nearly always associated with a nerve lesion of the same severity, resulting in highly demanding surgical interventions.

Young Men, Disability, Pain Syndrome

A total of 55% of patients are aged 15–25 years; 85% of the total are males. At least 70% have avulsions or total lesions and at least half of them have a disturbing pain syndrome (cf. the law of seven seventies [1–3]).

The Diagnostic Puzzle

For an analysis of the lesions we need the following information: the history, general and neurological examination, neurophysiological and radiological investigations. The history of trauma provides an estimate of the impact and circumstances of the trauma. A general examination is necessary to assess vital functions and to detect associated injuries. The neurological examination has to be very detailed: if the results are recorded on a chart, one can see the total neurological deficit at a glance (Fig. 1).

There is no doubt about the importance and the support of EMG, SNAP, and SSEP. Radiological investigations, consisting of plain X-ray, cervical myelography and computed tomography (CT) are also of the utmost value. CT is very reliable in detecting root avulsions and associated spinal cord lesions. Magnetic resonance imaging (MRI) is still far more appropriate for tumors. We often perform angiography to detect the vascular lesion and to visualize the vascular graft and the collateral circulation. Surgical exploration supported by preoperative neurophysiological and histological investigation can be highly relevant for the final diagnosis.

Creative Reconstructive Procedures for Improvement of Function

The treatment consists of several modalities depending on the nature, the topography, the severity, and the age of the lesion. For the neurosurgical intervention there are well-defined indications, such as an open lesion, a closed lesion with vascular insufficiency, or a compression by a hematoma or fracture. Also, if there is a severe lesion (degree 4, 5 or 6 according to Sunderland [4]) or no or only retarded recovery after 3–4 months, intervention is indicated. Severe early pain is suggestive of a (lower-root) avulsion. Finally, when there is uncertainty as to the degree of the lesion, one would consider exploration. There is a wide variety of surgical procedures. Sometimes a neurolysis is sufficient, but this is often part of the total surgical procedure. A nerve suture is seldom possible, more often we need grafting procedures. In most cases we use autologous thin grafts, preferably from the sural nerve. Other possibilities are a pedicled or free vascularized graft when we have to bridge a long distance or when there is a scarred wound bed. Reconstructions within the plexus are called intraplexal neurotizations, but in avulsion we have to look for a proximal stump outside the plexus, e.g., accessory nerve, cervical plexus, or intercostal nerves: an extraplexal neurotization. Sometimes there is no distal stump available, and in these cases we put the split graft into the muscle: nerve implantation. A nerve transposition can sometimes be useful. Vascularization procedures, e.g., with an omentum flap, can supplement the graft procedure. We abandoned the cervical laminectomy in order to establish an avulsion.

The coaptation is performed with fibrin glue, sometimes reinforced by 10 x 0 sutures.

There are several factors which influence and limit the quality of regeneration: the age of the patient, the age of the lesion, the length and the number of grafts, the unreachability of the intrinsic muscles. We should consider this in view of the most important goal of the overall treatment. The surgical procedures, primary and secondary, have to be directed at gaining functional results; priorities are then inevitable.

A Multidisciplinary Approach

In line with our view on these therapeutic measurements, we propagate the collaboration of the neurosurgeon with the rehabilitation specialists, the orthopedic and hand surgeons; and we enlist the support of neurophysiologists and radiologists.

The Highly Motivated Patient

It struck us during the follow-up period that we were dealing with a highly motivated group of patients in spite of sometimes poor results. Most of them resume their studies or work, or regain their daily activities. A persistent disturbing pain syndrome was found in five patients. We established a scoring system to evaluate the functional results after brachial plexus repair [1], with a follow-up period of at least 2 1/2 years (Table 2). Even in cases without any functional gain there will always be a better cosmetic aspect of the limb and a greater chance for improvement or disappearance of a severe pain syndrome [2, 3]. Extraplexal neurotizations result in a useful function (M3 or more) in 40%–50% of the patients. Direct muscle implantation yields a useful recovery in 60%–70% of the patients. Orthopedic and hand surgery increase these functional results.

In conclusion, the treatment of brachial plexus lesions is a challenge, worthwhile, and rewarding, but we must stress the need for early and overall treatment.

Table 2. Global results in brachial plexus repair

Pattern of the lesion	(*n*)	Gain[a]	Final result[b] (%)
Total avulsion	7	0–2	0–4
Avulsion C6–T1/C5 rupture	10	0–15	0–30
Avulsion C7–T1/C5C6 rupture	17	0–1	0–56
Avulsion C8T1/C5C6C7 rupture	3	2–10	24–76
Rupture C5C6C7C8T1	1	13	26
Rupture/avulsion C5C6(C7)	22	0–30	0–95
Retro-/infraclavicular lesions	14	5–36	28–96

[a] Evaluation of function of the upper limb is expressed in points. Normal function is 50 points. Total gain is the functional gain in points and is obtained by nerve repair alone.
[b] The final result consists of residual function, function gained by nerve surgery, and spontaneous regeneration. This is calculated in points and/or expressed as a percentage of the 50 points.

References

1. Alnot J, Narakas A (eds) (1989) Les paralysies du plexus brachial. Expansion Scientifique Francaise, Paris
2. Narakas A (1990) Brachial plexus injuries. In: (Plastic surgery, vol 7) The hand. Saunders, Philadelphia
3. Narakas A (1991) Neurotization in the treatment of brachial plexus injuries. In: Gelberman RH (ed) Operative nerve repair and reconstruction, vol 2. Lippincott, Philadelphia
4. Sunderland S (1978) Nerves and nerve injuries. Churchill Livingstone, Edinburgh

Findings and Results of 80 Surgical Revisions for Carpal Tunnel Syndrome

S. A. Rath[1], U. M. Mauer[1], and H. P. Richter[1]

Introduction

The carpal tunnel syndrome (CTS) is not only the most frequent peripheral nerve entrapment syndrome, but it also has a relatively high incidence, particularly in older women. In the face of the largely inadequate possibilities of conservative therapy, surgical treatment of CTS, which consists of decompressing the median nerve by severing the transverse carpal ligament, is a very effective method. It is a small operation which can be done under local anesthesia. However, failures of this apparently simple procedure occur. We would therefore like to present our experience with pre- and intraoperative findings as well as results of surgery for recurrent or residual CTS.

Material and Methods

The two main reasons for a second operation in patients with CTS must be clearly separated: whether symptoms recurred after a period of improvement – which is a true recurrence, or whether symptoms persisted in spite of surgery. The patient with recurrence has been pain-free or at least markedly improved after surgery, after some time pain and other symptoms recur. In the latter case, there has been no or only a minimal improvement with persisting or residual complaints following surgery despite a correct diagnosis.

In our own series of 1420 consecutive primary operations for CTS, of which a follow-up could be obtained in 1305 cases with an average observation time of 18 weeks (Table 1). In 6.5% of these 1305 an unsatisfactory result of median nerve decompressions was seen. In almost one-third of them (2.0%) we decided to operate again. In the majority of these patients (n = 22, 1.5%) it was considered necessary because of recurrent CTS, in the seven others (0.5%) because of persistent complaints.

One patient was operated on a third time because pain had recurred after several years.

In addition, 50 other patients, who had previously been operated on in another institution, underwent surgery for a second or even a third or fourth time. Of these

[1] Neurochirurgische Klinik, Universität Ulm, Bezirkskrankenhaus Günzburg, Ludwig-Heilmeyer-Straße 2, W-8870 Günzburg, FRG.

Advances in Neurosurgery, Vol. 21
R. Lorenz, M. Klinger, M. Brock (Eds.)

Table 1. Results following primary surgery for CTS

Status	(*n*)	%
No further symptoms, pain free	1188	91.0
No, only temporary, or minimal improvement,	85	6.5
of which		
– Secondary surgery for recurring CTS	22	1.7
– Surgical revision for persisting CTS	7	0.5

$n = 1305$; $t =$ average of 18 weeks.

26 suffered from residual complaints after primary median nerve decompression. Twenty of the remaining 24 patients had been operated on a second time, four a third, and one patient even a fourth time due to recurrent CTS.

Results

In 30 patients the value of the distal motor latency could be compared (Table 2). This is considered one of the main electrophysiological parameters in the diagnosis of CTS before the first and the second operation. In nearly the same number of patients either a clear improvement or a deterioration could be observed, independently of the history of recurring or persisting CTS. The distal motor latency therefore appears to be without significance once surgery has already been performed.

During our surgical revisions we found a scarring around the median nerve to be the main cause of recurring CTS. In every patient with persisting CTS the only, or at least an important, reason for compression of the median nerve was an incomplete severance of the transverse carpal ligament in the first operation (Table 3).

Table 2. Distal motor latency prior to the surgical revision as compared to findings before the first operation

Distal motor latency	Recurring CTS ($n = 23$)	Persisting CTS ($n = 7$)
Improved – 3.0 to –0.3	9	2
Unchanged – 0.2 to +0.2	5	1
Impaired + 0.3 to conduction block	9	4

Table 3. Intraoperative findings during surgical revisions in patients with CTS

	Recurring CTS ($n = 46$)	Persisting CTS ($n = 33$)
Scarring around median nerve	27	–
Scarring and incomplete severance of the transverse carpal ligament	10	12
Incomplete severance of the transverse carpal ligament	–	21
Neuroma	6	–
Other	3	–

Only 28 of 45 patients with recurring CTS hat no further symptoms after the surgical revision. In the postsurgical course ten more of these 45 patients developed a reflex sympathetic dystrophy. On the other hand, the patients with persisting CTS have rather good results after the surgical revisions (Table 4).

More patients with recurring symptoms than expected (13 patients) underwent an epineurectomy or an interfascicular neurolysis in the first operation on the carpal tunnel.

Discussion

In agreement with the literature [5, 8, 10] we found an incidence of 2% of surgical revisions after carpal tunnel decompression. Scarring in and around the nerve is the typical finding in patients with recurring CTS [1, 3]. In agreement with other authors [1–3] we found a worse outcome in these operations in contrast to patients with persisting CTS. In persisting CTS the result of the surgical revision is as good as that of a primary operation [1, 9]. The typical finding in patients with persisting CTS is an incomplete severance of the transverse carpal ligament [2, 9].

Table 4. Results in surgical revisions for CTS

	Recurring CTS ($n = 45$)	Persisting CTS ($n = 32$)
No further symptoms, pain-free	28	28
Complications	15	1
Reflex sympathetic dystrophy	10	1

$n = 80$; three patients lost for follow-up.

Internal neurolysis and other manipulations of the nerve are of no benefit in a primary operation [4, 6, 7, 9].

Conclusions

The distal motor latency of the median nerve – one of the main electrophysiological parameters in carpal tunnel syndrome – was found to be of no or of only minor value in patients with recurring or persisting CTS. The decision for another operation in such a patient is therefore based on an exact history and clinical examination.

In all cases of persisting complaints following median nerve decompression, an incomplete severance of the transverse carpal ligament was seen during the secondary surgery, in part associated with scarring around the nerve. A scar around the median nerve was found to be the main cause of recurrent CTS. We must stress the fact that in some patients with recurrent CTS a neuroma of the median nerve can be found, probably the result of a nerve lesion during the previous operation.

Postoperative results following secondary surgery were significantly better, and the complication rate was clearly lower in patients with persisting pain than in those with recurrent CTS. Therefore the conclusion for the first operation is that procedures on the nerve itself, in particular interfascicular neurolysis, should be avoided and restricted to exceptional cases. These procedures are not only unjustified in the "normal" CTS, but also carry the potential risk of scar formation within the nerve. In addition, the transverse carpal ligament should only be severed on its ulnar side where there is no danger of injuring branching nerves such as the thenar branch.

References

1. Antoniadis G, Richter H-P (1988) Carpaltunnelsyndrom – Intraoperative Befunde bei 45 Nachoperationen. In: Bock WJ, Schirmer M (eds) Komplikationen bei neurochirurgischen Eingriffen. Zuckerschwerdt, Munich pp 167–169
2. Büchler U, Goth D, Haußmann P, Lanz U, Martini AK, Wulle C (1983) Karpaltunnelsyndrom: Bericht über 56 Nachoperationen. Handchir Mikrochir Plast Chir 15 Suppl:3–12
3. Conolly WB (1978) Pitfalls in carpal tunnel decompression. Aust N Z J Surg 48:421–425
4. Holmgreen-Larsson H, Leszniewski W, Linden U, Rabow L, Thorling J (1985) Internal neurolysis or ligament division only in the carpal tunnel syndrome – results of a randomized study. Acta Neurochir (Wien) 74:118–121
5. Hybinette C-H, Mannerfelt L (1975) The carpal tunnel syndrome – retrospective study of 400 operated patients. Acta Orthop Scand 46:610–620
6. Lowry EL, Follender AB (1988) Interfascicular neurolysis in the severe carpal tunnel syndrome. Clin Orthop 227:251–254
7. MacDonald RI, Lichtman DM, Hanlon JJ, Wilson JN (1978) Complications of surgical release for carpal tunnel syndrome. J Hand Surg [Am] 3:70–76

8. Phalen GS (1966) The carpal-tunnel syndrome – seventeen years' experience in diagnosis and treatment of six hundred fifty-four hands. J Bone Surg [Am] 48:211–228
9. Richter H-P (1989) Therapeutische Möglichkeiten, Grundlagen und Richtlinien N. medianus. In: Tackmann W, Richter H-P, Stöhr M (eds) Kompressionssyndrome peripherer Nerven. Springer, Berlin Heidelberg New York, pp 66–79, 138–238
10. Yamaguchi DM, Lipscomb PR, Soule EH (1965) Carpal tunnel syndrome. Minn Med 48:22–33

Radial Nerve Lesions Associated with Fractures of the Humerus or Radius: Results of Surgical Treatment

S. Mirzai[1], A. Sepehrnia[1], G. Penkert[1], M. El Azm[1], and M. Samii[1]

Introduction

Components of the radial nerve arise from the spinal segments C5–T1. After its course through the axilla the radial nerve traverses the spiral groove of the humerus. It then turns abruptly forward round the lateral aspect of the humerus to pierce the lateral intermuscular septum. At the elbow, the radial nerve divides into two branches: the sensory superficial branch and the motoric deep branch [6, 8].

Owing to its proximity to the bone and tethering in the lateral intermuscular septum, the radial nerve is susceptible to injury [1, 13]. Injuries of radial nerve in association with fractures of the humerus or radius are frequent and the literature includes many cases [11, 13, 14]. The following data illustrate the importance of these injuries. The incidence of radial nerve involvement in fractures of the humerus varies between 2% and 16% [14]. There is a 60% rate of radial nerve involvement in nerve injuries associated with fractures and dislocations of long bones [5]. The radial nerve is injured more often than any other major nerve [1, 9, 14].

The present paper is a report on 54 patients operated upon for isolated radial nerve palsy associated with long bone fracture. All patients were operated on between 1978 and 1991 in our department. We report on etiology, operative treatment, and the results achieved with follow-up.

Clinical Material and Method

Seventy-nine patients with radial nerve disorders were reviewed at our department over a 13-year period (Table 1). Of these, 54 had radial nerve palsy complicating a fracture of the humerus or forearm. There were 45 males and nine females. The ages of the patients ranged from 1 to 78 years, with a mean of 27.6 years. The fracture incidence was about equal for the right and left side: 30 and 24, respectively. The radial nerve was most subject to injury in the mid-humeral region (28 cases). The fracture was located in the arm in the proximal third in 33 cases, in the middle third in 19 cases, and in the lower third in two cases. The nerve repair was performed in the first 4 months after trauma in 12 cases, from 5 to 8 months in 22

---

[1] Neurochirurgische Klinik, Krankenhaus Nordstadt, Haltenhoffstr. 41, W-3000 Hannover, FRG.

Advances in Neurosurgery, Vol. 21
R. Lorenz, M. Klinger, M. Brock (Eds.)

Table 1. Etiology of radial nerve injury in 79 patients operated on between 1978 and 1991

Etiology	Patients (n)
Bone fracture	54
Osteosynthesis	7
Gunshot wound	7
Penetrating wound	6
Stab wound	2
Laceration	2
Dog bite	1

cases, from 9 to 12 months in eight cases, and 13 months or over in the remaining 12 cases. In most patients, branches innervating the triceps were spared and more distal radial nerve fibers were damaged.

The notes from the postoperative controls were reviewed. A questionnaire considering the motor function of wrist and finger extensors was sent to all patients. The recovery of only the motor function of the nerve was evaluated. Radial nerve function was graded from MO (no movement) to M5 (normal power) according to Sunderland [14]. The sensation is of no functional importance in radial nerve injuries [6] and was not considered in the evaluation.

Radial nerve palsy associated with long bones fracture may be primary or secondary. Outcome data 40 patients with *isolated primary radial nerve lesion associated with a fracture* of the humerus or radius were available for the follow-up study. The average time interval between the injury and the operation was 11 months. In 11 patients an interfascicular neurolysis was performed; in 29 patients an interfascicular grafting was done. Graft length was 9.9 cm on the average, in five patients a defect of over 15-cm length was grafted.

Results

The results presented here are based on the notes from the postoperative controls 6–32 months after surgery and on a questionnaire considering the motoric function of the wrist and finger extensors received from 40 patients with *isolated primary radial nerve palsy associated with a fracture* of the humerus or the radius.

The length of follow-up varied from about 6 months to 13 years, on the average 4.6 years. Excellent or improved motor function occurred in 36 patients. A useful recovery (M3 or better) was achieved in 60% of cases. In four cases there was no evidence of recovery during the follow-up period (Fig. 1).

The location of the fracture or the age of the patient did not influence the postoperative outcome. The rate of recovery of nerve function after early nerve repair (within 4 months after the fracture) was superior to the results of delayed explo-

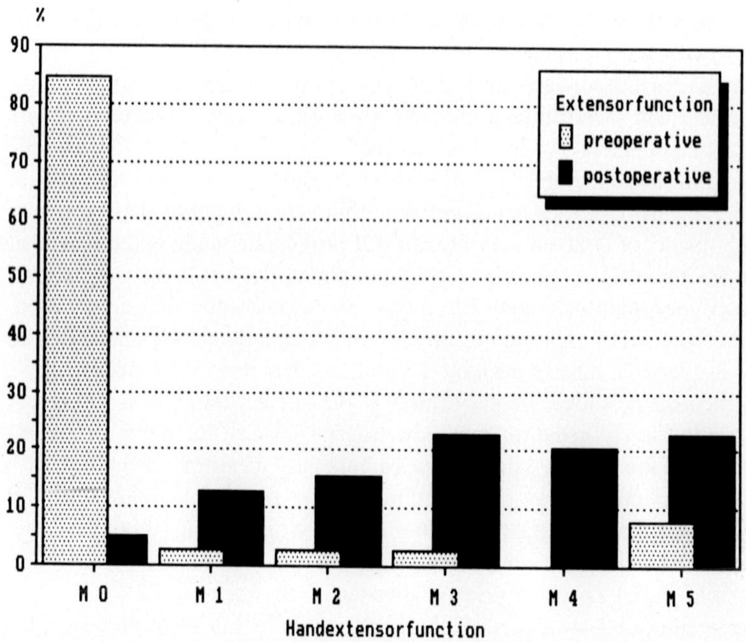

Fig. 1. Recovery of the function of wrist extensors. The function of wrist extensors pre- and postoperatively is demonstrated. Owing to the lesion of the posterior interosseous nerve, patients with preoperatively normal (M5) function of wrist extensors had only a paresis of finger extensors

ration. The patients with partial recovery of motoric function had a significantly longer time interval between injury and nerve repair than those with full recovery. The length of the nerve graft in combination with the interval between trauma and nerve repair seems to be decisive for the recovery of the motor function.

Discussion

Of all the major nerves in the body, the one most susceptible to injury by adjacent fractures is the radial nerve [7, 9, 14]. The radial nerve is most subject to injury in the long bone fractures at a level below the site where branches give off to the triceps. The incidence of radial nerve injuries associated with fracture of the humerus varies between 2% and 16% [14]. The majority of these injuries are varying levels of neurapraxia and will recover spontaneously [10]. Approximately 25% of the radial nerve injuries associated with closed fractures of the humerus will be lesions that require surgical treatment [14].

The length of time after fracture of long bones with associated radial nerve palsy before radial nerve exploration is justified has been a matter of some controversy [2–4, 10, 12]. Early versus delayed exploration is extensively discussed in the literature. Most authors agree that the radial nerve should be explored 3–4 months following a closed fracture if there has been no return of radial nerve function. Early exploration decreases the total period of disability [5].

After a fracture of the humerus or radius, conservative treatment remains indicated with clinical and electromyographical follow-up. If there is no clinical and electromyographical evidence of spontaneous recovery within 3–4 months after the fracture, the radial nerve should be explored. Our results showed that the rate of recovery of nerve function after nerve repair within 4 months after the fracture is superior to the results of delayed nerve repair. Of prognostic value is the length of time between fracture and nerve repair, which, in our study, was longer in patients with partial recovery than those with full recovery. A long study time interval between the injury and nerve exploration (on average 11 months in our study) causes a progressive irreversible muscle atrophy. If the nerve has undergone neuromatous degeneration, neurolysis should be performed. If the nerve continuity is disturbed, it should be grafted in the usual manner. The transposition of the nerve to the anteromedial aspect of the bone or joint cannot be generally recommended [15].

The use of splints prevents an overstretching of the extensor tendons and joint stiffness. When voluntary contractions have appeared, the splint should be discarded and a mechanical device substituted [14].

In conclusion, radial nerve injuries associated with fractures of long bones should be explored after 3–4 months, if there are no clinical or electromyographical signs of returning function.

References

1. Barton NJ (1973) Radial nerve lesions. Hand 5:200–208
2. Bleeker WA, Nijsten MWN, Duis HJ (1991) Treatment of humeral shaft fractures related to associated injuries. Acta Orthop Scand 62:148–153
3. Böstman O, Bakalim G, Vainionpää S, Wilppula E, Pätiälä H, Rokkanen P (1985) Immediate radial nerve palsy complicating fracture of the shaft of the humerus: when is early exploration justified? Injury 16:499–502
4. Böstman O, Bakalim G, Vainionpää S, Wilppula E, Pätiälä H, Rokkanen P (1986) Radial palsy in shaft fracture of the humerus. Acta Orthop Scand 57:316–319
5. Gurdjian ES, Smathers HM (1945) Peripheral nerve injury in fractures and dislocations of long bones. J Neurosurg 2:202–219
6. Haymaker W (1953) Peripheral nerve injuries: principles of diagnosis. Saunders, Philadelphia, pp 264–272
7. Kwasny O, Maier R (1991) Die Bedeutung von Nervenschäden bei der Oberarmfraktur. Unfallchirurg 94:461–467
8. Mumenthaler M, Schliack H (1987) Läsionen peripherer Nerven. Thieme, Stuttgart, pp 233–243
9. Omer GE, Spinner M (1980) Management of peripheral nerve problems. Saunders, Philadelphia, pp 502–506
10. Pollock FH, Drake D, Bovill EG, Day L, Trafton PG (1981) Treatment of radial neuropathy associated with fractures of the humerus. J Bone Joint Surg [Am] 63:239–243
11. Samardzic M, Grujicic D, Milinkovic ZB (1990) Radial nerve lesions associated with fractures of the humeral shaft. Injury 21:220–222
12. Shah JJ, Bhatti NA (1983) Radial nerve paralysis associated with fractures of the humerus. Clin Orthop 172:171–176

13. Stöhr M, Ritel H (1988) Nerven- und Nervenwurzelläsionen. VCH, Weinheim, pp 137–151
14. Sunderland S (1978) Nerves and nerve injuries. Churchill Livingstone, Edinburgh, pp 350, 820–839
15. Tscherne H, Ennker J, Flory PJ, Pahlow EU (1984) Verlagerung des N. Radialis bei Oberarmschaftbrüchen? Unfallheilkunde 87:7–12

Treatment Results of Anterior Submuscular Transposition and Medial Epicondylectomy for Ulnar Nerve Entrapment at the Elbow

H. Kolenda[1], B. Zimmerer[1], and K. Mursch[1]

Introduction

Superior success with the anterior submuscular transposition, compared to the subcutaneous transposition in the treatment of the ulnar nerve entrapment at the elbow, published by our department in 1974 and 1980 [3, 4] led us to apply this technique to any stage of this entrapment syndrome when the indication for operative therapy was given. Only 12 out of the 146 patients we operated on during the past 10 years were treated by medial epicondylectomy.

For the results presented here we reviewed the clinical histories of all these patients and evaluated more details of the pre- and postoperative history by means of a questionnaire. Excluding reoperations, 142 cases of primary operated ulnar nerve entrapments were analyzed. Eighty-one patients returned the questionnaire to us, the follow-up period being between 6 months and 9 years after the operation.

Results

Patients were between 6 and 74 years of age; 78% were male, most of them between 40 and 60 years of age. A total of 72% of our patients were manual workers and about 60% of them worked with mechanical stress on the arms and elbow joint. These workers bear a high risk of developing an ulnar palsy by the chronic tension the ulnar nerve is exposed to by an enlarged triceps muscle [1].

Pathogenesis

Besides working activities, degenerative alterations in 20%–30% or a luxation tendency of the nerve over the medial epicondylus in flexion of the joint in 37% of the patients caused mechanical stress for the ulnar nerve. The majority of the young patients and those working without mechanical stress on their arms developed symptoms after fractures or after operations for other reasons at the elbow joint (Fig. 1). Some showed a high degree of cubitus valgus or other lesions inducing an

---

[1] Neurochirurgische Klinik, Universität Göttingen, Robert-Koch-Str. 40, W-3400 Göttingen, FRG.

Advances in Neurosurgery, Vol. 21
R. Lorenz, M. Klinger, M. Brock (Eds.)

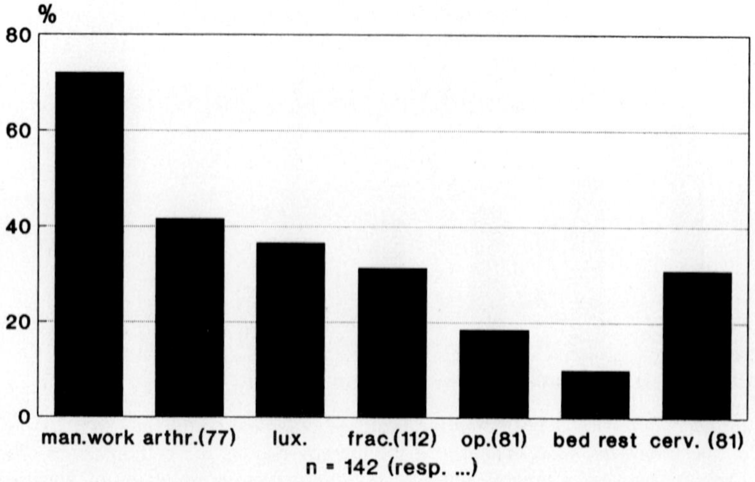

Fig. 1. In descending order, pathogenic factors for the ulnar nerve entrapment at the elbow are mentioned: manual work, arthrosis of elbow joint, tendency of luxation of the nerve, fractures near the joint, preceding operations at the elbow, preceding bed rest. The high incidence of accompanying cervical pain is of interest for differential diagnosis

increase of connective tissue. Finally, there were only two patients without any explicable "mechanical" reason for a cubital tunnel syndrome.

A high number of patients with accompanying neck pain have to be mentioned as cervical radiculopathy was the main differential diagnosis and the reason for further preoperative neurophysiological investigations by electroneurography or -myography.

Pre- and Postoperative Complaints

Adding a grade IV lesion to McGowan's staging system [5], we differentiated among the following grades of dysfunction:

Grade I: subjective disorders (*n* = 3; 2%)
Grade II: objective disorder, no atrophies (*n* = 49; 34.5%)
Grade III: severe neurological deficits (*n* = 82; 58%)
Grade IV: complete failure (*n* = 8; 5.5%)

Therefore about one third of the patients showed a slight deficit and two thirds had severe deficits with muscular atrophies. The analysis of the questionnaires demonstrated improvement, especially of the late sequelae of the ulnar nerve compression as paresis and atrophy after operative therapy (Fig. 2). While the sensitive innervation only partly improved, pain and paresthesia were nearly untouched by therapy.

These molesting sequelae of entrapment were nearly completely remitted in the cases operated by medial epicondylectomy (Fig. 3). In this context the high rate of

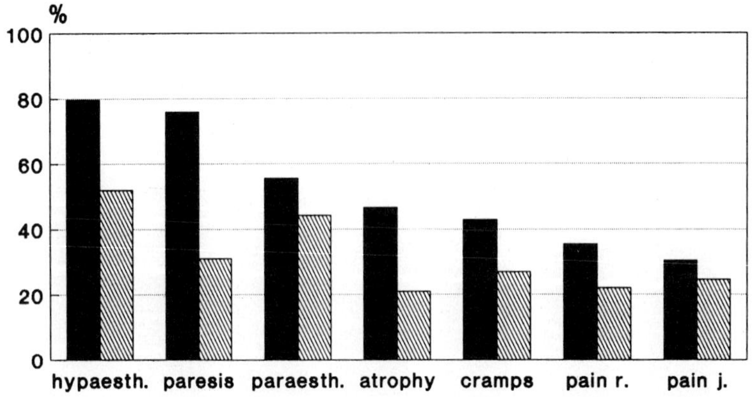

Fig. 2. Pre- (*solid columns*) and postoperative (*hatched columns*) complaints ($n = 79$) according to the questionnaires, independently of the therapy chosen, are demonstrated. The follow-up period was between 6 months and 9 years. *pain r*, pain in the region of sensitive innervation; *pain j*, local pain at the elbow joint

patients suffering from cramps in the forearm and hand muscles is to be outlined as it is seldom referred to in the literature and patients' histories.

Operative Results

Results of operative therapy were divided in to five degrees from –1 (worse) to +3 (healing) [6]. Follow-up values either from the patient's history or the questionnaire were available for 108 out of the 142 operations reviewed for this presentation; 18% of the patients showed bad results, 9% being worse and 9% being

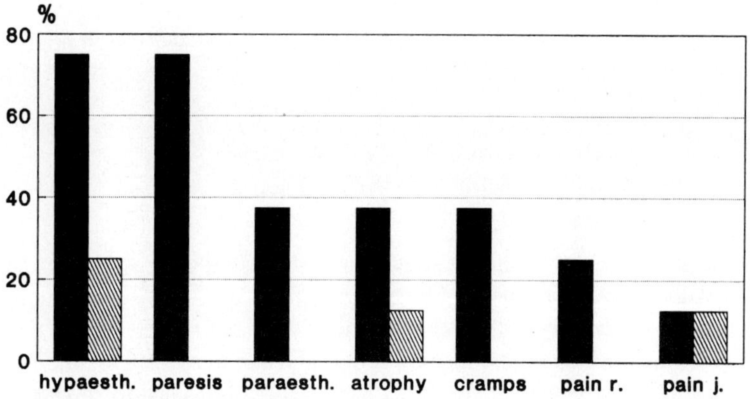

Fig. 3. Compared to Fig. 2 only pre- (*solid columns*) and postoperative (*hatched columns*) complaints of patients who underwent medial epicondylectomy are analyzed; follow-up intervals were between 5 and 6 years

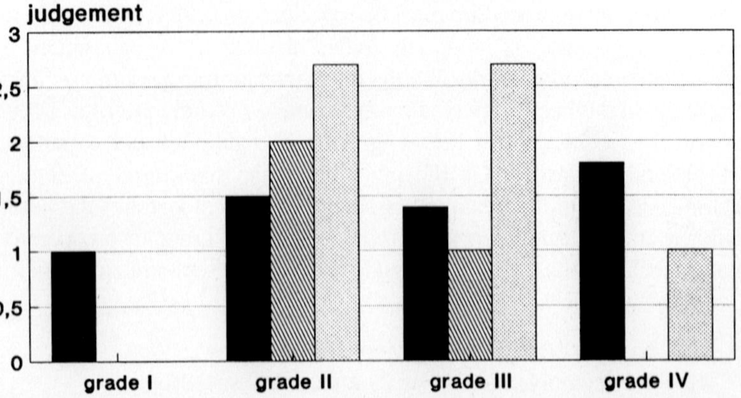

Fig. 4. Comparison of treatment results depending on preoperative grade of lesion and surgical technique chosen. *AST*, anterior submuscular transposition ($n = 91$), *AST + N*, AST + neurolysis ($n = 7$); *ME*, medial epicondylectomy ($n = 7$)

unchanged by operative therapy. The rest showed an improvement, but 21% were only slightly better. In 61% therapy was a success with 40% good results and 21% healing of symptoms.

With an average preoperative deficit of grade II, with 6 representing objective disorders with atrophies, the average result was +1.5, corresponding to a sufficient outcome.

According to Fig. 4, this outcome is caused by the deep volar transposition that resulted in a +1 to +2 outcome, independent of the grade of preoperative damage. A better correlation to the level of lesion is demonstrated by the seven patients operated on by medial epicondylectomy as well as by those seven cases in whom we combined anterior submuscular transposition with a neurolysis.

For grade II and even more so for grade III lesions, medial epicondylectomy showed an excellent outcome compared to that reached by deep volar transposition, while transposition was more successful in grade IV lesions.

Furthermore, results depended on duration of complaints, the patient's age, and the operating surgeon. The dependency on the surgeon may be due to individual technical modifications of operative therapy. According to a review article on operative therapy of cubital tunnel syndrome [2] it is, for example, an important difference whether anterior transposition is performed deeply intramuscularly or submuscularly, the submuscular technique being the more successful one.

Discussion

Mechanical stress of the ulnar nerve at the elbow joint induced by straining work activities or degenerative alterations at the cubital tunnel are responsible for the pathogenesis of the entrapment syndrome.

The aim of any operative procedure must be to reduce this stress and to give the nerve a chance to regenerate. As moderate grades of ulnar nerve entrapment respond well to medial epicondylectomy and the deep anterior transposition seems to cause a lesion at the nerve itself, reflected by the average outcome after this procedure, we suggest this technique for this range of cases although our experience with only 12 patients is limited. On the other hand, the superiority of anterior submuscular transposition in the treatment of severe cases demonstrates the necessity of applying operative techniques in correlation with the grade of preoperative dysfunction and mechanical causes of the syndrome. Our present strategy is as follows:

Grade I:	conservative therapy, possibly epicondylectomy
Grade II:	epicondylectomy, anterior subcutaneous transposition
Grade III:	anterior transposition or epicondylectomy
Grade IV:	anterior submuscular transposition, neurolysis

In order to make the decision between epicondylectomy or anterior transposition in grade II and III lesions, we examine pre- and intraoperative testing for luxation tendency of the ulnar nerve out of the cubital tunnel: if there is a tendency for luxation, epicondylectomy is performed. In patients without a luxation tendency, even in an intraoperative test, or with marked dystrophy of the nerve in the cubital tunnel, we prefer the anterior transposition, which in our clinic is carried out submuscularly. Microsurgical neurolysis is performed if the fascicular structure of the ulnar nerve cannot be confirmed in the exposed region.

References

1. Apfelberg DB, Larson SJ (1973) Dynamic anatomy of the ulnar nerve at the elbow. Plast Reconstr Surg 51:76–81
2. Dellon AL (1989) Review of treatment results for ulnar nerve entrapment at the elbow. J Hand Surg [Am] 14:688–700
3. Gerl A, Schlüter R (1980) Postoperative Kompression und Regeneration nach Ulnarisverlagerung. Zentralbl Neurochir 41:149–166
4. Gerl A, Thorwirth V (1974) Ergebnisse der Ulnarisverlagerung. Acta Neurochir (Wien) 30:227–246
5. McGowan AJ (1950) Results of transposition of ulnar nerve for traumatic ulnar neuritis. J Bone Joint Surg [Br] 32:293–301
6. Mooji JJA (1982) Ulnar nerve pathology at the elbow: the place of anterior transposition today. Acta Neurochir (Wien) 64:75–85

Ulnar Nerve Lesion During Lumbar Disc Operation

H. Wassmann[1] and D. Moskopp[1]

Introduction

This case report deals with a problem concerning an ulnar nerve lesion in dependence on positioning on the operating table during lumbar disc operation [8, 9, 11, 13, 18, 23–26]. The extent of informed consent in current legal use is discussed [6, 10, 14, 16, 19–22].

Report of the Case

A 38-year-old male patient underwent a lumbar disc operation at the level L 5/S 1 in the knee-elbow position in an out-of-town department. The procedure was uneventful and lasted 110 min. On the first postoperative morning the patient felt signs of a right-side accentuated ulnar nerve palsy while handling a knife for breakfast.

A neurological examination confirmed this suspicion. The ulnar nerve showed a habitual bilateral luxation on the medial epicondylus at the elbow. After 3 weeks, the EMG documented a bilateral ulnar nerve lesion with an accentuation on the right side.

After 1 year a bilateral ulnar nerve lesion showed signs of motor and sensitive deficit on the right side and of a sensitive deficit on the left side. Concurrent causes had been ruled out (i.e., cervical rib, cervical disc protrusion).

Legal Accusation

The patient sued his doctor on the basis that the information on the intraoperative positioning was insufficient. He said that the possibility of a peripheral nerve lesion had not been mentioned [4, 16, 18–25]. He argued that the ulnar nerve was damaged during the operation and affirmed that he had not been examined for his habitual luxation of the ulnar nerve. The doctor had to confess that he had neither performed the respective examination nor mentioned such a complication during the preoperative conversation.

[1] Klinik und Poliklinik für Neurochirurgie, Westfälische Wilhelms-Universität Münster, Albert-Schweitzer-Str. 33, W-4400 Münster, FRG.

Advances in Neurosurgery, Vol. 21
R. Lorenz, M. Klinger, M. Brock (Eds.)

Applied Anatomy of the Ulnar Nerve

The ulnar nerve has to change from the flexion side to the extension side on the medial upper arm before reaching the ulnar nerve sulcus on the medial epicondylus [2, 7, 15, 17]. It then enters the cubital tunnel [15]. The volume of this tunnel is reduced during flexion and here the nerve is prone to additional lesions [17].

A habitual dislocation of the nerve and riding over the medial epicondylus may produce a chronic ulnar nerve lesion [6]. The incidental percentage of a partial or complete habitual ulnar nerve dislocation varies from 4% to 16% [5, 15].

Incidence of the Perioperative Ulnar Nerve Lesion

Damage of the ulnar nerve plays the most important role of all perioperative lesions of peripheral nerves [10]. A habitual luxation at the elbow region was found in every third patient with a perioperative ulnar nerve lesion. The cubital tunnel is the most important point of this lesion [3].

For operative procedures in the supine position, a positioning of the forearm in the prone position was disadvantageous compared to the positioning with the forearm behind the head [26].

Discussion

The risk of a peripheral nerve lesion during a lumbar disc operation in the knee-elbow position is under 1% (Grumme, personal communication).

Nevertheless, it is judged to be a typical complication that has to be mentioned in the preoperative discussion. This was confirmed by a judge of the German Supreme Court (Bundesgerichtshof) [8, 21, 24]. The neurosurgeon is principally responsible for the positioning of the patient on the operation table. The anesthesiologist is only responsible for the positioning of the extremity on which he applies drugs and monitors vital parameters [1, 4, 5, 6, 8–14, 23, 25].

Conclusions

1. It is a advisible to inform the patient regarding the possibility of an intraoperative lesion of the ulnar and peroneal nerves resulting during the preoperative discussion from the positioning
2. All the patients on whom this operation will be performed should be examined for a habitual ulnar nerve dislocation on the medial epicondylus at the elbow region. If this variant is found, this has to be documented and the care in intraoperative positioning has to be increased.
3. To reduce the risk of an intraoperative ulnar nerve lesion, the forearms should be extended and supinated at the elbow during the knee-elbow position.

References

1. Anonymus (1987) Verantwortung für die prä-, intra- und postoperative Lagerung des Patienten – Vereinbarung des Berufsverbandes Deutscher Anästhesisten und des Berufsverbandes der Deutschen Chirurgen. Anasth Intensivmed 28:65
2. Apfelberg DB, Larson SJ (1973) Dynamic anatomy of the ulnar nerve at the elbow. Plast Reconstr Surg 51:76–81
3. Assmus H, Klug N, Kontopoulos P, Penzholz H (1974) Das Sulcus ulnaris Syndrom. Elektroneurographische Untersuchungen und Behandlungsergebnisse. J Neurol 208:109–122
4. Brahams D (1984) Ulnar nerve injury after general anaesthesia and intravenous infusion. Lancet 1:1306
5. Childress HM (1956) Recurrent ulnar nerve dislocation at the elbow. J Bone Joint Surg [Am] 38:978–984
6. Dawson DM, Krarup C (1989) Perioperative nerve lesions. Arch Neurol 46:1355–1360
7. Feindel W, Stratford J (1958) The role of the cubital tunnel in tardy ulnar palsy. Can J Surg 1:287–300
8. Herrmann J (1986) Aufklärung über mögliche Lagerungsschäden. Dtsch Med Wochenschr 111:273–274
9. Holfelder G, Uter P, Rausch E, Zierl O (1984) Vereinbarung zwischen dem Berufsverband Deutscher Anästhesisten und dem Berufsverband der Fachärzte für Orthopädie über die Zusammenarbeit bei der operativen Patientenversorgung. Anasth Intensivmed 25:464–466
10. Kroll DA, Caplan RA, Posner K, Ward RJ, Cheney FW (1990) Nerve injury associated with anesthesia. Anesthesiology 73:202–207
11. Localio RA, Lawthers AG, Brennan TA, Laird NM, Hebert LE, Peterson LM, Newhouse JP, Weiler PC, Hiatt HH (1991) Relation between malpractice claims and adverse events due to negligence. Results of the Harvard Medical Practice study. N Engl J Med 325:245–251
12. Mehdorn HM, Hoffmann B, Grote W (1990) Erfahrungen einer "Gutachterkommission für ärztliche Behandlungsfehler" mit Behandlungsfehlern im neurochirurgischen Fachgebiet. Adv Neurosurg 18:317–323
13. Müller-Osten W, Hempel K, Uter P, Opderbecke HW (1982) Vereinbarung über die Zusammenarbeit bei der operativen Patientenversorgung. Berufsverband Deutscher Anästhesisten, Berufsverband der Deutschen Chirurgen. In: Opderbecke HW, Weißauer W (eds) Entschließungen – Empfehlungen – Vereinbarungen. perimed, Erlangen, pp 39–42
14. Müller-Vahl H (1988) Komplikationen bei neurochirurgischen Eingriffen – Eine Übersicht aus Arzthaftpflichtverfahren. In: Bock WJ, Schirmer M (eds) Komplikationen bei neurochirurgischen Eingriffen. Zuckschwerdt, Munich, pp 170–175
15. Mumenthaler M, Schliack H (1987) Läsionen peripherer Nerven: Diagnostik und Therapie. Thieme, Stuttgart, pp 262–275
16. Nau HE, Gerhard H, Wiedemayer H, Reinhard V (1990) Eine seltene Komplikation nach Bandscheibenoperation in Knie-Ellenbogen-Lage. Adv Neurosurg 18:347–349
17. Rengachary SS (1985) Entrapment neuropathies. In: Wilkins RH, Rengachary SS (eds) Neurosurgery, vol 2. McGraw-Hill, New York, pp 1771–1795
18. Schindler H (1989) Arbeitsgebiet Operationssaal, 2nd edn. Enke, Stuttgart, pp 64, 65, 93, 94
19. Schirmer M (1988) Komplikationen der lumbalen Bandscheibenoperation In: Bock WJ, Schirmer M (eds) Komplikationen bei neurochirurgischen Eingriffen. Zuckschwerdt, Munich, pp 127–142
20. Sollmann DP (1988) Intra- und postoperative Komplikationen bei lumbalen Bandscheibenoperation. In: Bock WJ, Schirmer H (eds) Komplikationen bei neurochirurgischen Eingriffen. Zuckschwerdt, Munich, pp 143–149

21. Steffen E (1990) Neue Entwicklungsrichtlinien der BGH-Rechtsprechung zum Arzthaftungsrecht, 4th edn. RWS-Skript 137, p 88 (BDH Urteil vom 26.02.85 – VI ZR 124/83 NJW 1985, 2192 = VersR. 1985, 639, 640)
22. Stolke D, Seifert V, Dietz A (1990) Sorgfaltsmangel oder typische Komplikation – Auswertung der Begutachtung für die Schlichtungsstelle für Arzthaftpflichtfragen unter besonderer Berücksichtigung der Bandscheibenoperation. Adv Neurosurg 18:324–327
23. Weißauer W (1984) Anmerkung zur Vereinbarung zwischen dem Berufsverband Deutscher Anästhesisten und dem Berufsverband der Fachärzte für Orthopädie über die Zusammenarbeit bei der operativen Patientenversorgung. Anasth Intensivmed 25:467–427
24. Weißauer W (1985) Haftung für Lagerungsschäden. Urteil des Bundesgerichtshof vom 24. Januar 1984 – IV ZR 203/82. Anasth Intensivmed 26:65–69
25. Weißauer W (1987) Verantwortung für die Lagerung des Patienten – Zur Vereinbarung der Berufsverbände Deutscher Anästhesisten und der Deutschen Chirurgen. Anasth Intensivmed 28:66–67
26. Wey JM, Guinn GA (1985) Ulnar nerve injury with open-heart surgery. Ann Thorac Surg 39:358–360

Traumatic Lesions of the Lumbosacral Plexus: Microsurgical Treatment

A. Alexandre[1], G. Stevanato[1], F. Di Toma[2], F. Di Paola[2], F. Spigariol[3], and A. Carteri[1]

Introduction

In severely injured patients there is sometimes complete palsy of an inferior limb. This may be the expression of a lesion of the innervation of the limb at various anatomical levels; the cauda, nerve roots inside the foramina, different elements of the lumbosacral plexus, or the terminal branches may be involved. Traumatic lesions of the lumbosacral plexus are rarely reported in the literature. This is because (a) these are rare lesions, intraspinal aside from lesions of the cauda and of nerve roots and lesions of terminal branches, (b) the correct diagnosis is difficult since these anatomical structures are deep seated and not easily studied, even by modern diagnostic tools, and (c) the surgical approach is difficult since the microsurgical field is very deep, and the nerves are covered by large vessels and muscles very adherent to the spine. Diagnosis is difficult because the lesions are often multiple and are located in different anatomical sites: intra or extraspinal, pre-, intra-, or postplexal. The problem is complicated by the frequent association with severe bony lesions in the spine, lumbosacral junction, or coxofemoral articulation. The entailed problems of stability and their treatment may delay diagnosis and treatment of neural damage.

Patients and Methods

From 1987 up to now six patients have been operated on in our department for traumatic lesions of the lumbosacral plexus. Two young men and girl suffered a motorcycle road accident, with hyperabduction of one leg and traction – compression injury to the pelvis. In one of these a severe lesion of the brachial plexus had simultaneously developed. The other three persons suffered gunshot wound of the lumbosacral plexus during the revolution in Romania against Ceauşescu.

The diagnosis was based on (a) clinical demonstration of impaired function for innervation coming from a part or the entire territory of L3–S2, without sphincter impairment, (b) myelographic demonstration of the absence of radicular lesions, (c) CT demonstration of bone lesions, with hyperdense fibrotization of retroperitoneal tissues, and (d) EMG demonstration of impaired conduction of nerve fibers

[1] Division of Neurosurgery, Padova University, Treviso City Hospital, Treviso, Italy.
[2] Department of Radiology III, Treviso City Hospital, Treviso, Italy.
[3] Department of Radiology, Montebelluna Hospital, Montebelluna, Italy.

Advances in Neurosurgery, Vol. 21
R. Lorenz, M. Klinger, M. Brock (Eds.)

belonging to sciatic and femoral nerves, with preserved innervation for paravertebral muscles.

Surgery was performed by two approaches: either a lateral extraretroperitoneal approach or an anterior transperitoneal approach. The lateral lumbotomic extraperitoneal approach to the retroperitoneal space was apt to reach the lumber plexus and L2–4 contributions. The median laparotomic approach, going straight through the anterior and posterior peritoneal walls, was indicated to reach the more distal region of the sacral plexus, with L5–S5 components. The customary procedures of microsurgical neurolysis, as described by Millesi [4] were applied: epineurotomy, epineurectomy, and internal neurolysis were performed in a stepwise manner, as suggested by the severity of the damage and the extent of fibrotization in each individual case in each point of the plexuses. In the cases of gunshot lesions, sural nerve grafts were prepared and sutured or fixed by fibrin glue.

Results

In all these patients a clearcut improvement of the neural deficit was observed in the months following operation. M3 and M4 motor activity was obtained for femoral muscles and for semitendinosus, semimembranosus and biceps femoris muscles. Obviously the other muscles innervated by the sciatic nerve (anterior and posterior tibial components) are very distant from the site of the lesion and therefore not easily reached by regenerating axons. In any case, the improved motor control of the hip and proximal part of the leg allowed our patients to gain improved ability to move around and to use prothetic instruments.

Discussion

In the daily management of patients who have suffered traumatic injuries to several body areas, the lesion of the lumbosacral plexus may escape diagnosis for a long time. It is generally considered irreversible. As underlined by Narakas [5], when facing a complete palsy, it is not possible to reach a clinical differentiation between trunk interruption and anatomical continuity of fascicles since only root avulsion can be evidenced by myelography, computed tomography, and EMG. Myelography is helpful since traction applied to the lumbosacral plexus tears the arachnoid and dura, as in the case of brachial plexus injuries. Cerebrospinal fluid then leaks out along the roots into a cavity that becomes sealed off after dural and arachnoidal proliferation. The result is a traumatic meningocele, with a myelographic finding identical to that described in brachial plexus avulsions [6]. Post-traumatic retroperitoneal hemorrhage initially appears on computed tomography as a relatively high-density mass lesion obliterating the periaortic and perimuscular fat planes. The density, which initially is higher than that of muscles, decreases to a low-density mass weeks after [3], but fibrosis develops as a general increase in density, with less precise margins [1].

The indication for a precise surgical procedure may therefore remain difficult, but clinical results of neurolysis show that the intervention is worthwhile. We agree with the opinion of Brunelli [2] that the posterior approach is indicated when lesions of the cauda are present, and the anterior approach is indicated for purely plexal lesions. The extraperitoneal approach, which appears easier, allows a comfortable exposition of L3–L4 and L5 roots and femoral nerve, which can be traced down to the inguinal ligament. By this approach it is more difficult to come medially to the psoas muscle, behind the large iliac vessels, to L5-S1 and S2 components of the sacral plexus. This area is more clearly exposed by the median transperitoneal approach, which goes directly to the promontorium, that is the L5-S1 passage.

References

1. Alexandre A, Caretri A (1988) Il trattamento chirurgico delle lesioni traumatiche del plesso lombare. 37th congress of the Italian Neurosurgical Society, Treviso, 15–18 June
2. Brunelli G, Vigasio A (1986) Lumbar and sacral plexus surgery. Periph Nerve Repair Regen 4:21–25
3. Meyers MA (1976) Dynamic radiology of the abdomen: normal and pathologic anatomy. Springer, Berlin Heidelberg New York
4. Millesi H (1981) Internal neurolysis. In: Gorio A, Millesi H, Mingrino S (eds) Posttraumatic peripheral nerve regeneration. Raven, New York, pp 197–208
5. Narakas A (1986) Discussion and conclusions of the round table on sciatic nerve lesions of the G.A.M. Periph Nerve Repair Regen 4:75–76
6. Shapiro R (1977) Myelography. Year Book Medical Publishers, Chicago

Autologous Transplantation in Injury of Cauda Fibers: Results of a Reconstruction of Transected L5 Filaments in a Luxation Fracture L4/5

P. Knöringer[1] and E. Knöpfle[2]

Introduction

Since the methods of decompression, erection and stabilization of injuries in the spine of the trunk region are now developed [6–9], we decided to work more intensively on damages to the cauda equina. Damaged cauda fibers and peripheral nerves are subject to the same mechanisms of de- and regeneration. In their anatomical features, however, cauda fibers show the following differences compared with peripheral nerves: (a) cauda fibers are not surrounded by epineurium but are covered with a very thin perineural sheath, (b) cauda fibers are located in the cerebrospinal fluid and are surrounded by arachnoid and dural membranes, and (c) in contrast to many peripheral nerves, which are mixed, cauda fibers are always either purely motor or sensory filaments.

Experimental Work

A number of studies concerning end-to-end sutures or autologous transplantations are available on pigs, cats, and rats. These models have studied the innervation of the urinary bladder [1, 2, 3, 21]; severed motor or sensory filaments were reconstructed with an end-to-end suture, and the success of the procedure was tested. End-to-end sutures and autologous transplantations (from sensory cauda fibers taken from other filaments or from the peroneal nerve [13]) were performed on pigs for intradurally severed root filaments L5 and S1, and the effect of the suture was evaluated by light and electron microscopy [10, 11] and by electromyography [4, 5]. The microscopic examinations showed a regeneration rate of 50% for the motor filaments and one of 35% for the sensory filaments [16, 17]. This corresponds to Sunderland's findings [18–20] that the suture of injured peripheral nerves is associated with a more effective regeneration in motor fibers. Electromyography performed on pigs after end-to-end suture and autologous transplantation showed reinnervation in all animals [5].

---

[1] Neurochirurgische Klinik, Universität Ulm, Bezirkskrankenhaus Günzburg, Ludwig Heilmeyer-Str. 2, W-8870 Günzburg, FRG.
[2] Neurologische Klinik, Universität Ulm, Bezirkskrankenhaus, Ludwig-Heilmeyer-Str. 2, W-8870 Günzburg, FRG.

Advances in Neurosurgery, Vol. 21
R. Lorenz, M. Klinger, M. Brock (Eds.)

Clinical Work

During the treatment of spinal injuries, cauda fibers have been sutured repeatedly. While the reconstruction potential is reported, particularly in the Russian literature, intensive study of the available literature shows no exact follow-up reports with explicit success rates. Only Petrov [12] reported two successful cases of cauda fiber transplantation. However, this paper delivers only a very inaccurate description of one of the cases. This patient had a lesion at the level of the 4th lumbar vertebra with "resection of the damaged roots," transplanted with three 4-cm "grafts taken from the medial cutaneous brachial nerve." However, the recovery of bladder/rectal function after 60 days and the "progressive improvement of sensory and motor disturbances" after 80 days indicates that this was due to regeneration of decompressed root filaments rather than reinnervation following nerve grafting. Of the second case, we learn only that 8.5 cm had to be bridged. Thus this paper is of little help in evaluating the clinical prognosis following cauda fiber reconstruction.

Case Study

In a traffic accident on 21 July 1987, an 18-year-old patient suffered a luxation fracture L4/5 with incomplete cauda lesion from L4 and complete bilateral motor and sensory loss of the L5 root. The injury was treated elsewhere on 27 July 1987 by decompression laminectomy L5 with dural suture and stabilization with plate osteosynthesis and intertransversal fusion L4–S1. The luxation position was maintained because it was untreatable. Although all other disturbances subsequently disappeared, the motor and sensory loss of root L5 persisted, and the patient was admitted to our hospital on 11 August 1987. On admission we found a local, fistular wound infection with epidural abscess and spondylodiscitis L4/5 as well as a generally highly septic condition. The wound was revised on 26 August 1987, including removal of the epidural abscess, of infected bone tissue, spondylodiscitic tissue, implantation of a Septopal (Merck) chain L4/5, and the replacement of the unstable plates with an internal fixateur (Dick). The septopal chains were removed on 16 September 1987 and an intercorporal fusion with autologous hip bone was performed. The intradural revision showed a complete separation of the right motor and sensory root filament L5; the remaining filaments were intact (Fig. 1). Following excessive bilateral foraminotomy L4/5 (nonrelocated luxation), the distal root stumps were prepared in the right foramen. The defect size following resection of the compressed ends was 3.3 cm long (Fig. 2). Anatomical criteria permitted the unequivocal determination of the motor and sensory filaments. The defect was bridged with two 3.5-cm sural nerve grafts taken from the left leg. They were adapted with three sutures each of monofilament nylon 10 x 0 and additionally secured with fibrin sealant (Figs. 3, 4).

The patient initially had a complete Trendelenburg phenomenon (0/5 musculus gluteus medius), a 0/5 paralysis of the foot and toe extensor and anesthesia of the dermatoma L5. On follow-up on 8 March 1988, 8 months after the accident and 6

1 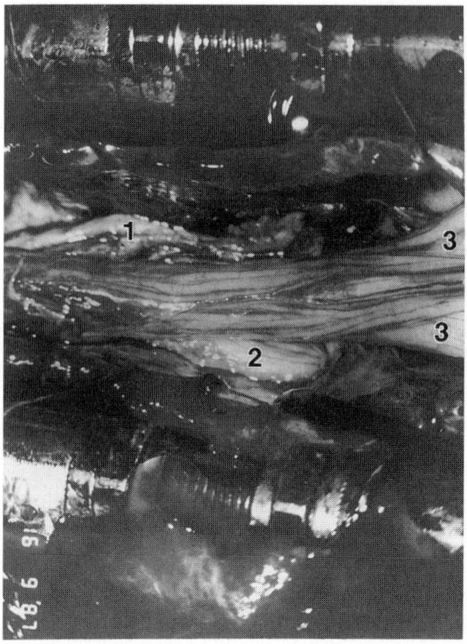

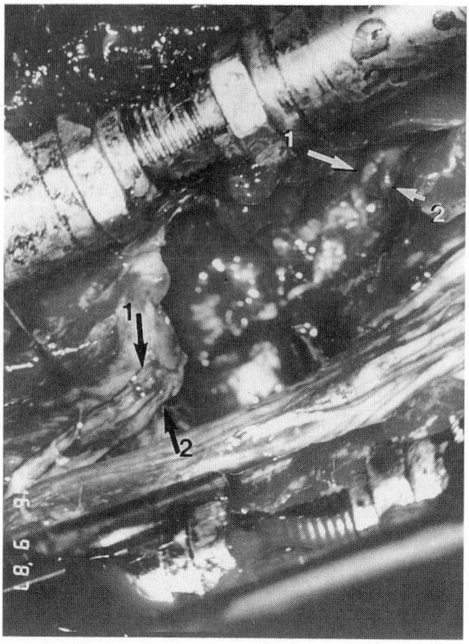 2

Fig. 1. The fracture is stabilized by internal fixateur (Dick); the dura is opened. *1*, transsected motor and sensory filament L5 of the right side; *2*, left L5 filaments; *3*, right and left S1 filaments

Fig. 2. The distal ends of the L5 filaments are visualized by foraminotomy (*arrows 1, 2* on the *right*). The crushed ends of the proximal and distal filaments are resected. *Arrows 1*, proximal and distal sensory L5 filament; *arrows 2*, proximal and distal L5 filament

months following grafting, the right musculus gluteus medius showed a strength of 3–4/5, whereas foot and toe elevation was 0/5. The dermatoma L5 showed distally pronounced, strong hypesthesia. Electromyography demonstrated spontaneous activity and reinnervation potentials in the musculus gluteus medius and only spontaneous activity in the musculus tibialis anterior. During follow-up on 1 September 1989, 23 months after transplantation, strength in the musculus gluteus medius was 4–5/5. The sensitivity in the dermatoma showed further improvement. There was no significant clinical or electromyographic change with regard to elevation of the foot or great toe.

On 17 September 1991, 4 years after transplantation, the strength in the musculus gluteus medius was 5/5, foot elevation was 1–2/5, and elevation of the big toe was 1/5. Discrete hypesthesia of the medial right foot and right great toe was found. Sensitivity to temperatures had returned to a lesser degree than the other two qualities. Electromyography no longer showed pathological spontaneous activity in the musculus gluteus medius, and voluntary innervation presented increased polyphasia with distinct lightening of the innervation pattern. Active denervation was present in the musculus tibialis anterior, but typical reinnervation potentials were now found for the first time.

3
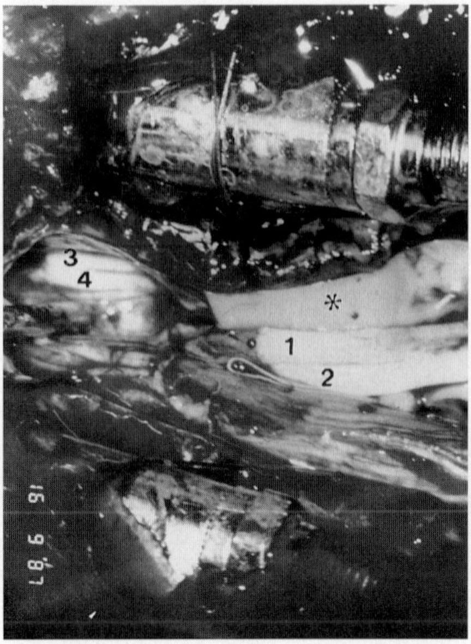

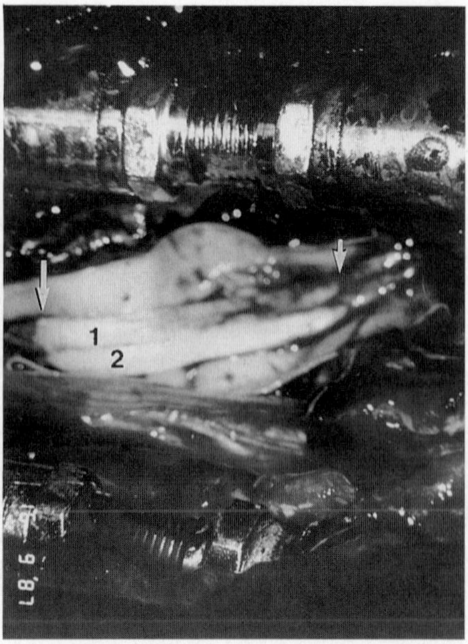

4

Fig. 3. Proximal suture line after transplantation with two sural nerve grafts, one for the motor, one for the sensory filament. *1*, nerve graft for the sensory L5 filament; *2*, nerve graft for the motor L5 filament; *3*, sensory L4 filament; *4*, motor L4 filament; * foil to facilitate suture

Fig. 4. Site after reconstruction of the L5 root. The length of each nerve graft is 3.5 cm. *1*, nerve graft for the sensory filament; *2*, nerve graft for the motor filament; *arrows*, proximal and distal ends of the nerve grafts

During the last follow-up on 5 May 1992, 4 years and 7 months after nerve grafting, no further clinical or electromyographic changes were found, so that this can be considered the final status.

Results

Autologous transplantation of the right motor and sensory root filament L5 at the level of the L4/5 interspace 2 months following injury reinstated normal functioning of the musculus gluteus medius and produced moderate improvement of foot and great toe elevator paralysis with slight improvement of the atrophy of the peroneal muscles. Esthesia and algesia in the L5 dermatoma was almost completely reconstituted. Sensitivity to temperature remained reduced in the distal dermatoma. This result must be considered an effect of the reconstruction of the L5 filaments and cannot be due to collateral innervation. This view is supported both by the timing of the recovery of motor function and by EMG findings. If one assumes 4 weeks for each bridging of the two suture sites and a growth velocity of 3 cm per month with a distance of the proximal suture site to the motor end-plate of the musculus gluteus of 11–12 cm, then a reinnervation of the muscle can be expected to occur within about 6 months. This was found both clinically and electromyographically. The reinnervation of the musculus tibialis anterior with a distance of 78 cm can be expected later than 2 years and 4 months. Accordingly, while no reinnervation of this muscle was found during follow-up on 1 September 1989, 1 year and 4 months after suture, this was present on 17 September 1991, 4 years after transplantation. Unfortunately, no follow-up was done in the intervening time, so that the exact date of reinnervation cannot be determined. According to the subjective impression of the patient, however, this event can be placed at the end of the second year following suture. Although there was clinical and electromyographic reinnervation, its effect was not decisive because the motor end-plates were too damaged after such a long denervation period [14]. The quality of sensory recovery can be regarded as very positive. This may be surprising considering the result of animal experiments, but the follow-up periods of the animal experiments were possibly too short and their clinical examination data difficult to interpret. However, there is sufficient clinical evidence that sensory end-organs have a longer survival time than the motor end-plates, so that the good recovery of sensory qualities can be explained even with a distance of up to 110 cm. Thus the sensitivity in the L5 dermatoma improved in the course of follow-up from proximal to distal, althout discrete hypesthesia and hypalgesia remained at the medial foot and the great toe.

Conclusions

Good partial success can be expected from end-to-end suture and autologous transplantation of severed cauda fibers. As expected, the proximal muscles have a much better chance of regeneration than the distal muscles due to the differences in the distance between the suture and site the motor end-plates. Reinnervation of the distal muscles is feasible 3–4 years following the procedure. The chances of reinnervation of the sensory qualities can be considered good even for long distances.

In the present case, determination of the corresponding motor and sensory stumps presented no difficulty. In more complicated cauda injuries, this may prove difficult to impossible. However, the problem may be solved by an appropriately extensive and clearly arranged site and meticulous intraoperative monitoring.

To improve the reinnervation results of the distal muscles, methods must be developed which allow the corresponding motor end-plate to survive long enough for the growing axon to reach it. One possibility is an implantable, continuous stimulator similar to a diaphragm pacemaker which could provide alternate physiological impulses from all sides to the nerve distal to the suture site.

References

1. Carlsson CA, Sundin T (1968) Reconstruction of severed ventral roots innervating the urinary bladder. An experimental study in cats. Scand J Urol Nephrol 2:199–210
2. Conzen MA (1978) Funktionsanalyse der Harnblase nach experimenteller Caudaläsion und operativer Wiederherstellung. Eine cystometrische Studie am Schwein. Inaugural Dissertation, University of Ulm
3. Conzen M, Sollmann H, Meier C (1981) Experimentelle Untersuchung der sakralen Blaseninnervation am Hausschwein (sus scrofa). Zbl Vet Med A 28:177–182
4. Conzen MA, Sollmann H (1982) Reinnervation of the urinary bladder after microsurgical reconstruction of transsected caudal fibres. An experimental study in pigs. Urol Res 10:141–144
5. Conzen M, Sollmann H (1985) Reinnervation after microsurgical repair of transsected cauda equina fibres. An electromyographic study. Neurochirurgia 28:6–7
6. Knöringer P (1987) Operative Frühbehandlung von Wirbelsäulen/Rückenmarksverletzungen im Bereich der Brust- und Lendenwirbelsäule. In: Bettag W (eds) Neurochirurgie in ausgewählten Kapiteln. Hippokrates, Stuttgart, pp 128–137
7. Knöringer P (1987) Zur Bedeutung traumatischer Bandscheibenvorfälle, raumfordernder Knochenfragmente und Duraläsionen bei Wirbelsäulen-Rückenmarksverletzungen. Hefte Unfallheilk 189:665–670
8. Knöringer P (1988) Neurochirurgische Indikationen bei Wirbelsäulenverletzungen. In: Hauptverband der gewerblichen Berufsgenossenschaften e.V. Bonn. Unfallmedizinische Tagungen der Landesverbände 68:81–94
9. Knöringer P (1989) Early surgical treatment of dorsal and lumbar spinal injuries. Advances in Neurotraumatology. Neurosurg Rev (Suppl 1) 12:536–547
10. Meier C, Sollmann H (1977) Regeneration of cauda equina fibres after transsection and end-to-end suture. Light and electron microscopic study in the pig. J Neurol 215:81–90
11. Meier C, Sollmann H (1978) Glial outgrowth and central-type myelination of regenerating axons in spinal nerve roots following transsection and suture: light and electron microscopic study in the pig. Neuropathol Appl Neurobiol 4:21–35
12. Petrov MA (1971) Transplantation of nerves and roots of the spinal cord. Reconstr Surg Traumatol 12:250–262
13. Radek A, Thomas PK, King RHM (1986) Perineurial differentiation in interchange grafts of rat peripheral nerve and spinal root. J Anat 147:207–217
14. Richter HP (1991) Reinnervation of skeletal muscle. A survey. Zbl Neurochir 52:109–117
15. Richter HP (1992) Transplantation von Nerven. Oto-Rhino-Laryngol Suppl 1:179–184
16. Sollmann H, Richter HP, Meier C (1977) Mikrochirurgische Rekonstruktion der Cauda equina als Behandlungsmöglichkeit bei Kaudaläsionen im Tierexperiment. Therapiewoche 27/41:7249–7250
17. Sollmann H, Richter HP, Meier C (1977) Microsurgical reconstruction of cauda equina fibres. Experimental study in the pig. In: Advances in neurosurgery, vol 4. Springer, Berlin Heidelberg, New York, pp 270–272
18. Sunderland S (1968) Nerves and nerve injuries. Livingstone, Edinburgh
19. Sunderland S, Bradley KC (1961a) Stress-strain phenomena in human peripheral nerve trunks. Brain 84:102–120
20. Sunderland S, Bradley KC (1961b) Stress-strain phenomena in human spinal nerve roots. Brain 84:120–124
21. Sundin T, Carlsson CA (1972) Reconstruction of severed dorsal roots innervating the urinary bladder. An experimental study in cats. Scand J Urol Nephrol 6:176–184

Factors To Be Considered in Nerve Anastomosis with Fibrin Adhesive

T. Herter[1] and P. Kreutzer[2]

Fibrin adhesives have already been used to a considerable extent in the treatment of intracranial nerves, solely because of the access conditions. However, where peripheral nerves are involved, the same surgeon will often continue to resort to conventional suture techniques although the problems associated with these are well known. In particular, the unavoidable traumatization of the nerves despite extremely elaborate techniques, the problem of suture granulomas despite the use of very fine sutures, and the impossibility of achieving a complete closure of the perineurium [7] with its resulting negative consequences have led to the need for an adhesive technique which, based on the pioneering work of Matras [6] and Kuderna [7], was used for the first time in 1974. However, the first failures with dehiscence of the joined regions were reported very soon after its introduction, with the putative causal factor being the fibrinolytic activity of tissue. To prevent this, a number of different antifibrinolytic agents were studied and aprotinin was finally selected for addition. However, the modified adhesive then led to a large number of fibroses. This situation, with premature dissociation on the one hand and fibrosis on the other, is still a problem today. The regeneration process can be permanently hindered by both these events. In view of this, it is not surprising that a number of surgeons still prefer conventional suture techniques, partly for reasons of caution, but perhaps also because they have no recommendations for the best approach with fibrin adhesives.

The initial step in an operation is to choose the anastomosis technique. One cannot rely on spontaneous adhesion since joined up tissue will separate once it becomes wet. Once a decision has been made to opt for a fibrin adhesive system, the next question is: which one?

The two adhesives currently on the market are those from Immuno (referred to here as A) and those from Behring (B). These differ not only in their ion concentration, but also mainly in Factor XIII content and in fibronectin concentration (Table 1). Adhesive A contains more Factor XIII, whereas adhesive B contains more fibronectin. It has been shown in animal studies [3, 5] that both substances promote fibrosis. The choice of adhesive could therefore only be made by direct experimental comparison. This revealed no statistically significant difference between A and B under the conditions stated [2].

[1] LV-Amt, Nordrhein-Westfalen, W-4400 Münster, FRG.
[2] Neurochirurgische Klinik und Poliklinik, Westfälische Wilhelms-Universität Münster, Albert-Schweitzer-Str. 33, W-4400 Münster, FRG.

Advances in Neurosurgery, Vol. 21
R. Lorenz, M. Klinger, M. Brock (Eds.)

Table 1. Composition of the two adhesives currently available commercially

		A[a]	B[b]
Total protein	(MG/ML)	80–120	99
Clottable protein	(MG/ML)	82	73
Fibrinogen	(MG/ML)	70–110	65–115
Factor XIII	(U/ML)	10–50	40–80
Fibronectin	5%–12%;2–9	MG/ML	Up to 2.9
In Examined Batches:	(MG/ML)	10.8–13.2	Max. 2.7
Constituents modifiable by the user			
Thrombin	(IU/ML)	4 or 500	400–600
Aprotinin	(KIU/ML)	3000	1000
CaCl2	(MMOL/L)	40	40

[a] Tissucol (Immuno).
[b] Beriplast (Behring).

The concentrations of Factor XIII and fibronectin can only be influenced by the choice of adhesive. However, the concentrations of thrombin and aprotinin can be determined by the user and special importance is therefore attached to these two.

The problems with fibroses commenced with the addition of aprotinin and it was therefore investigated for possible fibrosis-promoting properties (Herter and Windmann, unpublished results). The studies did not reveal any difference between the groups given two different aprotinin concentrations and a control group. Aprotinin appears only to exert an effect in conjunction with the fibrin adhesive system, by preventing the clot from breaking up. Kuderna [7] considered the optimal concentration to be 100 per milliliter kallikrein inactivator units (= 50 KIU/ml adhesive), which would lead to the anastomosis holding for approximately 4 days.

Thrombin is the second component which can be changed by the user. The concentration of thrombin determines the coagulation time and the cross-linking time. Thrombin was found to have a fibrosis-promoting effect in a comparable study (Herter and Windmann, unpublished results). It is therefore recommended that relatively low concentrations, such as 4 NIH-U/ml, be used. This precludes the use of ready-made double-injection systems or products which do not allow this concentration as an alternative, except where dilution is carried out by the user. In this case we recommend that the concentration be adjusted to approximately 1–2 NIH-U/ml.

The fibrin clot then envelops the nerves, at least at the site of anastomosis, like a sheath. If transplantation is carried out to reduce tension, then for the first few days the transplant can only be supplied with nutrient by diffusion. Penkert and Samii [8] presented microangiographies which showed that it took 3 days for vessels to be reconnected to each other. An important question is therefore whether the nutrient supply to the nerve is disturbed by the fibrin clot. In a test with the adhesive from Immuno A, no fibrosis-promoting effect was discernible with a fibrin adhesive cuff [4].

Table 2. Results of clinical comparisons carried out by Kuderna [7]

Outcome:	Good (%)	Fair (%)	Poor (%)
Transplantations with suture (n=51)	51	33	16
Transplantations with fibrin adhesive – total (n = 144)	53	37	10
Transplantations with fibrin adhesive – correct indication (n = 42)	71	29	–
Transplantations with fibrin adhesive and suture (n = 25)	72	12	16

The question of how a serially produced adhesive compares to a nerve suture from an experimental and clinical point of view was investigated by a direct comparison of both methods in the rat. Neither method proved superior in principle [1].

Numerous authors have also published the results of clincal comparisons in recent years. To our knowledge, Kuderna [7] has published the most comprehensive results, and these also suggest that, when applied correctly, there is no appreciable clinical difference between adhesives and sutures (Table 2).

Our current recommendations for the joining of nerves with fibrin adhesives, based on the advice of Kuderna [7] and our experience, are summarized in Table 3.

Table 3. Current recommendations for nerve joining with fibrin adhesives

1. A fibrin adhesive should only be used for tension-free anastomoses, i.e., for nerve transplants or replants with length reduction.
2. Where possible, adhesives should only be used in regions with longitudinal lateral structures.
3. With multifascicular nerves, a step-wise anastomosis is recommended for internal splinting purposes.
4. Care should be taken to ensure optimal coaptation and to avoid caliber fissures.
5. Proper mixing of the adhesive should be ensured.
6. An attempt should be made to tightly join up the perineurium, but without allowing adhesive to penetrate between the nerve stumps. No adhesion with surrounding areas.
7. The thrombin concentration should ideally be low – where possible below the 4 NIH/ml offered by one manufacturer.
8. Kuderna [2] recommends that the aprotinin concentration be diluted from 1000 or 3000 KIE to approximately 50 KIU/ml adhesive.
9. Immobilization is recommended for at least 3 weeks, with no concomitant tenorrhaphy.
10. Local cortisone application is not recommended and caution should be exercised in systemic use.

There are still some points to be resolved in respect of the aprotinin concentration: Kuderna [7] recommended a mere 100 KIU/ml whereas in animal tests we found no difference with one adhesive (B), and even when we used a concentration of 1000 KIU/ml we found an improvement with the other (Herter and Windmann, unpublished results). Differences in the fibrinolytic activity of tissue may play a role here and further studies are required. Current unterstanding indicates that a concentration of 1000 KIU/ml should not be exceeded.

In principle, we see no reasons for not using fibrin adhesives in nerve surgery, subject to the above preconditions. However, it cannot yet be conclusively stated that, as far as the end result is concerned, fibrin adhesive is superior. The technical simplicity of the use of fibrin adhesive can only mean an improvement in surgical standards and quality control.

References

1. Herter T (1989) Elektrophysiologischer Vergleich von geklebten und genähten Nervenanastomosen. Unfallchirurg 92:560–563
2. Herter T (1989) Gibt es eine Präferenz bei den Fibrinklebern für die Nervenanastomosierung? HNO 6:255–258
3. Herter T, Bennefeld H (1989) The influence of fibronectin and the fibrin adhesive on the fibrosing of a nerve anastomosis in the rat. Exp Med 189:321–329
4. Herter T, Schleep J, Windmann D (1989) Führen Fibrinklebermanschetten zur Fibrosierung von Nervenanatomosen? Neurochirurgia (Stuttg) 32:16–20
5. Herter T, Schleep J, Windmann D (1989) The influence of Factor XIII on the fibrosing of a nerve anastomosis in the rat. Exp Med 189:25–32
6. Matras H (1980) Die Entwicklung der "Fibrinklebung". Hefte Unfallheilkd 148:758–787
7. Kuderna H (1985) Die Fibrinklebung peripherer Nerven In: Nigst H (ed) Nervenwiederherstellung nach traumatischen Läsionen. Hippokrates, Stuttgart, pp 78–91
8. Penkert G, Samii M (1987) Zur Frage der Revaskularisation eines freien Nerventransplantates. 38th Annual Meeting of the German Society of Neurosurgeons, May 6, Münster

Alternatives to Autologous Nerve Grafting

H. Müller[1], T. Dombert[1], and H. Arnold[1]

It can be presumed that any materials interposed into traumatic nerve gaps serve only as guiding vehicles for regenerating axons growing toward the periphery, and many ideas about using guides or conduits (tubes) other than a piece of donor nerve have therefore been discussed. Reviews are provided by Weiss as early as 1944 [17] and recently by Fields Ellisman in 1989 [3] and by ourselves in 1992 [16]. Still, the procedure of microsurgical autologous nerve grafting remains the clinically routine method in dealing with peripheral nerve lesions caused by transection trauma and subsequent gap.

However, there may be some indications in at least rare clinical cases to look for alternatives to autologous nerve grafts. First, established surgical techniques applied primarily might have been unsuccessful. Secondly, there may be a lack of donor nerve material, for example in burns or plexus lesions. Another reason might be the occurrence of a systemic neurological disease, such as leprosy. In such a disease (which is rare in industrially developed countries but rather common elsewhere), all nerves are attacked, and no healthy autologous nerve is available for transplantation. Finally, the surgeon might deal with very distally located nerve lacerations, for example, concerning digital nerves. These (sensory) nerves are prone to regenerate very successfully, i.e., regardless of the technique that was chosen.

What are the present alternatives to autologous nerve grafts? A summary of the currently available methods was presented by the participants in Millesi's symposium in Vienna in 1991 "Peripheral Nerve Surgery Today" [10]. Strauch et al. reported on the use of autologous vein transplants and Glasby et al. on autologous muscle basal lamina. The rule of laminin-containing biosubstrates in promoting axonal regeneration has also been the subject of some of our own papers recently [12–15]. Mackinnon et al. reported on one clinical case of transplantation of a fresh nerve allograft in a patient with an extended sciatic nerve lesion. The patient subsequently received immunosuppressive therapy. So far, no significant clinical success has been observed in this single case. On the other end of the scale, nonbiogenic tubular implants have also been tried. Dellon et al. used bioresorbable polyglycolic acid (Dexon) tubes, while Lundborg [6] prefers nondegradable inert synthetic implants.

Of the alternative methods mentioned, the silicone chamber model developed by Lundborg et al. [5] has allowed the most extensive and reproducible

[1] Klinik für Neurochirurgie, Medizinischen Universität zu Lübeck, Ratzeburger Allee 160, W-2400 Lübeck, FRG.

Advances in Neurosurgery, Vol. 21
R. Lorenz, M. Klinger, M. Brock (Eds.)

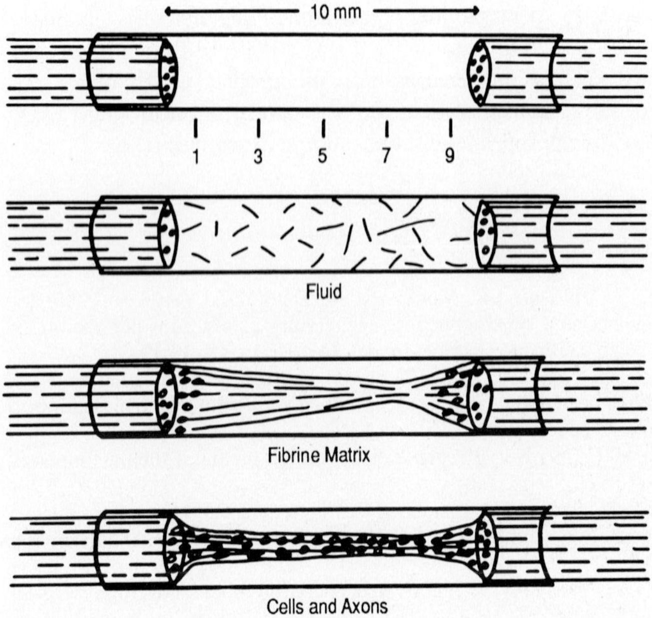

Fig. 1. Spatial-temporal progress of cellular events within silicone regeneration chambers

experimental studies so far. First, within such a regeneration chamber model, the spatial-temporal progress of the regenerative events can be studied in vivo on the cellular and perhaps even molecular level (Fig. 1) [18]. Furthermore, the chamber contents can be collected and studied for neurotrophic activity [4]. Finally, the ongoing regeneration process can be manipulated experimentally. The first attempts at doing so were performed by providing such chambers with artificial matrices

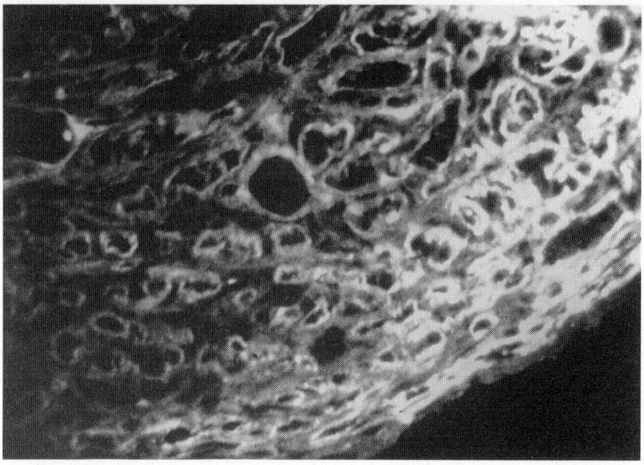

Fig. 2. Immunostain for laminin of a mature nerve regenerating

[19], supplying protentially neurotrophic biochemical agents, for example, extracellular matrix proteins such as laminin [8, 9, 11] and prefilling with laminin-containing biosubstrates such as placenta-amnion membrane [1]. Evidence that laminin must be one of the crucial factors during the regeneration progress [2, 7] can also be demonstrated by appropriate immunostaining procedures (Fig. 2).

References

1. Danielsen N, Müller H, Williams LR, Manthorpe M, Davis GE, Varon S (1988) Rat amnion membrane matrix as a substratum for regenerating axons from peripheral and central neurons: effects in a silicone chamber model. Dev Brain Res 39:39–50
2. Davis GE, Manthorpe M, Engvall E, Varon S (1985) Isolation and characterization of rat schwannoma neurite promoting factor: evidence that the factor contains laminin. J Neurosci 5:2662–2671
3. Fields RD, Ellisman M (1989) Nerve regeneration through artificial tubular implants. Prog Neurobiol 33:87–134
4. Longo FM, Manthorpe M, Skaper SD, Lundborg G, Varon S (1983) Neuronotrophic activities accummulate in vivo within silicone nerve regeneration chambers. Brain Res 261:109–117
5. Lundborg G, Longo FM, Varon S (1982) Nerve regeneration model and trophic factors in vivo. Brain Res 232:157–161
6. Lundborg G (1991) Clinical use of tubes for nerve repair. Peripheral Nerve Surgery Today. Vienna, Nov. 23–26
7. Manthorpe M, Engvall E, Ruoslahti E, Longo FM, Davis GE, Varon S (1983) Laminin promotes neuritic regeneration from cultured peripheral and central neurons. J Cell Biol 97:1882–1890
8. Müller H (1988) Further evaluation of the effects of laminin, testosterone, ganglioside GM1, and catalase on early growth in rat nerve regeneration chambers. Exp Neurol 101:228–233
9. Müller H (1990) Biochemical manipulation of the microenvironment in experimental nerve regeneration chambers. In: Samii M (ed) Peripheral nerve lesions, Springer, Berlin Heidelberg New York, pp 81–87
10. Millesi H (1991) International symposium: Peripheral Nerve Surgery Today. Turning point or continuous development? Vienna, Nov 23–26
11. Müller H, Williams LR, Varon S (1986) Nerve regeneration chamber: evaluation of exogenous agents applied by multiple injections. Brain Res 413:320–326
12. Müller H, Dombert T, Arnold H (1991) Experimental nerve regeneration: what do axons like to grow on? Peripheral Nerve Surgery Today. Vienna, Nov. 23–26
13. Müller H, Dombert T, Arnold H (1992) Experimental peripheral nerve regeneration: interposition of placenta-amnion membrane and umbilical cord versus autologous transplantation. Adv Neurosurg 20:376–380
14. Müller H, Dombert T, Terzis AJA, Arnold H (1992) Microsurgical peripheral nerve regeneration experiments: axonal growth on laminin-containing substrates. 11th Congress of the International Microsurgical Society Rhodos, June 21–26
15. Müller H, Dombert T, Arnold H (1992) Non-neural laminin containing biosubstrates as regenerative matrices for axons in vivo. 4th European Meeting on Neuropathology Berlin, July 14–19
16. Müller H, Dombert T, Arnold H (1992) Tubular nerve prostheses of non-neural origin: Historical and current concepts. Neuron (in press)
17. Weiss P (1944) The technology of nerve regeneration: a review. Sutureless tubulation and related methods of nerve repair. J Neurosurg 1:400–450

18. Williams LR, Longo FM, Powell HC, Lundborg G, Varon S (1983) Spatial-temporal progress of peripheral nerve regeneration within a silicone chamber: parameters for a bioassay. J Comp Neurol 218:460–470
19. Williams LR, Danielsen N, Müller H, Varon S (1987) Exogenous matrix precursors promote functional nerve regeneration across a 15 mm gap within a silicone chamber in the rat. J Comp Neurol 264:284–290

Motor Unit Reorganization After End-to-end Repair of an Experimentally Injured Peripheral Nerve

A. C. Nacimiento[1], A. Mautes[1], and H. Jaksche[1]

A previous study from this laboratory showed that changes in histochemical profile and morphometry of an affected muscle are reliable indicators as well as predictors of reinnervation processes over time following experimental peripheral nerve crush injury [1]. This approach was applied in the present study, which addresses changes evolving after end-to-end repair.

Sprague-Dawley rats of 250–300 g in body weight were used. The right peroneal nerve was sharply transected 10 mm distal to its point of muscle entry and subsequently repaired by coaptation with three 10–0 nylon perineurial stitches. Reinnervation changes were examined in the extensor digitorum longus (EDL), a fast-twitch muscle. Thick (10 µm) frozen serial cross sections were processed for histochemical typing and morphometry of single fibers, on the basis of their myofibrillar ATPase (pH 4.3) and succinate dehydrogenase (SDH) enzyme activities. Three muscle fiber types can be thus functionally identified: (a) type I, slow oxidative (SO); (b) type IIA, fast oxidative glycolytic (FOG); (c) type IIB, fast glycolytic (FG) [2, 7]. EDL histochemical profile (fiber type composition and size distribution), and morphometry (total fiber count and cross-sectional area) were assessed on both sides in normal animals, and 15, 30, and 60 days after repair in operated animals by computer-assisted quantification. Measurements were statistically evaluated by one-way analysis of variance over time, and Student's t-test between sides.

Fiber type composition showed on both sides an additional group generated by type conversion (Fig. 1).

Relative to its SDH-oxidative capacity, this type was intermediate (SDH INT) between the purely glycolytic (FG) and the mixed glycolytic oxidative groups. SDH INT appeared 15 days after repair, and increased considerably 30 and 60 days later. Topographically, the homogeneous checkerboard pattern of normal muscle shifted on the repaired side to a heterogeneous, clustered one, which persisted for the duration of the observations (60 days). The unoperated side did not show this shift.

The cross-sectional area increased over time on both sides and in all fiber types (Fig. 2). Changes on the operated side 15 days after repair, a time point in which denervation effects are expected to be still pronounced, were fiber type dependent. There was a large, significant decrease in the glycolytic group (FG), and a clear but

[1] Neurochirurgisches Forschungslaboratorium, Medizinische Fakultät, Universität des Saarlandes, W-6650 Homburg/Saar, FRG.

Advances in Neurosurgery, Vol. 21
R. Lorenz, M. Klinger, M. Brock (Eds.)

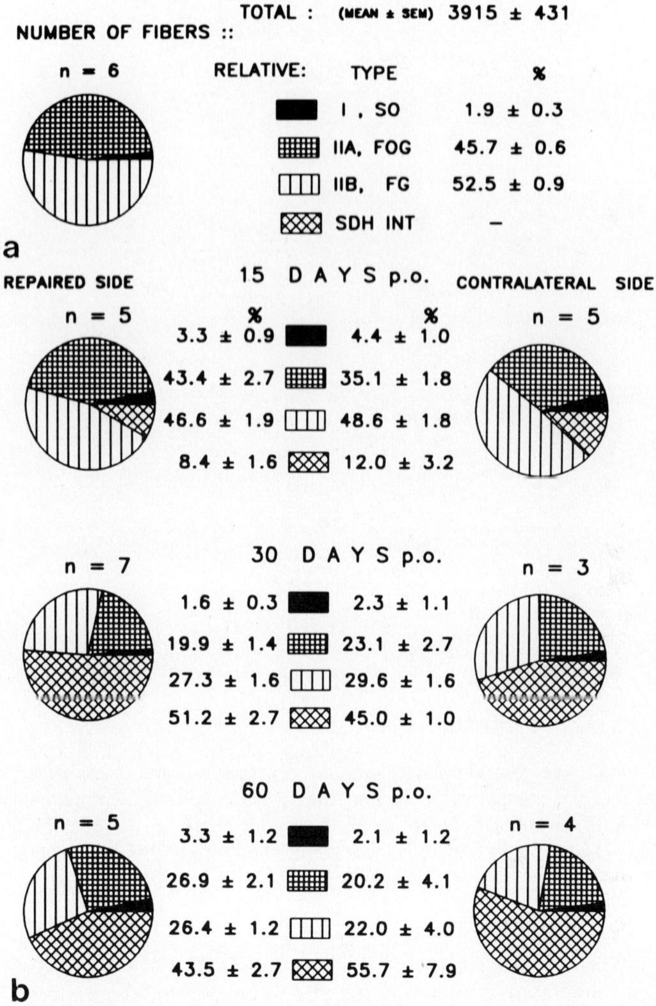

Fig. 1. a, b. *Fiber type composition of EDL muscle.* **a** Normal muscle; **b** after peroneal nerve end-to-end repair. *SO*, slow oxidative; *FOG*, fast oxidative glycolytic; *FG*, fast glycolytic; *SDH INT* succinate dehydrogenase intermediate. There were no statistical differences between sides. Fiber type conversion to SDH INT, encroached the FG and FOG groups, thus displacing the normal profile toward a four-type pattern on both repaired and unoperated sides

not significant decrease in the mixed oxidative glycolytic one (FOG), whereas the SO group remained unaltered. Thus, the highest vulnerability to axotomy appeared to be selectively confined to the group characterizing the physiological fast-twitch property of EDL [5].

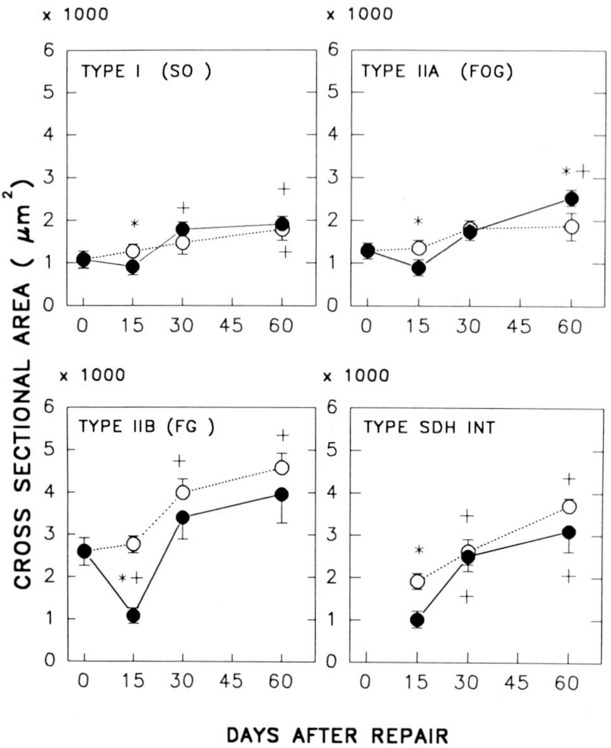

Fig. 2. *Size changes over time t* = 0, normal muscle; *solid circles* repaired side; *open circles*, unoperated side; *asterisks* $p \leq .05$, comparison between sides; *crosses*, $p \leq .05$, comparison vs. normal muscle. Note significant size decrease at 15 days after repair in the glycolytic group. Final size (60 days) was similar in both sides, but significantly higher than in normal muscle

Distribution of size over time after repair displayed a marked and progressive fiber type-dependent rearrangement as shown in the three-dimensional diagrams of Fig. 3. The most remarkable changes were observed in the glycolytic group: its normally even distribution (see $t = 0$) shifted on the repaired side into a wide-band frequency pattern encompassing a continuum from small to large fiber sizes. Contralaterally there was only a discrete regrouping around the middle-size range. The SDH INT group showed a similar, but less marked tendency.

In the oxidative groups (FOG and SO) there was on both sides an increase in frequency of middle-sized fibers, which was, however, clearly limited in range.

Under normal functional demands, motor unit types are histochemically and physiologically stable [3, 6]. This stability, however, may be readily upset by conditions which lead to a restructuring of motor units such as, for example, nerve cross section [3]. The present results indicate that during reinnervation after nerve repair changes ensue which may produce a profound and long-lasting destabilization of motor unit organization. This was signalled by a vigorous fiber type con-

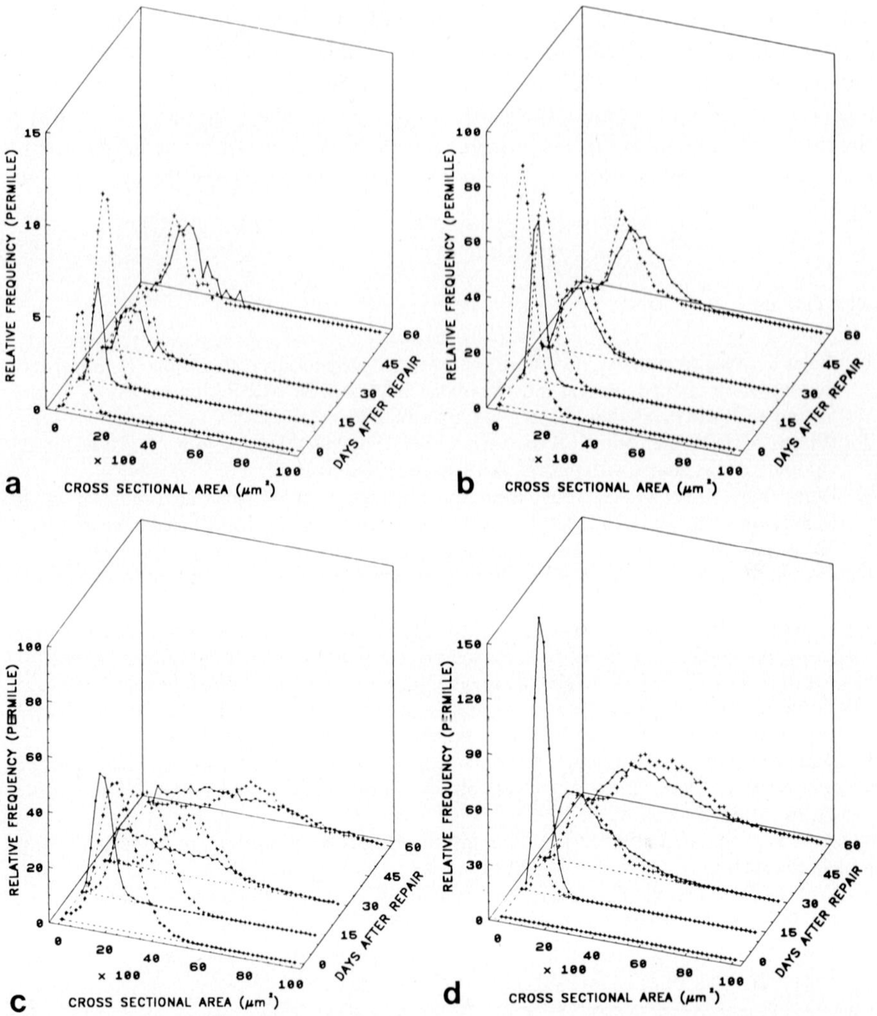

Fig. 3. a–d. *Three-dimensional profiles of size distribution of fiber types over time after repair.* **a** Type I (SO); **b** type IIA (FOG); **c** type IIB (FG); **d** type SDH INT. *Squares,* repaired side; *crosses,* contralateral side. $t = 0$, normal distribution, with the following cross-sectional maxima ± SEM: type I–SO: 1072 ± 106 μm²; type IIA–FOG: 1283 ± 124 μm²; type IIB–FG: 2590 ± 326 μm². Note redistribution of fiber size in all types 60 days after repair, with the FG group being most affected

version activity in the glycolytic range, which in turn produced a pronounced scattering in size distribution. These changes may be attributed to a polyneuronal reinnervation of the affected muscle fibers. Multiple innervation of muscle is normal in neonate animals [2]. Later, elimination of excess connections leads to the single innervating axon pattern of the adult. Thus, reinnervation after repair seems to bring about a regression to the immature motor unit organization form. After repair, type-matching [3, 8] (all fibers in a motor unit belong to the same type) and place-matching [9] (somatotopic projection of motor columns to muscle fiber groups) are unstable and vulnerable. Inherent to this is inaccuracy in guidance of regenerating axons to their targets [4]. Improving accuracy of target recognition should enhance chances for successful reconnection after nerve repair. Searching for ways to accomplish this is of prime importance for improving the clinical quality of nerve repair.

References

1. Adler G, Nacimiento AC (1990) Experimental peripheral crush lesion. II. Short-term reinnervation changes in fast muscle fibers. In: Samii M (ed) Peripheral nerve lesions. Springer, Berlin Heidelberg New York, pp 189–196
2. Brooke MH, Williamson E, Kaiser KK (1971) The behaviour of four fiber types in developing and reinnervated muscle. Arch Neurol 25:360–366
3. Burke RE (1981) Motor units: anatomy, physiology and functional organisation. In: Handbook of physiology, sect 1, vol 2. American Physiological Society, Bethesda, pp 345–422
4. Fawcett W, Keynes RJ (1990) Peripheral nerve regeneration. Annu Rev Neurosci 13:43–60
5. Hashimoto H, Mautes A, Nacimiento AC (1991) Peripheral nerve graft repair changes size and histochemical profile of affected muscle fibers. Soc Neurosci Abstr 17:98.5
6. Nacimiento AC, Marx C (1990) Experimental peripheral nerve crush lesion. I. Posttraumatic metabolic responses of spinal motoneurones over time. In: Samii M (ed) Peripheral nerve lesions. Springer, Berlin Heidelberg New York, pp 175–188
7. Peter JB, Barnard RJ, Edgerton VR, Gillespie CA, Stempel KE (1972) Metabolic profiles of three fiber types of skeletal muscle in guinea pigs and rabbits. Biochemistry 11:2627–2633
8. Pette D, Vrbová G (1985) Neural control of phenotypic expression in mammalian muscle fibers. Muscle Nerve 8:676–689
9. Weinert DM, Jaksche H, Ludt H, Nacimiento AC (1989) Plasticity of a spinal motoneuron nucleus after peripheral nerve graft repair. Soc Neurosci Abstr. 15:127.1

Differential Localization of the Nerve Growth Factor Receptor in Tumors of the Peripheral Nervous System

R. Schober[1] and K. T. Vogeley[1]

Introduction

The nerve growth factor is a polypeptide that plays an important role in the differentiation and maintenance of sympathetic neurons and, generally, of cells deriving from the neural crest [4]. The biological actions of the nerve growth factor are initiated by specific binding to one of the nerve growth factor receptors (NGF-R) on the surface of the target cell. Tumors expressing NGF-R include phaeochromocytomas, melanomas, and tumors of the peripheral nervous system, as already described by several authors [1, 2, 6, 7, 9, 10, 16, 20]. In most of these studies, however, the results were recorded without taking into account the various tissue components and the often heterogeneous tumor subtypes. We have therefore analyzed the histological distribution of NGF-R in more detail in a variety of peripheral nervous system tumors including control material from normal nerves. The specificity of the immunoreaction was monitored by simultaneous Western blot analysis in several cases.

Material and Methods

The material comprised 34 surgically removed tumors and, in addition, normal peripheral nerves (brachial plexus, sciatic nerve, and median nerve) from two autopsy cases. Details of their classification and site as well of the immunohistochemical procedures are to be found in a concurrent report on vascular permeability changes [12]. In this study, the monoclonal antibody ME20–4 (Amersham-Buchler, Brunswick, FRG) was used in a dilution of 1:25 on paraffin sections in all and on frozen sections in a number of cases. In addition, a panel of other primary antibodies including anti-S-100 (DAKO, Hamburg, FRG; dilution of 1:2000) was applied.

Western blotting was performed with protein preparations from three neurinomas, three neurofibromas, and one normal sciatic nerve according to standard methods, details of which are described elsewhere [8].

[1] Abteilung Neuropathologie, Medizinische Einrichtungen der Heinrich-Heine-Universität, Moorenstraße 5, W-4000 Düsseldorf 1, FRG.

Advances in Neurosurgery, Vol. 21
R. Lorenz, M. Klinger, M. Brock (Eds.)

Results

Nerve growth factor receptor immunoreactivity was present in all normal nerves but was confined to the inner cell layers of the perineurium. In addition to the perineurial staining, there was a consistent decoration of the outer circumference of blood vessels, presumably corresponding to pericytes. Perineurial staining was also observed in traumatic neuromas (Fig. 1a). The cells forming the sheath of Henle were clearly and consistently positive in contrast to the endoneurium of the sprouting miniature fascicles.

In tumors of the peripheral nervous system, the results varied, depending on the material used for immunostaining. On cryostat sections, benign neurinomas, neurofibromas, and ganglioneuromas in their neuromatous portions showed a generally positive reaction. The regional staining intensity varied only slightly, e.g., the palisading areas of neurinomas were more strongly stained than the loosely structured reticular areas. Using paraffin section, these regional differences were accentuated. Preferential decoration of subcapsular or subperineurial and of perivascular tumor areas was a consistent finding in benign peripheral nervous system tumors. Anaplastic peripheral nerve sheath tumors showed very little subcapsular and perivascular staining and otherwise were generally negative. Pronounced regional differences in NGF-R staining were present in several special tumor cases. In one spinal and one dermal neurofibroma with focal tactile body differentiation, these organelles were strongly stained (Fig. 1b). Other areas with a diffuse growth pattern were negative for NGF-R, while the immunoreaction for S-100 was uniformly positive in these tumors. A plexiform neurofibroma with onion bulb formations and intratumoral microneurinomas showed a preferential staining of the outer capsule-like cell layers of the microtumors (Fig. 1c). This case may also be designated as symmetrical neurofibroma and is described in more detail elsewhere [13]. A lipofibromatous hamartoma of the median nerve, details of which have already been published [11], showed exclusive staining of the broadened and proliferating perineurial septae (Fig. 1d). The intrafascicular and intratumoral Schwann cells were decorated by S-100, resulting in a staining pattern reciprocal to NGF-R.

The Western blots uniformly showed the 75-kD band characteristic for the low-affinity NGF-R, although the intensity of immunostaining markedly differed from specimen to specimen (Fig. 2).

Fig. 1a-d. Immunohistochemistry of NGF-R (PAP method, counterstained with hematoxylin). **a** Traumatic neuroma, showing a positive reaction confined to the sheath cells of miniature fascicles, while the nerve of origin (*below*) is negative. **b** Neurofibroma type III with diffuse infiltration of adipose tissue (*below*), showing strong and almost exclusive immunoreactivity of tactile corpuscles. **c** Symmetrical neurofibroma, showing preferential staining of the outer circumference of neoplastic onion bulbs and microneurinomas. **d** Lipofibromatous hamartoma of median nerve, showing immunoreactivity of the proliferating perineurium only. **a, b,** x 160; **c** x 110; **d** x 40

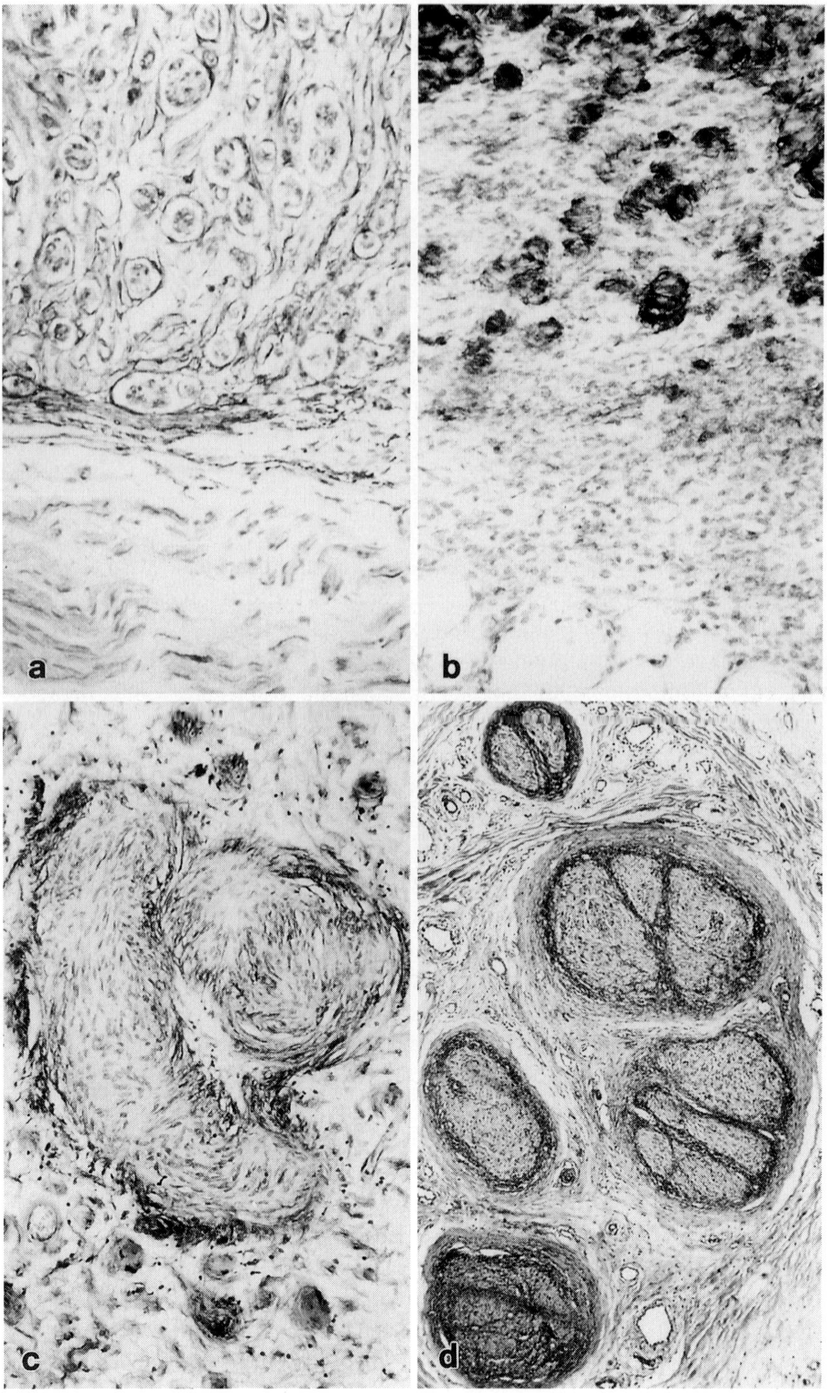
a
b
c
d

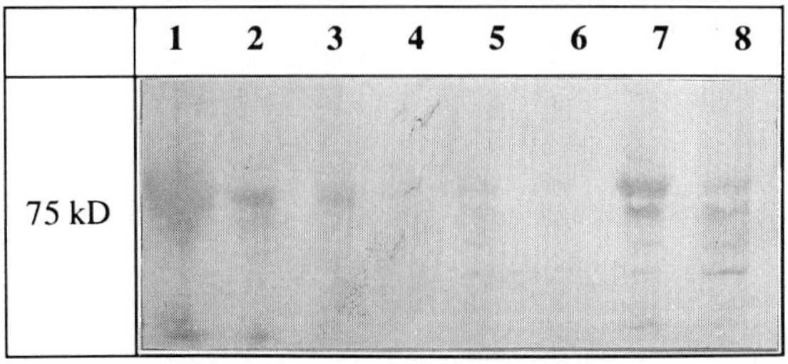

Fig. 2. Western blot, demonstrating the characteristic band for the low affinity NGF-R of 75 kD, with immunoreactivity differing from specimen to specimen. Bands of lower molecular weight represent proteolytic fragments. *1*, Normal sciatic nerve (S 269/92); *2*, neurinoma (NP 614/89); *3*, neurinoma (NP 636/89); *4*, neurinoma (NP 291/90); *5*, neurinoma (NP 795/89); *6*, neurofibroma (NP 1226/91); *7*, neurofibroma (NP 713/91); *8*, neurofibroma (NP 7/90)

Discussion

The results of this study show that NGF-R in peripheral nervous system tumors is preferentially localized in perivascular areas and in sheath structures analogous to the perineurium. This is particularly well demonstrated in certain special and rare tumor types, e.g., the lipofibromatous hamartoma of the median nerve and the symmetrical neurofibroma. Our findings in neoplastic lesions are well compatible with the decoration by NGF-R of the inner perineurial layers of normal nerve, and of the perineurium of the miniature fascicles in traumatic neuromas [2, 3, 14, 20]. Other authors report a negative reaction in normal nerve, reversing to positivity after nerve transection in the distal stump only [15]. Although the specificity of the immunoreaction has been proven by Western blot analysis in the present study, such differences may be explained by the use of different primary antibodies.

The inner layer of the perineurium is composed of highly specialized cells constituting the principal substrates of the blood-nerve barrier. It is therefore not surprising that anaplastic peripheral nerve sheath tumors in which the tumor cells are largely undifferentiated generally do not express NGF-R. This result is also in line with experimental investigations demonstrating a differentiating and a reverse transforming effect of nerve growth factor, the ligand of NGF-R, on human neurogenic tumor cell lines in vitro [19].

In type III neurofibromas with tactile body differentiation, the histogenesis of these specialized structures is still controversial. Arguments have been presented both for a perineurial derivation on fine structural grounds [18], and for a Schwann cell derivation on the basis of their immunoreactivity for S-100 [17]. The positive reaction for NGF-R as demonstrated in the present study would favor the former, but further criteria seem necessary to resolve this debate unequivocally.

Perineurial tissue structures have been shown to react with antibodies to the epithelial membrane antigen (EMA) obtained by immunization to human milk protein [5]. It appears that the monoclonal antibody ME20–4 against NGF-R, although not specific, is of additional use as a marker for a subset of normal perineurial cells and their neoplastic counterparts in tumors of the peripheral nervous system.

References

1. Baker DL, Molenaar WM, Trojanowski JQ, Evans AE, Ross AH, Rorke LB, Packer RJ, Lee VM-Y, Pleasure D (1991) Nerve growth factor receptor expression in peripheral and central neuroectodermal tumors, other pediatric brain tumors, and during development of the adrenal gland. Am J Pathol 139:115–122
2. Chesa PG, Rettig WJ, Thomson TM, Old LJ, Melamed MR (1988) Immunohistochemical analysis of nerve growth factor receptor expression in normal and malignant human tissues. J Histochem Cytochem 36:383–389
3. Kerkhoff H, Jennekens FGI, Troost D, Veldman H (1991) Nerve growth factor receptor immunostaining in the spinal cord and peripheral nerves in amyotrophic lateral sclerosis. Acta Neuropathol (Berl) 81:649–656
4. Levi-Montalcini R (1987) The nerve growth factor 35 years later. Science 237:1154–1162
5. Perentes E, Rubinstein LJ (1987) Recent applications on immunoperoxidase histochemistry in human neurooncology. An update. Arch Pathol Lab Med 111:796–812
6. Perosio PM, Brooks JJ (1988) Expression of nerve growth factor receptor in paraffin-embedded soft tissue tumors. Am J Pathol 132:152–160
7. Prior R, Reifenberger G, Wechsler W (1989) Nerve growth factor receptor in tumours of the human nervous system. Immunohistochemical analysis of receptor expression and tumour growth fraction. Pathol Res Pract 135:332–338
8. Reifenberger G (1991) Immunhistochemie der Tumoren des Nervensystems. Springer, Berlin Heidelberg New York, pp 35–36
9. Riopelle RJ, Haliotis T, Roder JC (1983) Nerve growth factor receptors of human tumors of neural crest origin: characterization of binding site heterogeneity and alteration by theophylline. Cancer Res 43:5184–5189
10. Ross AH, Grob P, Bothwell M, Elder DE, Ernst CS, Marano N, Ghrist BFD, Slemp CC, Herlyn M, Atkinson B, Koprowski H (1984) Characterization of nerve growth factor receptor in neural crest tumors using monoclonal antibodies. Proc Natl Acad Sci USA 81:6681–6685
11. Schober R, Nicola N, Wechsler W (1985) Kasuistischer Beitrag zum lipofibromatösen Hamartom des Nervus medianus: neuropathologischer Bericht von zwei Fällen. Acta Neuropathol (Berl) 66:18–23
12. Schober R, Vogeley KT, Urich H, Hölzle E, Wechsler W (1992) Vascular permeability changes in tumours of the peripheral nervous system. Virchows Arch [A] 420:59–64
13. Schober R, Reifenberger G, Kremer G, Urich H (1992) Symmetrical neurofibroma with Schwann cell predominance and focal formation of microneurinomas. Acta Neuropathol (Berl)
14. Sobue G, Yasuda T, Mitsuma T, Ross AH, Pleasure D (1988) Expression of nerve growth factor receptor in human peripheral neuropathies. Ann Neurol 24:64–72
15. Taniuchi M, Clark HB, Johnson EM Jr (1986) Induction of nerve growth factor receptor in Schwann cells after axotomy. Proc Natl Acad Sci USA 83:4094–4098
16. Thompson SJ, Schatteman GC, Gown AM, Bothwell M (1989) A monoclonal antibody against nerve growth factor receptor. Immunohistochemical analysis of normal and neoplastic human tissue. Am J Clin Pathol 92:415–423
17. Watabe K, Kumanishi T, Ikuta F, Oyake Y (1983) Tactile-like corpuscles in neurofibromas: Immunohistochemical demonstration of S-100 protein. Acta Neuropathol (Berl) 61:173–177

18. Weiser G (1978) Neurofibrom und Perineuralzelle. Elektronenoptische Untersuchung an 9 Neurofibromen. Virchows Arch [A] 379:73–83
19. Yaeger MJ, Koestner A, Marushige K, Marushige Y (1991) The reverse transforming effects of nerve growth factor on five human neurogenic tumor cell lines: in vitro results. Acta Neuropathol (Berl) 83:72–80
20. Yasuda T, Sobue G, Mitsuma T, Takahashi A, Hashizume Y (1989) Nerve growth factor receptor immunoreactivity in human benign peripheral nerve sheath tumor. Acta Neuropathol (Berl) 77:591–598

The Ansa Cervicalis Hypoglossal – Facial Anastomosis for Indirect Facial Nerve Reconstruction

H. H. Steiner[1], M. S. von Haken[1], H. G. Steiner Milz[1], F. K. Albert[1], and J. Hamer[1]

Introduction

Since the introduction of the indirect facial nerve reconstruction using accessory nerve by Drobnik [5] in 1879, a variety of donor nerves have been used. Anastomosis with the glossopharyngeal nerve [2, 19] and the phrenic nerve [8] were soon abandoned; the hypoglossal nerve was the one used most [11, 13, 14, 15]. The present study intends to show the efficiency of indirect facial nerve anastomosis with the ansa cervicalis of the hypoglossal nerve.

Clinical Material and Methods

In the years between 1986 and 1991 we carried out facial nerve reconstruction with the ansa cervicalis. Twenty-one patients (11 male, ten female) were operated on. The average age was 41.5 years (between 21 and 65 years), mean follow-up was 1.8 years (from 0.5 up to 4.5 years). In 18 patients, the cause of the facial nerve deficit was intracisternal; in three patients it was due to an intratemporal lesion.

The operative approach followed the usual technique (see Fig. 1), as described by other authors [15, 17].

Results

Ranking of postoperative results was mainly oriented according to clinical recovery of facial nerve function. On the one hand, we examined the normalization of resting tone, on the other, the capacity of the active mimic innervation.

In the periorbital region we found the palpebral aperture to be satisfactory (no more than 12 mm) in seven patients. In the case of a further six patients there was a sufficient symmetry with a palpebral aperture that did not exceed 14 mm. Active lid closure (minimum 80%) was possible in nine patients. Six patients were even able to frown using their forehead. Unsatisfactory active lid closure was seen in six patients.

Excellent recovery of perioral resting tone was found in 14 patients and, achieving a symmetric position of the mouth, an additional four patients showed sufficient

---

[1] Neurochirurgische Klinik, Universität Heidelberg, Im Neuenheimer Feld 400, W-6900 Heidelberg, FRG.

Advances in Neurosurgery, Vol. 21
R. Lorenz, M. Klinger, M. Brock (Eds.)

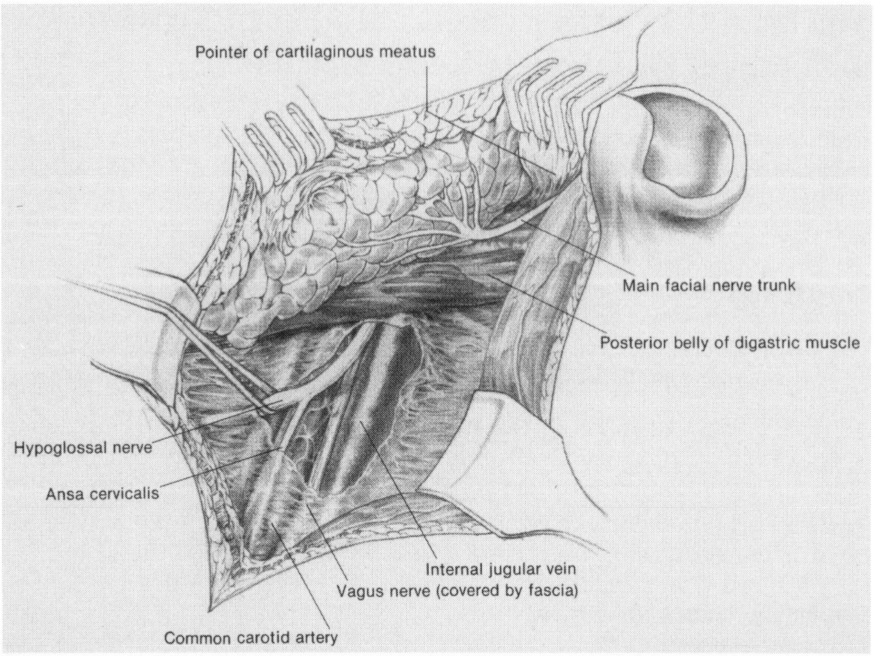

Fig. 1. Operative site. Landmarks to find the facial nerve are the posterior belly of digastric muscle, the anterior edge of sternocleidomastoid muscle, and the pointer of the cartilaginous auditory canal. The hypoglossal nerve, or the ansa cervicalis, can be easily identified inferior to the digastric muscle at the level of the bifurcation of the carotid artery. (From [17])

symmetry. The results of the active innervation in the perioral region were excellent in 14 patients, with nearly complete exposition of teeth. Only three patients had unsatisfactory active perioral motility.

Table 1. Operative results in the periorbital region (n = 21) (ranking group)

Operative results	(n)	(%)
Normal palpebral aperture, complete closure of eye lids, frowning possible (very good results)	6	29
Excellent/good resting tone and motility (good results)	3	14
Sufficient motility (satisfactory results)	6	28.5
Unsatisfactory motility (unsatisfactory results)	6	28.5

Table 2. Operative results in the perioral region ($n = 21$) (ranking group)

Operative results	(n)	(%)
Symmetric position of the mouth and excellent/good motility (very good and good results)	14	66
Asymmetric position of the mouth and good motility (satisfactory results)	4	19
Unsatisfactory resting tone and motility (unsatisfactory results)	3	15

Generally the restitution of perioral muscle groups proved to be more satisfactory than in the periorbital region. On the other hand, the results of the periorbital region should not be underestimated, especially with regard to functional results, as sufficient lid closure covering the cornea was found in no fewer than 15 patients. A summary of operative results is shown in Tables 1 and 2. Complications were not observed. There is a definite positive correlation between the time of surgery after the lesion and the operative results (Fig. 2).

Discussion

As early as 1903, improvement of facial symmetry and active motility was described by Körte [13] for the hypoglossal – facial anastomosis. Favorable outcome regarding the perioral region was described in as many as 60% of cases [1, 3, 6, 7, 9, 12, 16]. The chances of recovery in the forehead and periorbital region are generally estimated to be less favorable [1, 4, 6, 9, 17]. A study by Stennert [18] shows a tendency towards normalization of the muscle tonus at a rate of 70% in

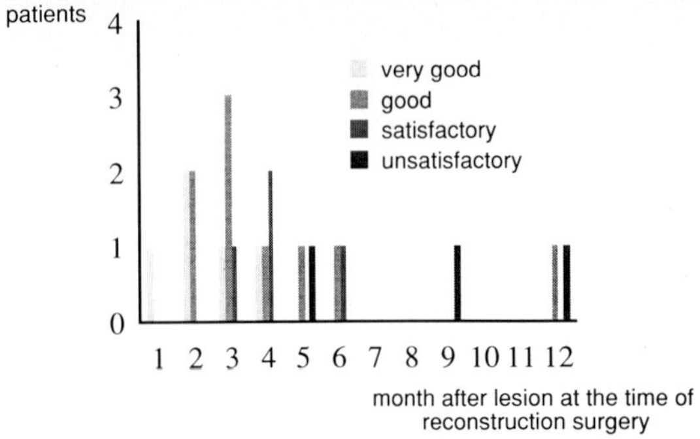

Fig. 2. Correlation between operative results regarding motility in the perioral region and the timespan from the lesion of the facial nerve to reconstruction surgery. The columns represent our ranking groups for postoperative results as shown in Table 2

the perioral area and 10% in the periorbital area. Accordingly, the active innervation in the perioral region was very satisfactory with an exposition of teeth in 50% of cases. A sufficient closure of the eye lids could be demonstrated in 35% of patients [18].

A disadvantage of the hypoglossal – facial anastomosis lies in the relatively high rate of synkinetic facial movements. It has been described as being as high as 80% in the perioral region by other authors [4, 18]. Following recent findings, the hemiparalysis of the tongue is also a major handicap for patients [10]. The results of ansa cervicalis hypoglossal – facial anastomosis are as successful as anastomosis with the main hypoglossal nerve trunk. In the region of the forehead and periorbital region, results from ansa cervicalis anastomosis are superior, as can be seen in a comparison with other data [18]. When using ansa cervicalis, impairing synkinetic facial movements after tongue innervation are less frequently observed. In our patients we could only observe this phenomenon in one case. An obvious advantage is the lack of neurological deficit by using the ansa cervicalis as the donor nerve.

Owing to the fact that results from the use of ansa cervicalis in the indirect reconstruction of the facial nerve proved to be favorable, we abandoned the use of the main hypoglossal nerve trunk. There were only three cases where an anastomosis with rudimentary ansa cervicalis was not possible. Since early reconstruction showed best results in our study, we prefer early surgery when the interruption of facial nerve continuity is evident.

References

1. Alexander E, Davis CH (1954) Correction of peripheral paralysis of the facial nerve by hypoglossal facial anastomosis. South Med J 47:299–302
2. Ballence CA (1924) An address on the results obtained in some experiments in which the facial and recurrent laryngeal nerves were anastomosed with other nerves. Br Med J 2:349–354
3. Coleman CC (1940) Results of facio-hypoglossal anastomosis in the treatment of facial paralysis. Ann Surg 3:958–970
4. Conley J, Baker CD (1979) Hypoglossal-facial nerve anastomosis for reinnervation of the paralyzed face. Plast Reconstr Surg 63:63–72
5. Drobnik T (1879) Facial palsy. Richter, Würzburg
6. Evans DM (1974) Hypoglosso-facial anastomosis in the treatment of facial palsy. Br J Plast Surg 27:252–257
7. Falbe-Hansen J, Hermann S (1967) Hypoglosso-facial anastomosis. Acta Neurol Scand 43:472–478
8. Hardy RC, Perret G, Meyers R (1957) Phrenicofacial nerve anastomosis for facial paralysis. J Neursurg 14:400–404
9. Hitselberger WE (1974) Hypoglossal-facial-anastomosis. Otolaryngol Clin North Am 7:545–550
10. Jeske J, Rauhut F (1992) Klinische und elektrophysiologische Langzeitergebnisse bei Patienten mit Hypoglossus – Facialisanastomosen. 43rd annual meeting of the Deutsche Gesellschaft für Neurochirurgie, Frankfort
11. Kautzky R (1956) Die periphere Fazialislähmung und ihre Behandlung mittels Nervenpfropfung. Fortschr Kiefer Gesichtschir 2:119–126

12. Kessler H, Moldaver J, Pool JL (1959) Hypoglossal-facial anastomosis for treatment of facial paralysis. Neurology (Minneap) 9:118–125
13. Körte W (1903) Ein Fall von Nervenpfropfung des N. Facialis auf den N. Hypoglossus. Dtsch Med Wochenschr 29:293–295
14. Metelka M (1966) Anastomoza N VII – N XII lepenim plazmou. Cesk Neurol 29:305–310
15. Miehlke A (1979) Fazialislähmungen. In: Berendes J, Link R, Zöllner F (eds) Hals-Nasen-Ohrenheilkunde in Praxis und Klinik. Thieme, Stuttgart
16. Nisch F (1973) Ergebnisse bei Fazialis-Hypoglossus Anastomosen. Neurol Med Psychol (Leipz) 25:488–493
17. Samii M, Draf W (1989) Facial nerve and skull base surgery. In: Samii M, Draf W (eds) Surgery of the skull base. Springer, Berlin Heidelberg New York, pp 474–507
18. Stennert E (1979) I. Hypoglossal facial anastomosis: its significance for modern facial surgery. II. Combined approach in extratemporal facial nerve reconstruction. Clin Plast Surg 6:471–486
19. Watson-Williams E (1927) Glossopharyngeal facial nerve anastomosis. Proc R Soc Med 20:1439–1442

Lesions of the Accessory Nerve in Its Extracranial Course

A. Sepehrnia[1], W. Bini[1], and M. Samii[1]

Introduction

Iatrogenic lesions of the accessory nerve in its extracranial course are extraordinarily frequent. The primary causes are either lymph node biopsies or other procedures performed in the lateral cervical triangle behind the border of the sternocleidomastoid muscle. Other less frequent nonsurgical causes reported in the literature include: injections, Trendelenburg position, radiotherapy, trauma and insect bites.

On the deep cervical fascia, over the levator scapulae muscle, the accessory nerve courses to the trapezius muscle along the lateral cervical region. It is precisely in this area that the nerve is only protected by the superficial cervical fascia. Along this course and topography one finds also the superficial lymph nodes.

Symptoms

The clinical picture corresponding to an accesory nerve palsy is characterized by sternocleidomastoid and upper trapezius muscle deficit. The altered voluntary motor function is manifested by not being able to lift the shoulder. Furthermore, the elevation of the shoulder joint is reduced. In cases in which the upper portion of the trapezius is also involved, lateral abduction of the shoulder is possible only through the deltoid muscle. Strength is reduced to one third and the abduction reaches only 90°. In almost all patients there is marked pain. Shoulder and upper arm pain are usually the primary complaint. Hanging of the shoulder can also cause an associated lesion of the ligaments with traction of the brachial plexus, causing irradiating pain and paresthesia. Other reported symptoms are local pain and altered sensation in the lateral cervical region. This can be due to the involvement of one or more sensitive branches of the cervical plexus with neuroma formation.

Differential diagnostic problems may lead to false interpretation of the complaints and labeling the patient as having cervical disc disease.

---

[1] Neurochirurgische Klinik, Krankenhaus Nordstadt, Haltenhoffstr. 41, W-3000 Hannover, FRG.

Advances in Neurosurgery, Vol. 21
R. Lorenz, M. Klinger, M. Brock (Eds.)

Therapy

When confronted with a slight palsy, a conservative attitude should be adopted at first with physiotherapy to strengthen the synergistic muscles. Nevertheless, when a marked palsy is evident without signs of reinnervation of the corresponding muscles 3 months after the lesion, surgical exposure/intervention is indicated and, in our opinion, constitutes, the method of choice.

Surgical Technique

The skin incision usually involves the pre-existing scar. The exposure of the accessory nerve is performed at first distally and then proximally to the area of lesion, that is, we identify the nerve in its healthy portions, avoiding initially the scar tissue/segment. As orientation we use the known topographical landmarks of the lateral cervical triangle. On the posterior border of the sternocleidomastoid muscle we first identify the punctum nervosum with its individual nerve structures and then localize the accessory nerve. The distal portion can usually be found at the level of the upper border of the trapezius muscle. Further preparation of the scar tissue must be carried out with extreme care in order to preserve continuity. If this is the case, a microsurgical neurolysis is indicated; if, on the other hand, there is loss of continuity the defect must be bridged using an autologous nerve transplant harvested, for example, from the sural nerve.

In those patients in whom the affected muscles are so atrophic that even with nerve reconstruction techniques we foresee unsatisfactory results, orthopedic procedures to improve the functional status are considered and discussed with the patient.

Material and Method

Since 1977, 40 patients with accessory nerve lesions have been treated in our clinic. The mechanisms responsible for these lesions are summarized in Table 1. Seventy-five percent had a lymph node removal. In 27 cases there was loss of continuity, and in 12 patients we performed a microneurolysis. In one case, besides a

Table 1. Etiology of 40 accessory nerve lesions treated in Nordstadt Hospital (1977–1991)

Lymph node extirpation (lateral cervical triangle)	30
Penetrating wounds, trauma	5
Lymph node extirpation (mandible)	1
Atheroma removal (posterior border of sternocleidomastoid muscle)	1
Cyst removal (lateral cervical region)	1
Hematoma evacuation	1
Brachial plexus biopsy (NF 1 patient)	1

Table 2. Results of treatment

Patient	Very good	Good	Moderately good	Moderately bad	No improvement	Not examined	Graft length (cm)	Time between lesion and operation (month)	Interruption of continuity
Microneurolysis									
2	+							20	
1						+		8 1/2	
5					+			32	
6	+							4	
10[a]	+							4 1/2	
12	+							5	
13	+							5	
15	+							26	
17	+							2 1/2	
26	+							1 1/2	
35					+			3	
38		+						6	
4						+	5.0	5	+
8[b]	+						3.5	10	+
9						+	2.5	5 1/2	
11[b]	+						4.0	14	+
14					+		3.0	7	
16	+						3.0	7	+
18				+			2.0	8	+
19[b]		+					10.0	3	+
21						+	5.0	8	+
22					+		10.0	3	+
23				+			6.0	9	+
24				+			8.0	2	+
25	+						–	8	+

Microneurolysis							
27[b]			+		1.5	3 1/2	+
28	+				8.0	6	–[c]
29	+				4.0	6	+
30[b]		+			5.0	36	+
31				+	4.0	3 1/2	+
32			+		4.0	8	+
33		+			12.0	10 1/2	+
34[b]	+				5.0	10	+
37				+	3.0	72	+
39	+				2.5	2 1/2	+
40	+				4.0	14	+
3			+			3	
7	+					6	
36	+					2 1/2	
20[d]				+			

[a] Microneurolysis and end-to-end anastomosis of a fascicle.
[b] Residual innervation by cervical branches.
[c] Cicatricial plate.
[d] Sewing of the nerve stump into the trapezius muscle.

neurolysis, we also performed an end-to-end coaptation of a solitary fascicle from the main trunk. Three patients received an end-to-end coaptation, in 24 we transplanted, and in one we positioned the nerve stump in the trapezius muscle without reconstruction. We were able to have a complete follow-up in 36 cases.

Results and Discussion

The most frequently observed lesion of the accessory nerve is iatrogenic in nature, after lymph node extirpations or biopsy procedures performed in the lateral neck region. The prognosis regarding spontaneous regeneration/recuperation has been considered as very poor. The indication for a surgical procedure should be a result of clinical and electrophysiological criteria, event though experience has shown that there is quite often little correlation between intraoperative findings and preoperative electromyographic data. This is probably due to the many anatomical variations and the anastomosis of the accessory nerve with cervical motor branches. Even in longstanding lesions (1–3 years) we favor an operation if there is still pathological spontaneous activity in the recordings in the form of fibrillations and positive "steil" waves. Nevertheless, the most favorable results are achieved when surgery is done within the first year. The type of procedure (microneurolysis, end-to-end coaptation, or transplantation) depends on the degree of lesioning, as observed intraoperatively. Microsurgical techniques and sound topographical orientation are key points for achieving good results. We have summed up our follow-up results in Table 2.

References

1. Ballantyne AJ, Guinn GA (1966) Reduction of shoulder disability after neck dissection. Am J Surg 112:662–665
2. Becker GD, Parell GJ (1979) Technique of preserving the spinal acessory nerve during radical neck dissection. Laryngoscope 89:827–831
3. Bushe KA (1971) Mikrochirurgische Maßnahmen zur Funktionsrückkehr nach Accessoriuslähmung durch Lymphdrüsenextirpation am Hals. Unfallheilkunde 107:213–219
4. Carenfelt C, Eliasson K (1980) Occurrence, duration and prognosis of unexpected accessory nerve paresis in radical neck dissection. Acta Otolaryngol 90:470–473
5. Dunn AW (1974) Trapezius paralysis after minor surgical procedures in the posterior triangle. South Med J 67:312–315
6. Gordon SL et al (1977) Accessory nerve function after surgical procedures in the posterior triangle. Arch Surg 112:264–268
7. Hagenah R, Kosak M, Freckmann N (1983) Anatomic topographical relationship of the intraspinal accessory root to the upper cervical roots and to the vessels of the cranial cervical region. Acta Anat 115:158–167
8. Hausamen JE, Samii M, Schmidseder R (1976) Indication and technique for the reconstruction of nerve defects in the head and neck. J Max Fac Surg 2:159–167
9. Hausamen JE, Samii M, Schmidseder R (1976) Autologe Nerventransplantation zur Überbrückung von Nervenenddefekten in Kiefer- und Gesichtsbereich. Fortschr Kiefer Gesichtschir 20:118–120

10. Lang J (1981) Neuroanatomie der Nn. accessorius and hypoglossus. Arch Oto Rhino Laryngol 231:1–69
11. Müller-Vahl H, Schliack H (1982) Accessoriuslähmungen nach ärztlichen Eingriffen am Hals. Dtsch Arztebl 22:23–27
12. Müller-Vahl H (1983) Accessoriuslähmungen. Akt Neurol 10:18–23
13. Norden A (1946) Peripheral injuries to the spinal accessory nerve. Acta Chir Scand 94:515–532
14. Olarte M, Adams D (1977) Accessory nerve palsy. J Neurol Neurosurg Psychat 40:1113–1116
15. Penzholz H (1970) Läsionen des N. accessorius am Hals und ihre Behandlung. Therapiewoche 13:534–536
16. Samii M (1973) Interfaszikuläre autologe Nerventransplantation. Dtsch Arzteblatt 19:1257–1262
17. Samii M (1980) Fascicular peripheral nerve repair. Modern techniques in surgery, Neurosurgery, vol 17. Futura, Mount Kisco, NY
18. Samii M (1981) Operative treatment of accessory nerve lesions. In: Samii M, Jannetta (eds) The cranial nerves. Springer, Berlin Heidelberg New York
19. Sikken I, Höltje WJ, (1980) Die Rekonstruktion des Nervus Accessorius nach radikaler Neck dissection Dtsch. Z Mund Kiefer Gesichts Chir 4:36–39
20. Stearns MP, Shaeen OH (1981) Preservation of the accessory nerve in block dissection of the neck. J Laryngol Otol 95:1141–1148
21. Strelka J (1978) Anatomicke Variacie Nervus Accessorius Cesk Oto laryngol 27:222–226
22. Wright TA (1975) Accessory spinal nerve injuries. Clin Orthop 108:13–18

Results of Surgical Treatment of Meralgia Paresthetica

S. Mirzai[1], A. Sepehrnia[1], M. El Azm[1], G. Penkert[1], and M. Samii[1]

Introduction

Meralgia paresthetica, a common nerve entrapment syndrome [14], is an isolated disturbance of the sensation in the distribution area of the lateral femoral cutaneous nerve. This syndrome, characterized by pain, burning, tingling, numbness, and/or a variety of other paresthesias in the anterolateral area of the thigh, was first described by Bernhardt in 1895 [2] and named meralgia paresthetica by Roth in the same year [19]. Also in the same year, Sigmund Freud [7], who suffered from meralgia paresthetica, described his own affliction.

The purely sensory nerve is derived from the second and third lumbar root. The lateral femoral cutaneous nerve usually passes through and emerges from the lateral aspect of the psoas muscle as a single trunk which descends across the iliac muscle before turning toward the anterior superior iliac spine. It emerges through an opening in or behind the lateral attachment of the inguinal ligament at the anterior superior iliac spine. The nerve angulates sharply downward into the thigh just medial to the anterior superior iliac spine. It emerges medial to the origin of the sartorius muscle and pierces the fascia lata approximately 5 cm below the inguinal ligament [4, 14].

This report describes the results of the surgical treatment of 30 patients operated on in our department between 1978 and 1992. Nonsurgical and surgical management of meralgia paresthetica will be briefly discussed.

Clinical Material

Between 1978 and 1992 30 patients with meralgia paresthetica were operated on in our clinic. The female to male ratio was 2:1. Age of patients at the time of surgery ranged from 33 to 71 years (average ± SD 48.2 ± 9 years). The duration of the symptoms ranged from 1 month to 15 years with an average of 3.4 years. The disease affected the right side more often than the left side (21 and seven patients, respectively); bilateral cases were in the minority (two patients). Twenty-nine patients were available for the follow-up study.

The average postoperative follow-up period was 5.8 years. Four patients had a previous operation or trauma in the inguinal area on the same side.

---

[1] Neurochirurgische Klinik, Krankenhaus Nordstadt, Haltenhoffstr. 41, W-3000 Hannover, FRG.

Advances in Neurosurgery, Vol. 21
R. Lorenz, M. Klinger, M. Brock (Eds.)

Twenty-eight patients complained of pain, 13 of numbness. Neurological examination revealed hypesthesia in 25 patients, hypalgesia in ten patients and hyperpathia or dysesthesia in four. In at least 18 patients it was possible to reproduce the pain distribution by deep digital pressure just medial to the anterior superior iliac spine. The diagnosis was confirmed with the relief of pain obtained by injecting the nerve locally with an anesthetic agent. In atypical cases a disc prolapse, spinal stenosis, and neoplastic diseases of the spine or abdomen were excluded radiologically.

Treatment

If the diagnosis was confirmed and the patient did not improve with conservative treatment, surgical therapy was indicated. In 30 cases surgery was performed. With the patient under general anesthesia, a 4-cm oblique skin incision was performed parallel and 1 cm inferior to the lateral extent of the inguinal ligament (Fig. 1). The fascia lata was incised in the same direction. The nerve could be identified in most cases medial from the anterior superior iliac spine and the origin of the sartorius muscle and under the inguinal ligament (Fig. 2). Depending on the intraoperative findings, a local decompression (division of the upper margin of the ligament) and/or a neurolysis was performed. Only in one single case was the nerve sectioned. We have not performed rerouting procedures. We performed a neurolysis in four patients, local decompression in six patients and local decompression and

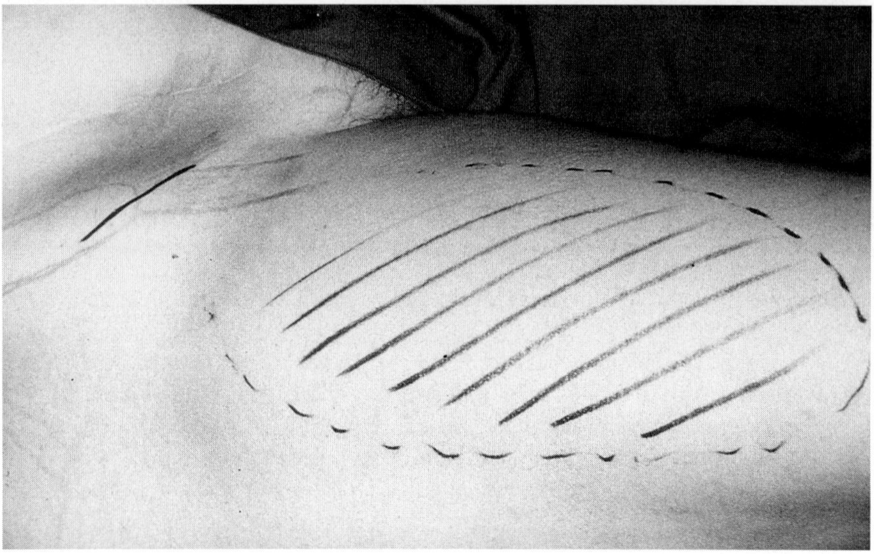

Fig. 1. Skin incision parallel and 1 cm inferior to the lateral attachment of the inguinal ligament on anterior superior iliac spine (*right*). The nerve can mostly be identified in the angle between the lateral part of the inguinal ligament and the sartorius muscle. The hypesthetic area on the thigh is marked

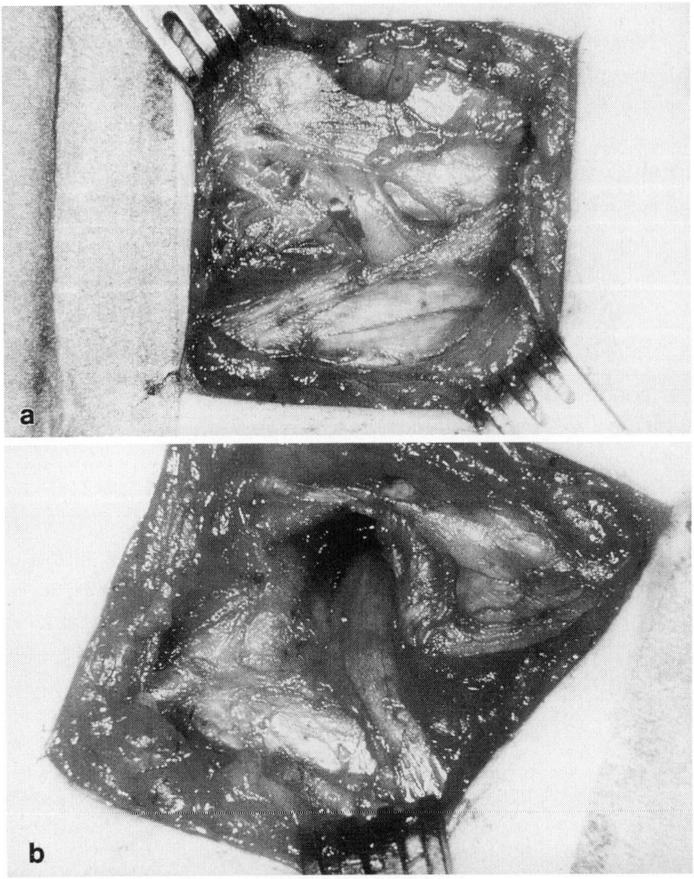

Fig. 2 Compression of the lateral femoral cutaneous nerve under the inguinal ligament (**a**). After partial division of the inguinal ligament and neurolysis the nerve is decompressed (**b**)

neurolysis in 18 patients. Only in one patient, who had had a previous local decompression without improvement of the symptoms, was the nerve resected within the scar tissue.

In four patients the nerve was found in scar tissue and was neurolysed. In one patient the nerve passed over the anterior superior iliac spine rather than medial to it and was compressed by the bone. In the remaining 25 patients the nerve appeared to pass through a split in the inguinal ligament at its attachment to the anterior superior iliac spine or under the inguinal ligament and was compressed there. In six patients a significant enlargement or pseudoganglion was present in the area of the nerve where it passed under the inguinal ligament.

Table 1. Results of surgery ($n = 29$)

Operation	Outcome Good (n)	Improved (n)	Recurrence (n)
Decompression and neurolysis	16	1	1
Decompression	1	3	2
Neurolysis	2	1	1
Section	–	1	–

Results

Immediately after the operation all patients were pain free. All patients were examined postoperatively, and a questionnaire was conceived for a further long-term, follow-up (average follow-up period 5.8 years). Nineteen patients remained symptom free. Six patients reported a significant improvement of the symptoms, only after prolonged walking or in extreme hip extension did they notice pain in the distribution area of the nerve.

At long-term follow-up we documented that four patients were again symptomatic a few months to years after surgery. In these cases we could not find any other underlying pathology responsible for the recurrence. Compared to other patients, these particular patients had had a significantly longer duration of symptoms and more previous operations with scarring in the inguinal region. In one the nerve was later sectioned and a clinical improvement resulted; the symptoms did not disappear totally, however. In another patient of this group, the nerve was sectioned later elsewhere, but this procedure also did not bring any relief (Table 1).

Discussion

Since the original descriptions of Bernhardt [2] and Roth [19] in 1895, many clinical reviews have been published on meralgia paresthetica [3, 9, 13, 14, 20, 22]. Controversy exists in the literature as to the etiology of the syndrome. Over 80 possible etiologies have been described [4]. It is often seen in obesity, during pregnancy, and after trauma or operations in the inguinal region. Familial occurrence [15], occupational causes, [8] and coexistence with spinal stenosis [10, 11] have been reported.

The correct diagnosis of meralgia paresthetica can be safely inferred in most cases from the patient's history alone. When a neuropathy is present, the region is extremely tender to deep palpation. Somatosensory evoked potentials are a useful tool to confirm a suspected diagnosis [6, 17]. A careful neurological, physical, and radiological examination is therefore required to rule out other causes such as spinal, intra-abdominal, and pelvic pathology or surgical procedures that may have involved the nerve [18, 20, 21].

Meralgia paresthetica is not a rare disease and it may be completely incapacitating.

Patients should be reassured that the affliction is benign and not symptomatic of a more serious neurological disorder [13]. In the early stages, conservative treatment is indicated, with attempts being made to eliminate obvious causes, e.g., removal of tight binders, braces, and corsets, and weight reduction [20]. The use of ice packs and injection of local anesthetic agents together with steroids can provide lasting relief [22]. Epidural injection of dexamethasone at the level L3/4 is described in the literature [10]. The use of transcutaneous electrical nerve stimulation (TENS) can be helpful during pregnancy [5].

Surgical therapy should only be resorted to in patients with persistent or severe pain, and only a minority of patients need surgical treatment [22]. The disease was first treated surgically by Hager in 1885 [12]. Since then different methods for surgical relief of meralgia paresthetica have been used with varying results. As an operative approach, the suprainguinal as well as infrainguinal ligament approaches are performed with good results [1, 9]. The operations available include: incision of the posterior band of the split ligament, incision of the thigh band of fascia iliaca, simple section of the nerve above or below the inguinal ligament, transposition of the nerve, and neurolysis [1, 9, 14, 21, 22]. Successes have been documented for each of these procedures. However, difficulty in identifying the nerve at operation and/or performing adequate decompression may lead to surgical failure. Sectioned nerves can produce annoying numbness in the region of sensory innervation and often develop painful neuromas that could be more troublesome than the meralgia [21]. In conclusion, the results of this study with its long follow-up period indicate that local decompression and neurolysis via the infrainguinal ligament approach is a good alternative to single procedures such as neurolysis, decompression, section, or transposition.

References

1. Aldrich EF, van den Heever CM (1989) Suprainguinal ligament approach for surgical treatment of meralgia paresthetica. J Neurosurg 70:492–494
2. Bernhardt M (1895) Ueber isoliert im Gebiete des N. cutaneus femoris externus vorkommende Parästhesien. Neurol Centralbl 14:242–244
3. Bollinger A (1961) Die Meralgia parasthetica: klinisches Bild und Pathogenese anhand von 158 eigenen Fällen. Schweiz Arch Neurol Psychiatr 87:58–102
4. Edelson JG, Nathan H (1977) Meralgia paresthetica. An anatomical interpretation. Clin Orthop 122:255–264
5. Fisher AP (1987) Transcutaneous electrical nerve stimulation in meralgia paraesthetica of pregnancy. Br J Obstet Gynaecol 94:603–604
6. Flügel KA, Sturm U, Skiba N (1984) Somatosensibel evozierte Potentiale nach Stimulation des N. cutaneus femoris lateralis bei Normalpersonen und Patienten mit Meralgia paraesthetica. Z EEG EMG 15:88–93
7. Freud S (1895) Ueber die Bernhardt'sche Sensibilitätsstörung am Oberschenkel. Neurol Centralbl 14:491–492
8. Garcia-Albea E, Palomo F, Tejeiro J, Cabrera F (1990) Occupational meralgia paresthetica. J Neurol Neurosurg Psychiatry 53:708

9. Ghent WR (1961) Further studies on meralgia paresthetica. Can Med Assoc J 85:871–875
10. Guo-Xiang J, Wei-Dong X (1988) Meralgia paraesthetica of spinal origin. J Bone Joint Surg [Br] 70:843–844
11. Guo-Xiang J, Wei-Dong X, Ai-Hao W (1988) Spinal stenosis with meralgia paraesthetica. J Bone Joint Surg [Br] 70:272–273
12. Hager W (1885) Neuralgia femoris, resection des Nerv. cutan. femoris anterior externus, Heilung. Dtsch Med Wochenschr 11:218–219
13. Jones RK (1974) Meralgia paresthetica as a cause of leg discomfort. Can Med Assoc J 111:541–542
14. Keegan JJ, Holyoke EA (1962) Meralgia paresthetica. An anatomical and surgical study. J Neurosurg 19:341–345
15. Malin JP (1979) Familial meralgia paresthetica with an autosomal dominant trait. J Neurol 221:133–136
16. Mumenthaler M, Schliack H (1987) Läsionen peripherer Nerven. Thieme, Stuttgart, pp 309–312
17. Riggs JE, Chamberlain SM, Gutierrez AR, Gutmann L (1986) Dermatomal somatosensory evoked potentials in meralgia paresthetica. Arch Neurol 43:1101–1102
18. Rinkel GJE, Wokke JHJ (1990) Meralgia paraesthetica as the first symptom of a metastatic tumor in the lumbar spine. 92:365–367
19. Roth WK (1985) Meralgia paraesthetica. Med Obozr (Moskau) 43:678
20. Stevens H (1957) Meralgia paresthetica. Arch Neurol Psychiatry 77:557–574
21. Sunderland S (1978) Nerves and nerve injuries. Churchill Livingstone, Edinburgh, pp 1007–1010
22. Williams PH, Terzil KP (1991) Management of meralgia paresthetica. J Neurosurg 74:76–80

Serum Neuron-Specific Enolase in Ischemic Brain Damage

M. Horn[1], W. Schlote[2], F. Seger[2], and G. Oremek[3]

Introduction

Neuron-specific enolase (NSE) represents the y,y isoenzyme of the dimeric protein enolase which is a soluble enzyme of the glycolytical pathway. Physiologically, NSE is specifically present in neuronal cytoplasm and dendrites, and in cells of the amine precursor uptake and decarboxylation (APUD) cell system [5]. Since patients suffering from APUDomas, neuroblastomas, or small cell carcinoma of the lung show elevated NSE titers in serum, NSE has been clinically established as a diagnostic and prognostic marker in such neoplasms [1, 5, 8]. However, recently obtained immunohistochemical findings of a decrease in neuronal NSE immunoreactivity in experimental animals and humans following transient cerebral ischemia suggested cytoplasmic NSE loss due to ischemia [3, 6]. Previous studies have shown intracellular compounds, especially NSE, to accumulate in the extracellular fluid and cerebrospinal fluid (CSF) after ischemia [7]. The present study was performed in order to clarify if neuronal NSE release in ischemic brain damage is accompanied by an increase of NSE levels in serum. Therefore, serum NSE was measured at various times after experimental transient forebrain ischemia followed by histological evaluation of ischemic neuronal damage.

Material and Methods

Forebrain ischemia was induced in adult Mongolian gerbils (*Meriones unguiculatus*) of either sex, 50–70 g in weight, by occlusion of both common carotid arteries (BCO). After induction of anesthesia with 2% halothane in 70% nitrogen and 30% oxygen, a midline skin incision was made and both commoncarotid arteries were exposed. BCO was performed by the use of Biemer clips (FD 562, Aesculap). After 5 min ($n = 30$) or 15 min ($n = 30$), respectively, brains were recirculated spontaneously by removal of clips. After suturing of the skin incision, animals were allowed to survive for 8 h, 12 h, 24 h, 48 h, 72 h, or 96 h, respectively. Blood sam-

[1] Neurologisches Institut (Edinger-Institut), Universität Frankfurt, Deutschordenstr. 46, W-6000 Frankfurt/M. 71, FRG.
[2] Neurochirurgische Klinik, Universität Würzburg, Josef-Schneider-Str. 11, W 8700 Würzburg, FRG.
[3] Abteilung Klinische Chemie, Universität Frankfurt, Deutschordenstr. 46, W-6000 Frankfurt/M. 71, FRG.

Advances in Neurosurgery, Vol. 21
R. Lorenz, M. Klinger, M. Brock (Eds.)

ples were taken by transdiaphragmatic puncture. Serum NSE was measured using an enzyme immunoassay technique (Roche) in nonischemic controls, in sham-operated animals, and in both ischemic groups prior to transcardiac perfusion fixation. Histologically, paraffin-embedded coronal brain sections including the dorsal hippocampus (1.4–1.7 mm posterior to the bregma) were investigated with regard to stigmata of ischemic neuronal damage. In each case, the density of unaffected selective vulnerable CA1 neurons was evaluated by morphometrical measurement.

Results

Sham-Operated and Normal Control Animals. Brains of sham-operated animals ($n = 12$) showed absence of ischemic neuronal damage and normal neuronal density in hippocampus CA1. In both sham-operated animals and nonischemic controls ($n = 20$) NSE serum titers were below 10 μg/ml (mean ± standard deviation: 6.16 ± 2.63).

Five-Minute BCO. Brief forebrain ischemia resulted in an average increase of NSE serum levels to about the threefold of control within 24-h of reperfusion (mean ± standard deviation: 19.0 ± 4.5 ng/ml). A slow decrease was observed between 72 h and 96 h following ischemia (Fig. 1). On the other hand, ischemic cell

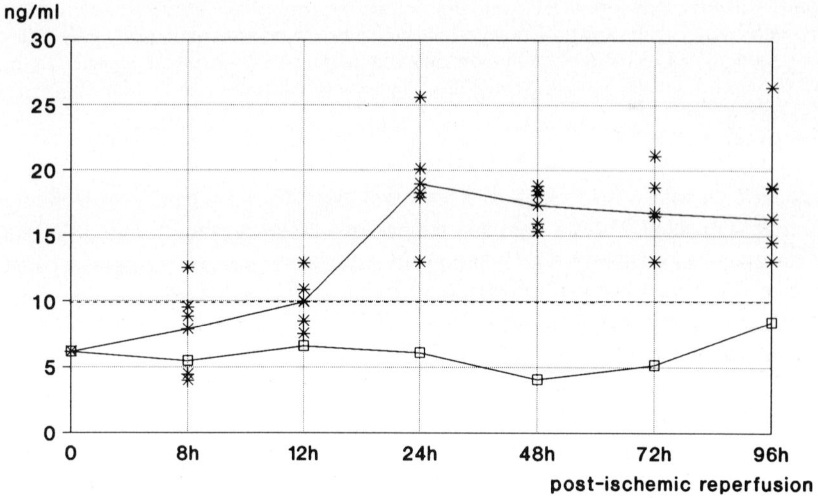

Fig. 1. Time course of NSE serum levels in gerbils submitted to 5 min bilateral carotid occlusion *(asterisks)* or in sham-operated controls (*squares*), respectively. Each item represents an individual value (*asterisk*) or the mean of two animals (*square*). NSE serum titers in both nonischemic and sham-operated animals were 6.16 ± 2.63 ng/ml. Therefore the value of 10.0 ng/ml was regarded as the upper limit of normal range. At 24 h, 48 h, 72 h, and 96 h levels of serum NSE in ischemic animals were significantly different from control, whereas maximal levels were detected 24 h post ischemia

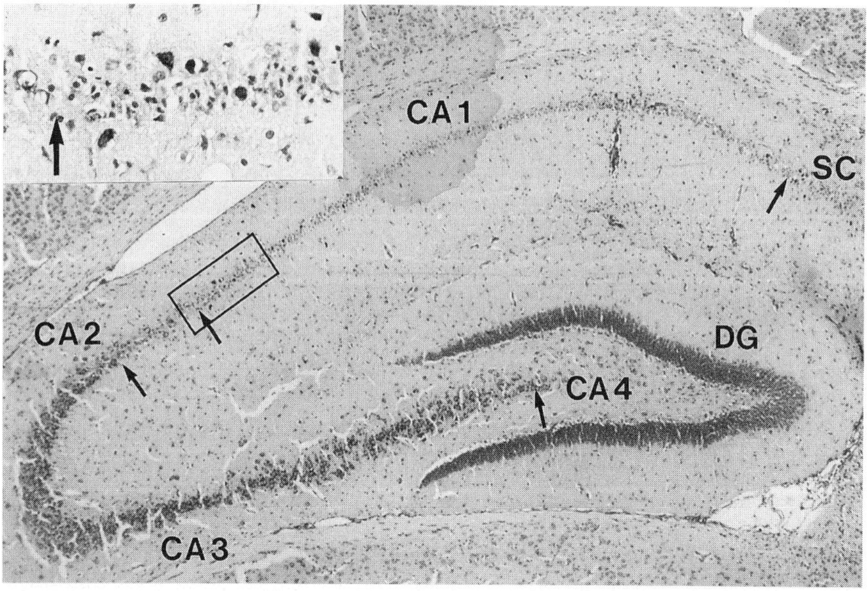

Fig. 2. Low-power microphotograph showing the dorsal hippocampus of the Mongolian gerbil 96 h following 5 min forebrain ischemia. Approximated borders of subfields CA1, CA2, CA3, and CA4 are indicated by *arrows* (*SC*, subiculum; *DG*, dentate gyrus). Definite manifestation of the ischemic lesion is restricted to the selectively vulnerable CA1 subfield which is subtotally destroyed. The border region between CA1 and CA2 is marked by a *rectangle* which is shown in detail at high-power microscopy at the *upper left*. Most CA1 pyramidal cells are pyknotic accompanied by perineuronal microvacuolation. Only a few neurons show minor ischemic alteration and, therefore, are not irreversibly damaged. On the very *left*, morphologically well-preserved CA2 neurons are shown. Cresyl violet stain, 1:80 or 1:300 (inset)

change first became visible 24 h post ischemia and was restricted to selectively vulnerable hippocampal CA1 neurons. Neuronal necrosis appeared after 48 h and was completed by 96 h survival, resulting in subtotal destruction of the CA1 cell layer (Fig. 2). Thus, a significant diminution of histologically unaffected neurons was observed after 48 h post-ischemic reperfusion.

Fifteen-Minute BCO. In animals submitted to severe forebrain ischemia, NSE serum titers were already elevated by 8 h survival (mean ± standard deviation: 15.2 ± 3.6 ng/ml). Within 48 h reperfusion a striking increase of serum NSE occurred (mean ± standard deviation: 132.4 ± 44.2 ng/ml). Levels decreased by 72 h survival, but were significantly elevated even after 96 h (Fig. 3). Following 24 h survival, histology of the hippocampal subfield CA1 showed a progressive reduction in neuronal density. In contrast to brains of the 5 min BCO group, the majority of animals submitted to 15 min BCO revealed ischemic brain lesions extending to the whole hippocampus inconstantly involving CA3 neurons (Fig. 4).

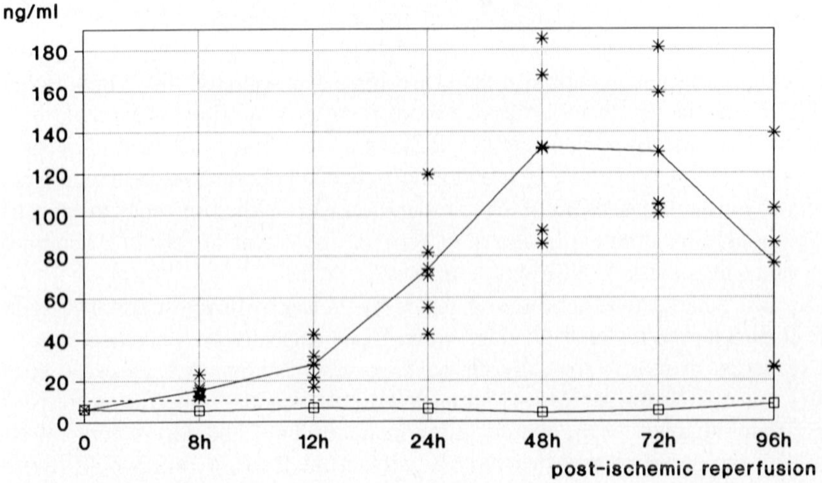

Fig. 3. Time course of NSE serum levels in gerbils submitted to 15 min bilateral carotid occlusion *(asterisks)* or in sham-operated controls (*squares*), respectively, Each item represents an individual value (*asterisk*) or the mean of two animals (*square*). Significantly higher levels were found in ischemic animals than in controls as early as 8 h following ischemia. Maximal values were detected at 48 h and 72 h. Levels were significantly elevated even by 96 h survival

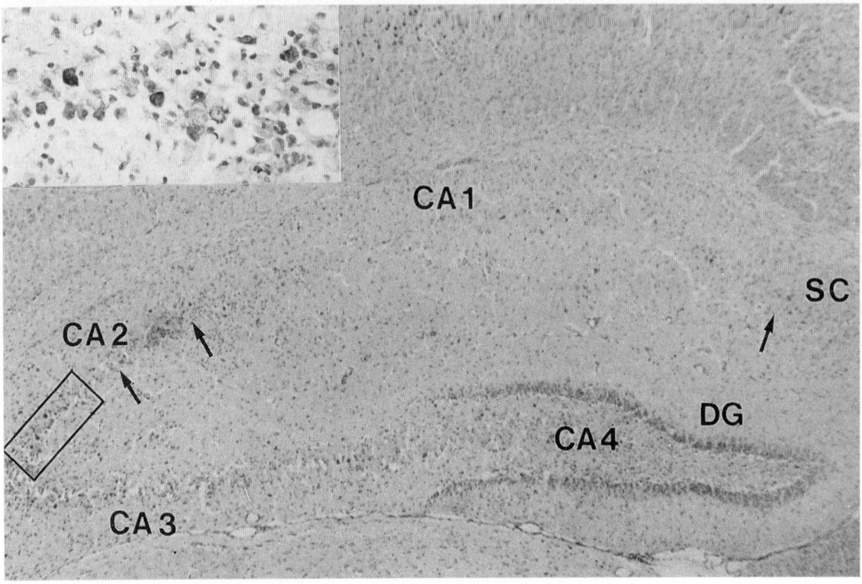

Fig. 4. Fifteen-minute forebrain ischemia followed by 96 h survival result in neuronal lesions extending to the whole hippocampus. The CA1 subfield is completely destroyed, whereas the majority of neurons in CA2 and CA4 show ischemic neuronal necrosis. Even relatively resistant CA3 subfield and granule cells of the dentate gyrus (*DG*) are involved in the ischemic lesion. Part of CA3 is marked by a *rectangle* and shown in detail at high-power microscopy at the upper *left*. Microvacuolation of the CA3 cell layer and subtotal loss of neurons are found. *SC*, subiculum. Cresyl violet stain, 1:80 or 1:300 (*inset*)

Discussion

Numerous experimental studies in the gerbil have demonstrated that 5 min global cerebral ischemia reproducibly causes necrosis only in selective vulnerable hippocampal CA1 neurons [4]. Therefore, BCO of 5 min duration seemed to be suitable for testing the sensitivity of monitoring ischemic brain lesions by serum NSE detection. Furthermore, BCO of 15 min duration was applied in order to investigate a possible quantitative relationship between the extent of resulting neuronal injury and a hypothesized NSE serum increase.

Elevated NSE serum titers were detected by 24 h reperfusion following 5 min BCO or by 8 h reperfusion following 15 min BCO, respectively, whereas a significant reduction of morphologically unsuspicious CA1 neurons was observed after 48 h (5 min BCO) or after 24 h (15 min BCO) post-ischemic reperfusion, respectively. Data obtained by the present study including brief and severe cerebral ischemia in the gerbil clearly indicate a significant increase of serum NSE levels prior to relevant changes within hippocampal neuronal density. Defects of the neuronal plasma membrane related to ischemia obviously cause release of cytoplasmic NSE into the neuropil. Accumulation of NSE in the CSF and ischemia-induced disruption of the blood-brain barrier finally result in an increase of NSE levels in serum. This pathophysiological concept is supported by immunohistochemical findings of cytoplasmic *NSE diminution* in both gerbil and human following cerebral ischemia [3, 6]. On the other hand, experimental findings in rat CSF following four-vessel occlusion and clinical data on CSF in patients with stroke indicate *increased NSE levels* [2, 7].

As elevation of NSE serum levels preceded ischemic neuronal necrosis in the gerbil hippocampus, it is expected that measurement of serum NSE could be a valuable tool in clinical detection of early ischemic brain damage. Especially global cerebral ischemia, i.e., patients resuscitated from cardiac arrest, is suggested to be accompanied by elevated NSE serum titers. Moreover, serum NSE detection may be useful as a tool in diagnosis and as a predictor of outcome in neuronal injury of different etiology such as stroke, vasospasm due to subarachnoid hemorrhage, or even craniocerebral trauma. Suitable clinicopathological studies are needed to confirm the present experimental findings of post-ischemic NSE serum changes in the human.

References

1. Cooper EH (1985) Neuron specific enolase a marker of (small cell) cancers of neuronal and neuroendocrine origin. Biomed Pharmacother 39:165–166
2. Hay E, Royds JA, Aelwyn G, Davies-Jones B, Lewtas NA, Timperly WR, Taylor CB (1984) Cerebrospinal fluid enolase in stroke. J Neurol Neurosurg Psychiatry 47:724–729
3. Horn M, Lang C, Schlote W (1991) Delayed neuronal death caused by cardiac arrest in man. Clin Neuropathol 10:270
4. Kirino T, Sano K (1984) Selective vulnerability in the gerbil hippocampus following transient ischemia. Acta Neuropathol (Berl) 62:201–208

5. Marangos PJ (1991) Neuron specific enolase as a clinical tool in neurologic and endocrine deseases. In: Gratzl M, Langley K (eds) Markers of neural and endocrine cells. VCH, Weinheim, pp 181–189
6. Matsumoto M, Yamamoto K, Homburger HA, Yanagihara T (1987) Early detection of cerebral ischemic damage and repair process in the gerbil by use of an immunohistochemical technique. Mayo Clin Proc 62:460–472
7. Steinberg R, Gueniau C, Scarna H, Keller A, Worcel M, Pujol JF (1984) Experimental brain ischemia: neuron-specific enolase level in cerebrospinal fluid as an index of neuronal damage. J Neurochem 43:19–24
8. Wielders JPM, Bartels CT, Bank CMC, Meek JCE, van Dieijen-Visser MP, Brombacher PJ (1991) The diagnostic value of neuron-specific enolase and carcino-embryonic antigen analyses in patients with carcinoma of the lung. J Clin Chem Biochem 28:225–231

Preliminiary Experience with Three-Dimensional Magnetic Resonance Angiography in the Identification of Intracranial Aneurysms

G. Siepmann[1], F. E. Zanella[1], N. Freckmann[1], and J. Bunke[1]

Introduction

The development of magnetic resonance angiography (MRA) during recent years led to a new, noninvasive method of imaging blood vessels [1, 2, 4]. Previous reports demonstrated the possibility of studying the anatomy and pathology of intracranial vasculature using a three-dimensional gradient-echo sequence (3D-MRA) [5, 6, 8, 10]. This technique can be used in addition to routine MR studies of the brain parenchyma without administration of contrast agents. The examination time varies between 7 and 12 min depending on the number of partitions. The purpose of this study was to determine sensitivity and specificity of 3D-MRA in comparison with intraarterial digital subtraction angiography (IADSA).

Material and Methods

Fifteen patients suffering from intracranial aneurysm were studied by IADSA and MRA within the last 6 months. The aneurysms were located in the internal carotid artery ($n = 5$), the middle cerebral artery ($n = 4$), the ophthalmic artery ($n = 2$), the vertebral artery ($n = 2$), the basilar artery ($n = 1$), and the posterior communicating artery ($n = 1$). Six of these patients were examined because of a subarachnoid hemorrhage, five revealed signs and symptoms of mass effect, and four demonstrated aneurysms incidentally shown on computed tomographic scans. There were four giant intracranial aneurysms, three located in the internal carotid artery and one at the tip of the basilar artery.

Magnetic resonance imaging was performed with a 0.5 Tesla system (Gyroscan, Philips) using a circular polarized head coil. At first routine spin-echo (SE) MR imaging of the brain was performed with multiecho T2-weighted axial (TR/TE = 2000/30100 ms) and T1-weighted axial (TR/TE = 500/30 ms) pulse sequences. The MRA examination based on a FFE 3D inflow sequence with low flip angle (TR/TE = 33/9 ms, flip 20°, field of view 230 mm). The volume slab was oriented axially to cover the circle of Willis, and we chose imaging volumes with 64 partitions ranging in thickness from 1.0 to 1.2 mm. Imaging time was 7.15 min for 64 partitions. Afterwards datasets were reconstructed on a Sun-based worksta-

[1] Abteilung Neuroradiologie, Universitätskrankenhaus Eppendorf, Martinistr. 52, W-2000 Hamburg, FRG.

Advances in Neurosurgery, Vol. 21
R. Lorenz, M. Klinger, M. Brock (Eds.)

tion (Gyroview, Philips) by means of a ray-tracing technique which incorporates a maximal intensity projection for better details. All patients underwent IADSA (Polytron, Siemens), which included anteroposterior, lateral, and oblique views.

Results

There was a good correlation between MRA and IADSA in 11 of 15 patients with intracranial aneurysms (Figs. 1–4). However, aneurysms smaller than 5 mm could not be detected by MRA. Examination of the four giant aneurysms showed that the slow flow part was poorly visualized. Furthermore, it was difficult to differentiate turbulences from thrombotic material in aneurysm. In five patients MRA was unable to identify the neck of the aneurysm and to demonstrate the relationship of the aneurysm to smaller vessels in the neighborhood. In patients suffering from subarachnoidal hemorrhage ($n = 6$), structures characterized by short T1, such as older coagulated blood, also appeared bright in MRA.

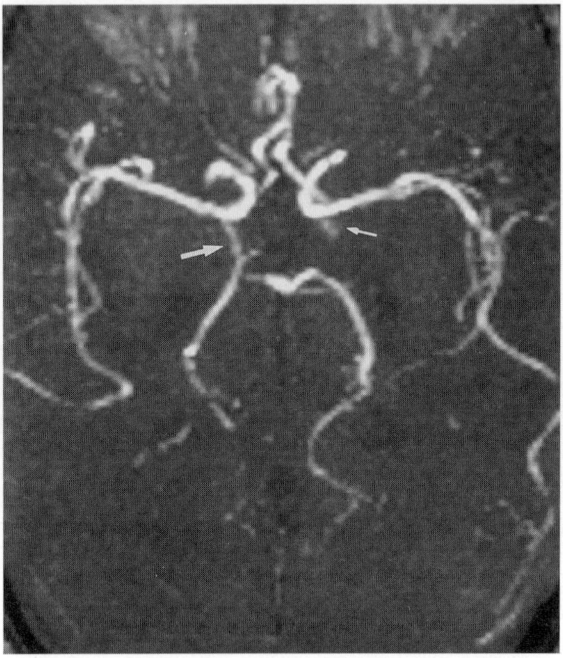

Fig. 1. Three-dimensional MRA at the level of the circle of Willis demonstrates a small aneurysm of the left posterior communicating artery (*small arrow*). Good visualization of the right posterior communicating artery (*large arrow*)

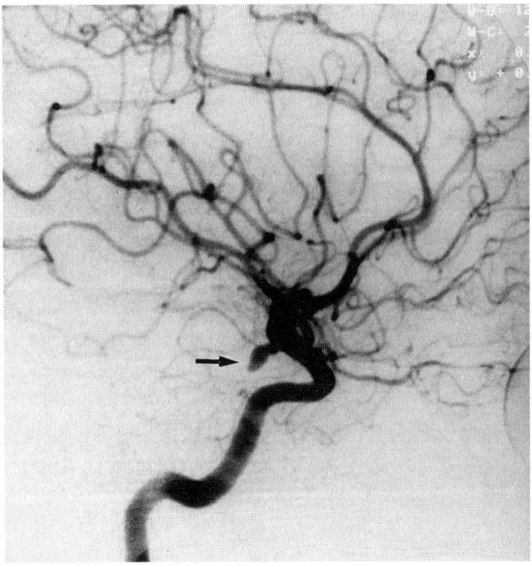

Fig. 2. Same patient as in Fig. 1: corresponding IADSA study

Discussion

Development of a gradient-echo 3D volume MRA technique leads to accurate, reproducible images of the intracranial circulation. This method can be used in addition to traditional SE sequences. The advantages of MRA include noninvasiveness and the ability to manipulate data, especially when 3D acquisitions have been obtained and multiple reconstructions in different planes can be done. The main disadvantage of this technique was the nonvisualization of aneurysms smaller than 5 mm. Additional problems and limitations of MRA were demonstrated in the four cases of giant aneurysms. The slowly flowing part in these aneurysms was poorly visualized owing to the saturation of the moving spins residing for too long within the excited volume. This is one of the reasons why the size of these aneurysms is underestimated in MRA. Another difficulty is the differentiation between turbulences and thrombotic material within the aneurysm. Both lead to signal loss and only a combination of MRA and conventional MR imaging of the brain allows a correct diagnosis [6, 7, 9]. The limitation of resolution in MRA leads to a nonidentification of the aneurysm neck and smaller vessels in the neighborhood in some cases. At the present time, important information in the preoperation planning of intracerebral aneurysms cannot be solved by MRA alone. The sensitivity and specifity of conventional angiography is still superior and cannot be replaced by MRA in these cases.

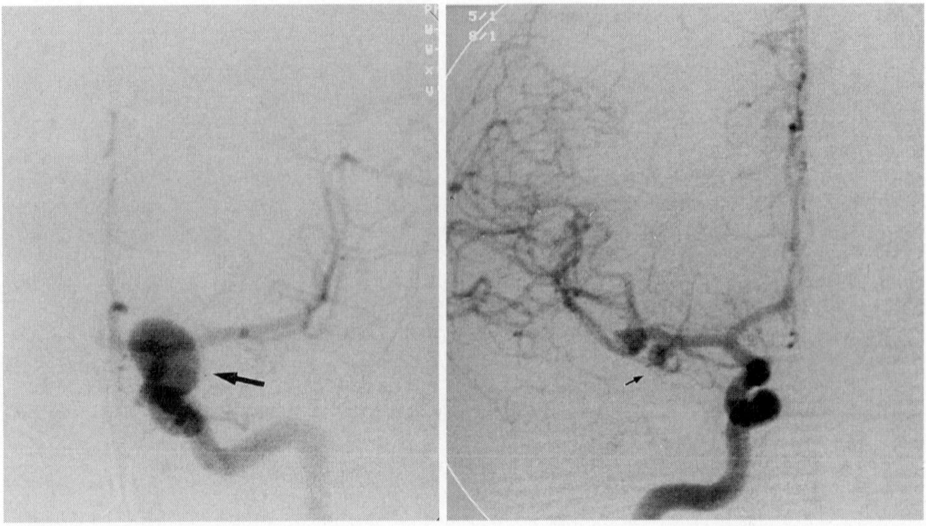

Fig. 3. Conventional angiography reveals a large aneurysm of the left carotid artery (*large arrow*). A smaller aneurysm in the right M1 segment of the middle cerebral artery (*small arrow*) is seen as an incidental finding

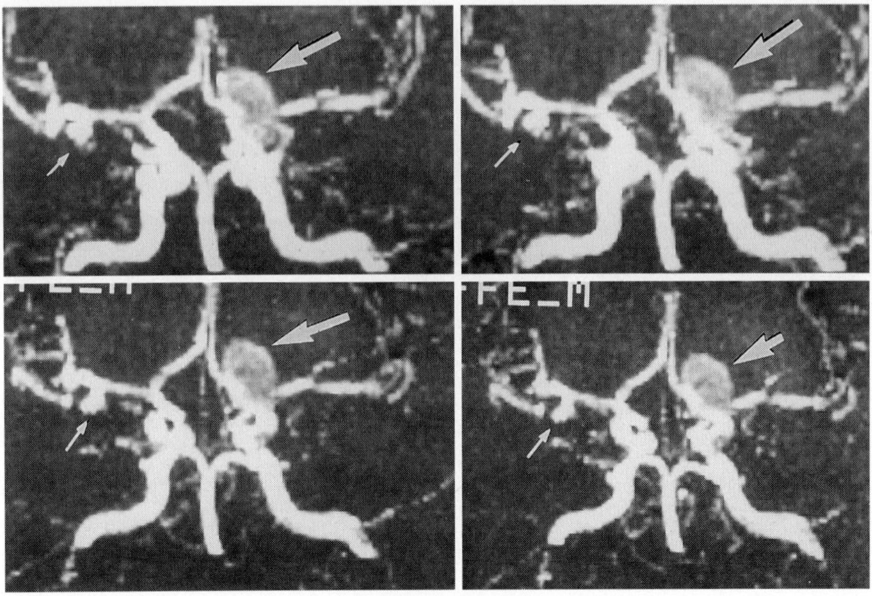

Fig. 4. MRA is also able to demonstrate both aneurysms (*large arrows,* aneurysm of the left carotid artery: *small arrow,* aneurysm of the middle cerebral artery)

References

1. Dumoulin CL, Hart HR (1986) Magnetic resonance angiography. Radiology 161:717–720
2. Edelmann RR, Mattle HP, Atkinson DJ et al. (1990) MR angiography. AJR Am J Roentgenol 154:937–946
3. Gustorf-Aeckerle R, Kraft R, Volle E et al. (1992) 3D-MR-Angiographie zur Aneurysmadiagnostik bei akuter SAB. Klin Neuroradiol 2:1–5
4. Laub GA, Kaiser WA (1988) MR angiography with gradient motion refocussing. J Comput Assist Tomogr 12(3):378–382
5. Masaryk TJ, Modic MT, Ross JS et al. (1989) Intracranial circulation: preliminary clinical results with three dimensional volume MR angiography. Radiology 171:793–799
6. Masaryk TJ, Modic MT, Ruggieri DM et al. (1989) Three dimensional (volume) gradient echo imaging of the carotid bifurcation: preliminary clinical experience. Radiology 171:801–806
7. Olsen WL, Brant-Zawadzki M, Hodes J et al. (1987) Giant intracranial aneurysms. MR imaging. Radiology 163:431–435
8. Ostertun B, Gieseke J, Steudel A et al. (1990) Klinische Anwendung der MR-Angiographie mit 2D und 3D Inflow-Techniken. Röntgenstrahlen 64:14
9. Ross GS, Masaryk TJ, Modic MT et al. (1990) Intracranial aneurysm: evaluation by MR angiography. AJNR 11:449–455
10. Ruggieri PM, Laub GA, Masaryk TJ et al. (1989) Intracranial circulation: pulse-sequence considerations in three-dimensional (volume) MR-angiography. Radiology 171:785–791

Transarticular C1–C2 Screw Fixation Combined with Fusion of the Craniocervical Junction in Arthritic Patients

A. Montazem[1], J. Schalm[2], and W. Tressel[3]

Introduction

In arthritic patients with involvement of the cervical spine and atlantoaxial instability, treatment is usually by fusion of C1 and C2 with a cerclage [10]. The selection of patients for surgery is usually based on the extent of atlanto-dens mobility. Magnetic resonance imaging (MRI) of the craniocervical junction further clarifies the indication for surgery [1, 4]. Even when there seems to be no major instability, the spinal canal of the upper cervical spine is often narrowed by proliferated connective tissue and rheumatic pannus around the dens and atlas [2, 6, 9]. MRI will demonstrate the presence of such alterations and thus confirm the indication for surgery. The stabilizing procedures (C1, C2 cerclage) used up to now failed to produce satisfactory results because they leave the two vertebrae fixed in only one plane of motion. By combining two surgical procedures we attempt to obtain three-dimensional stability.

Methods

For stabilization in all three planes of motion we use transarticular C2–C1 screw fixation (from the arch of C2 into the lateral mass of C1 on both sides) in combination with traditional occipitocervical fusion with an interposed autogenic bone graft. Screw fixation has the advantage that it allows immediate intraoperative reduction and fixation of the C1–C2 joint even if the arch of the atlas is eroded.

Since subsequent MRI follow-ups are required [1], we have developed titanium compression screws with titanium washers to ensure undisturbed imaging postoperatively.

For the stabilization of the upper cervical spine in the vertical plane (atlantoaxial impaction), we perform a fusion from CO to C2 using a corticocancellous iliac crest graft. With a titanium wire cerclage the graft is tightly fixed to the occiput, C1, and C2. Additional cancellous bone is packed on both sides of the

[1] Abteilung Neurochirurgie, Zentralklinikum Augsburg, Stenglinstr., W-8900 Augsburg, FRG.
[2] Klinik für Medizinische Rheumatologie, Zentralklinikum Augsburg, Stenglinstr., W-8900 Augsburg, FRG.
[3] Hessingsche orthopädische Kliniken, Zentrum für orthopädische Rheumatologie und Rehabilitation, Hessingstr. 17, W-8900 Augsburg, FRG.

Advances in Neurosurgery, Vol. 21
R. Lorenz, M. Klinger, M. Brock (Eds.)

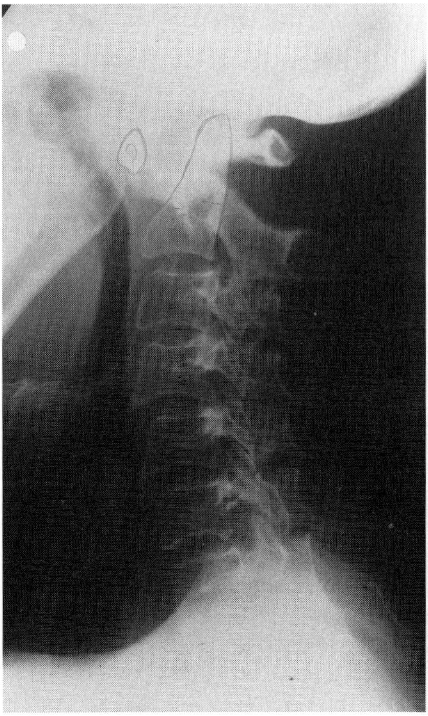

Fig. 1. Horizontal instability

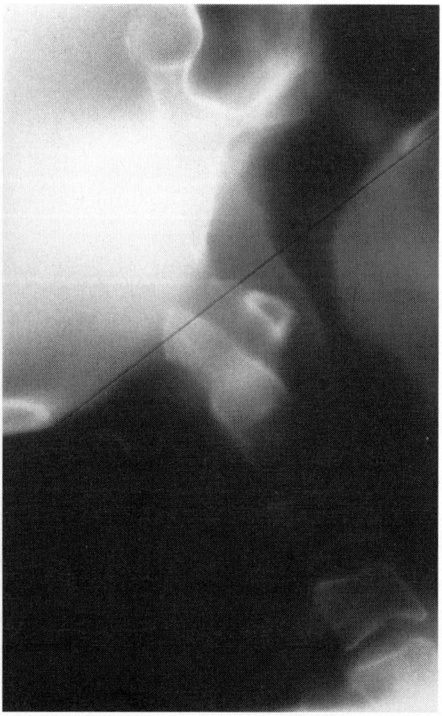

Fig. 2. Vertical instability (atlantoaxial impaction)

3 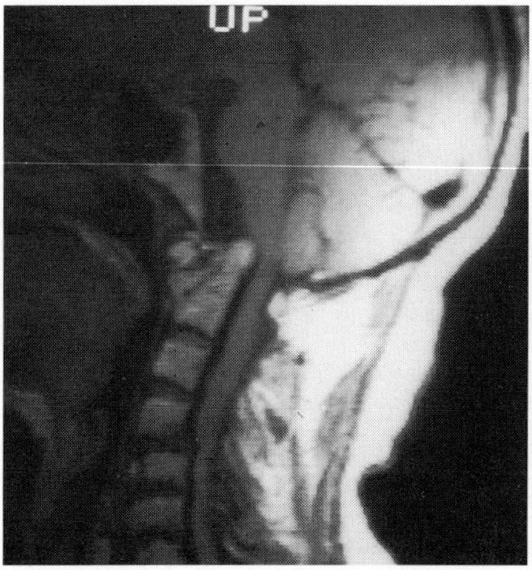

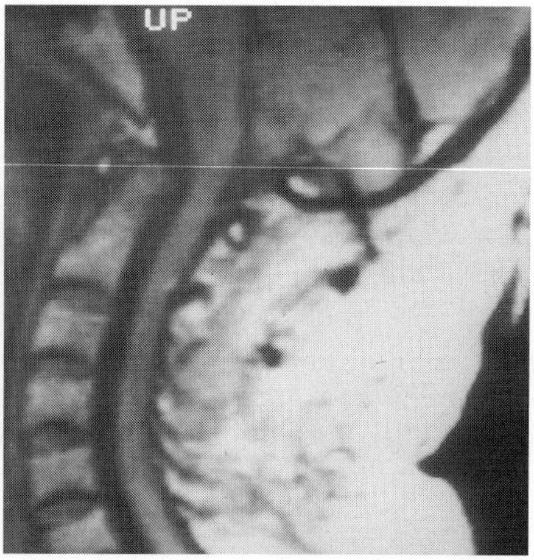 4

Fig. 3. Preoperative MRI – compression of cervical cord due to thickening of the atlanto-dens joint

Fig. 4. Postoperative MRI – no artefact with titanium compression screws

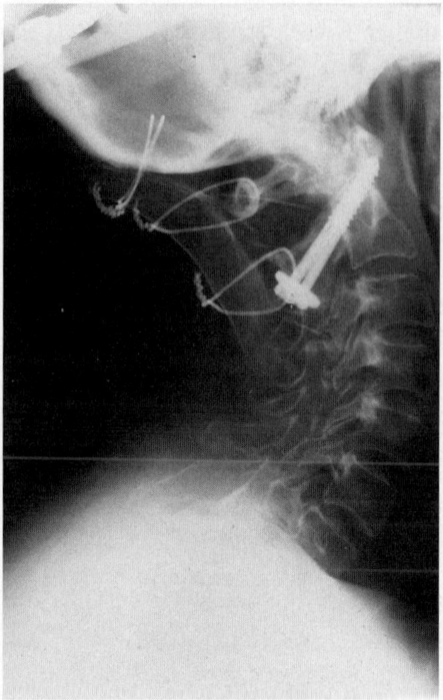

Fig. 5. Transarticular C2–C1 screw fixation combined with C0–C3 fusion

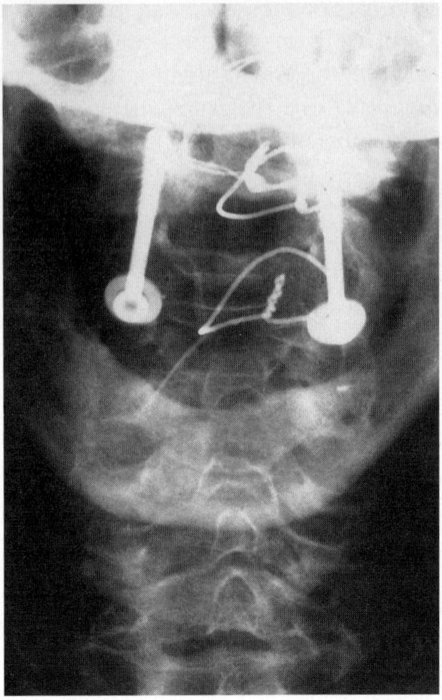

Fig. 6. AP view

full thickness graft. Postoperatively, the patient is fully mobilized following application of a halo orthosis, which is removed after 5 weeks, at the earliest, and not without a radiographic checkup [2, 5–7, 11].

Results and Patient Population

In the past 5 years we operated on 64 arthritic patients with severe deformity and various patterns of cervical spine instability. In 21 patients occipitocervical fusion (C0, C1, C2) with autogenic bone graft and wire cerclage was performed alone. Since March 1989 we have additionally performed transarticular screw fixation of C1 and C2 in a total of 43 patients.

Regular follow-ups revealed no recurrence of the instability. After surgery, no atlantoaxial impaction was seen to develop or, if already pre-existing, to progress. MRI checkups were possible only in the patients operated after March 1991; that was the time that we started to use titanium screws.

Discussion: Merits and Drawbacks of this Method as Against Other Surgical Procedures

For the operator performing a transarticular C1, C2 screw fixation, it is important to aim at the lateral mass of C1 at a correct angle between vertebral artery, C2, root and dural sac. Drilling in the squamous part of the occipital bone may result in an opening of the dura, and subsequently a CSF fistula may form. Because of the potential of subsequent hemorrhage at the occiput, the possibility of a surgical revision of the posterior fossa must be accommodated [6]. The average length of the procedure of 2.5 hours is considerably more than that of a simple C1, C2 wire cerclage [6].

Apart from superficial wound healing disorders in five patients, we observed no complications in our patients. Compromised C2 roots or circulatory disorders of the vertebral artery were not seen.

The merit of this rather complex procedure is that it allows immediate stabilization in all three planes of motion [3]. In the patients treated with transarticular screw fixation so far there has been neither the development of an atlantoaxial impaction nor a recurrence of instability. Simple wire cerclage, however, is rather frequently associated with a recurrence of instability due to fracture of the arch of C1, particulary when the arch is already eroded [4–6].

Conclusion and Summary

A total of 64 patients with instability of the upper cervical spine due to rheumatoid arthritis required surgical treatment. Using transarticular C1, C2 screw fixation combined with occipitocervical fusion a three-dimensional stabilization of the upper cervical spine is achieved. This method offers considerable advantages over the commonly used C1, C2 wire cerclage. All patients were subjected to regular follow-ups, which revealed no recurrence of instability.

References

1. Brattstroem H (1986) Die Halswirbelsäule bei Polyarthritis. Radiologie, Indikationen zur Operation und Ergebnisse. Orthopade 15 (4):291–296
2. Goldi I (1984) A synopsis of surgery for rheumatoid arthritis (excluding the hand). Clin Orthop 191:185–192
3. Kankaanpaeae U, Santavirta S (1985) Cervical spine involvement in rheumatoid arthritis. Ann Chir Gynaecol Suppl 198:117–121
4. Kirk AP, Patel U, Phillips H, Cardoe N (1987) Cervical myelopathy complicating multiple joint replacement in rheumatoid disease. Br J Rheumatol 26(4):275–278
5. Lesoin F, Combelles G, Bouasakao N, Cama A, Delandsheer JM, Jomin MA (1984) Use of acrylic prosthesis in cervical spina pathology (report of 45 cases). Acta Neurochir (Wien) 71(1–2):141–149
6. Lesoin F, Duquesnoy B, Destee A, Leys D, Rousseaux M, Carini S, Verier A, Jomin M (1985) Cervical neurological complications of rheumatoid arthritis. Surgical treatment, techniques and indications. Acta Neurochir (Wien) 78(3–4):91–97
7. Lesoin F, Jomin M, Pellerin P, Pruvo JP, Carini S, Servato R, Rousseaux M (1986) Transclival transcervical approach to the upper cervical spine and clivus. Acta Neurochir (Wien) 80(3–4):100–104
8. Lipson SJ (1989) Rheumatoid arthritis in the cervical spine. Clin Orthop 239:121–127
9. Santavirta S, Sandelin J, Slaetis P (1985) Posterior atlanto-axial subluxation in rheumatoid arthritis. Acta Orthop Scand 56(4):298–301
10. Schleich A, Albrecht HJ, Nusselt L, Rave O, Weller E, Westerburg KW (1985) Zur Risikobeurteilung occipito-cervicaler Dislokation bei entzündlich-rheumatischen Krankheiten. Z Rheumatol 44(3):120–132
11. Swann M (1983) Surgical treatment of the cervical spine in rheumatoid arthritis. Ann Acad Med Singapore 12(2):233–242

Strategy of Endovascular Treatment of Mixed Plexiform and Fistulous Intracranial Arteriovenous Malformations

H. C. Nahser[1] and D. Kühne[1]

In the endovascular treatment of cerebral arteriovenous malformations, which in the majority of cases is performed preoperatively or before radiosurgery, those angiomas in which direct fistulas are combined with more plexiform elements within the nidus have a special importance. When an embolization is performed using polymerizing fluids, there is the danger that they may pass the nidus through the fistula and block the venous outlet of the angioma. The sudden change of hemodynamics may lead to severe hemorrhagic complications. After a careful selective analysis by means of microcatheterization of the different feeding vessels, the direct fistulas should first be eliminated by particular substances of suitable size.

Patients

In 15 cases out of 116 patients treated for large complex cerebral arteriovenous malformations, this constellation was found in superselective angiography. The fistulous components were blocked in several stages. In three patients the direct fistulas were occluded with a latex balloon, which was mounted on a tracker catheter. The system was advanced to the exact anatomical location of the arteriovenous fistula, filled with isotonic contrast media, and then detached. In one patient with several larger fistulas, one was occluded with a balloon and the remaining fistulas with coils. In the other 12 patients coils were used exclusively to achieve an exact occlusion of the fistula site. This was followed by embolization of the feeders of plexiform compartments with liquids (bucrylate). In one patient there was a complete obliteration of the angioma as visualized by angiography and nuclear magnetic resonance (NMR). In all other cases with remaining nidus, consecutive surgery or radiosurgery was instituted. As a complication 1 h after balloon occlusion of a broad fistulous connection, we recorded in one patient a parietal lobar hematoma manifesting initially with complete hemiparesis and aphasia. After reabsorption of the hematoma no neurological sequela persisted. In the case of a young woman in whom the angioma had manifested with seizures and in whom coils were selected for closure of a single large fistula within the nidus, we recorded an initial migration of two coils to the main draining hemispherical vein of the angioma. Choosing larger coils which kept their position, the fistula was

[1] Abteilung für Neuroradiologie, Alfried-Krupp-Krankenhaus, Alfried-Krupp-Str. 21, W-4300 Essen, FRG.

Advances in Neurosurgery, Vol. 21
R. Lorenz, M. Klinger, M. Brock (Eds.)

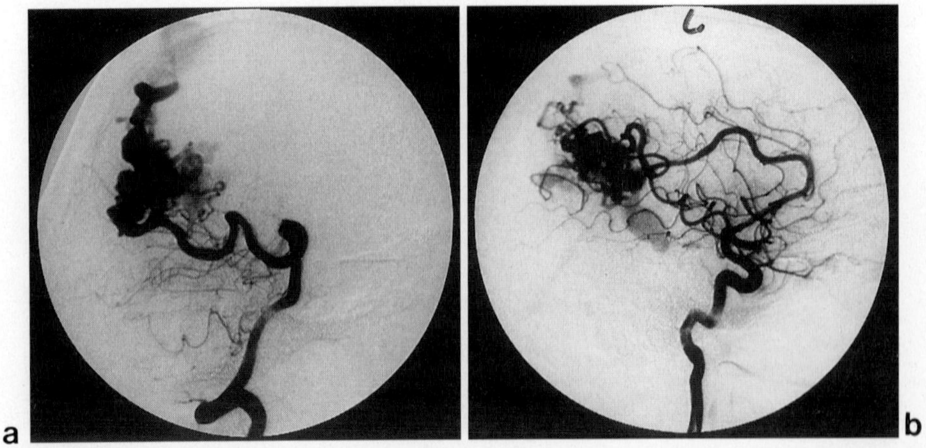

Fig. 1a,b. The parietal angioma in this 29-year-old woman was symptomatic with seizures. Main feeding branches were recruited from the posterior cerebral (**a**) and the anterior cerebral artery (**b**)

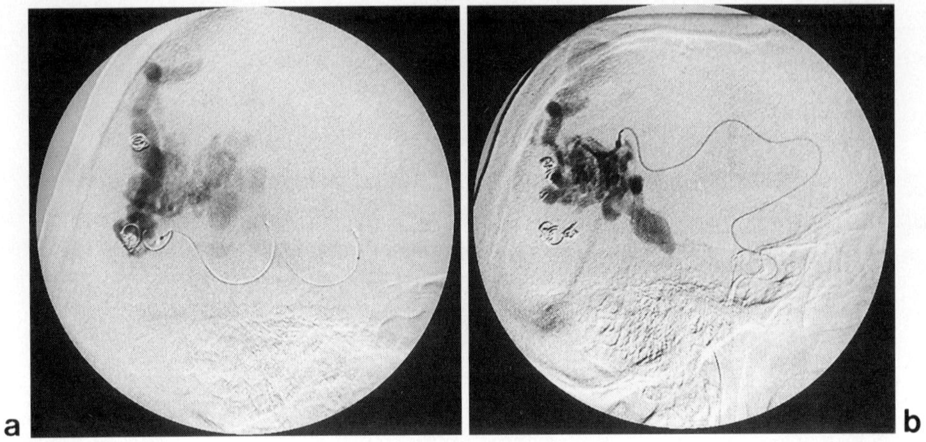

Fig. 2a,b. Microcatheterization and superselective angiography disclosed the fistulous parietooccipital posterior branch (**a**) and the more plexiform pericalosal branch (**b**). The fistula site was occluded with several coils, but two coils, which had been too small, were lost into the single main draining vein but did not lead to an obstruction of the venous outlet (**a**). In the next step embolization of the plexiform compartment was performed with bucrylate (**b**)

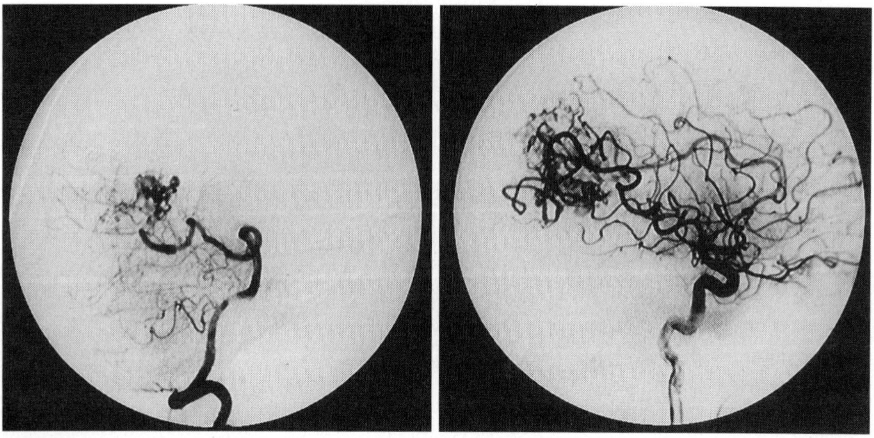

a b

Fig. 3a,b. After this two-step approach there is marked reduction of influx to the angioma and reduction of the size of the nidus (**a** lateral vertebral, **b** lateral left carotid) so that radiosurgery could be instituted in patient who had no neurological deficits

ocluded gradually. There was no thrombosis of the single main draining vein and the plexiform compartments could then be embolized with bucrylate in the next stage.

Discussion

In cerebral arteriovenous malformations with a combination of larger fistulous and plexiform elements, stepwise obliteration of the fistulas with larger particular substances, which is instituted first of all, is able to reduce the danger of bleeding throughout the neuroradiological interventional treatment. To diminish further risks which can be attributed to the abrupt change in hemodynamics after fistula closure, detachable balloon coils offer the possibility of closing the fistula more gradually so that surrounding blood vessels can adjust to the new flow situation. Although balloons can be positioned more exactly to the lesion site than coils, the detachment maneuver of coils is more secure. When there is a migration of a few coils which are too small, this does not lead to a thrombosis within draining veins.

Proliferation Rate in Meningiomas: Validity of Ki-67 and Proliferation-Associated Nuclear Antigen Labeling Indices

C. Lang[1], W. Hirschberger[1], and W. Schlote[1]

Introduction

In meningiomas the proliferation index determined with Ki-67 antibody is usually regarded as a reliable criterion of the biological behavior of this tumor entity, as far as it is based on cell proliferation activity. Since its first description by Gerdes et al. in 1983 [3], several studies on the proliferation rate of brain tumors have reported Ki-67 labeling indices (LI) of about 1% or even less than 1% in benign meningiomas, i.e., tumors without any atypical histological findings [2, 5, 8].

Recently, deviating results have been reported, leading to uncertainty as to Ki-67 LI and its value to predict proliferation potential of meningiomas [1].

In the present study, a series of meningiomas of various subtypes and hemangiopericytomas of meninges were investigated with regard to localization, clinical data, recurrences, and atypical histology to find an explanation for these discrepancies. Recently another monoclonal antibody raised against a proliferation-associated nuclear antigen (PCNA) has been developed [7], providing the possibility for labeling proliferating cells even in paraffin-embedded tissue. PCNA is known as an auxiliary protein for DNA polymerase δ which is correlated with the S phase of the cell cycle, whereas Ki-67 labels all phases of the cell cycle except G_0. Therefore, we compared Ki-67 and PCNA LIs in order to explore its role as another proliferation marker.

Material and Methods

A total of 47 meningiomas, including eight recurrent tumors from the meningothelial, fibroblastic, angioblastic, transitional, psammomatous, anaplastic type, and six hemangiopericytomas of the meninges were studied. Frozen sections of surgical biopsies of about 5–7 μm were incubated with Ki-67 monoclonal antibody (Dianova, Hamburg) and after undergoing a modified alkaline phosphatase anti-alkaline phosphatase technique (APAAP), the slides were slightly counterstained with Meyer's hemalum. Human tonsil was used, as positive control; negative controls were treated as above, but omitting the primary antibody. Using the avidin-biotin complex method, PCNA immunostaining (Dako, Denmark) was performed on corresponding areas in paraffin sections of ten meningiomas.

---

[1] Neurologisches Institut (Edinger-Institut), Universität Frankfurt, Deutschordenstr. 46, W-6000 Frankfurt/M. 71, FRG.

Advances in Neurosurgery, Vol. 21
R. Lorenz, M. Klinger, M. Brock (Eds.)

The percentage of Ki-67 or PCNA-positive cells, respectively, was determined with the aid of a semi-automated opto-manual microcomputer device (MOP-Videoplan, Kontron) equipped with a digitizer tablet. Depending on the distribution and density of the tumor cells, a total of at least 1200 cells was counted per tissue sample using an ocular grid defining an area of 0.08 mm^2 at magnification x 400; 15–20 fields of view were evaluated by an automatically guided zig-zag movement. The median and range of labeled cells of each tumor were documented.

Results

According to their site of origin three recurrent meningiomas out of 18 were located on the convexity, two of eight recurred in the middle fossa, and one of seven each in the posterior and anterior fossa, respectively. Ki-67 LI was below 1% in meningothelial, angioblastic, fibroblastic, and psammomatous meningiomas, even in three recurrent tumors. The transitional type revealed 1.41% positive cells, including two recurrences with LIs of 1.90% and 3.58% showing atypical histological features such as increased number of mitoses and polymorphism. In anaplastic meningiomas Ki-67 LI was 9.29%, representing a sharp separation between benign and anaplastic tumors. The distribution of proliferating cells in hemangiopericytomas was variable with a mean LI of 2.49%, whereby the youngest patient, a 29-year-old woman, showed a LI of 7.11% (Table 1).

In all meningiomas unexpectedly high values for PCNA labeling were observed compared to Ki-67 labeling (Fig. 1). Furthermore, the tumor cells revealed a higher variety in expression of the antigen which is reflected by a different PCNA staining pattern. This phenomenon renders the distinction of labeled from nonlabeled cells difficult. The PCNA LI ranged from 13.05% to 63.27% in benign tumors, and to 64.51% and 71.13%, respectively, in two anaplastic meningiomas (Fig. 2).

Discussion

Since current diagnostic criteria such as mitotic figures, polymorphism, or cellularity only allow a vague prediction of the proliferative potential of slowly growing

Table 1. Ki-67 labeling index in meningiomas

Histology	Number	Recurrence	Median (%)	Range (%)
Meningothelial	15	1	0.82	0.00–14.02
Angioblastic	2	–	0.85	0.00–5.00
Fibroblastic	10	1	0.62	0.00–5.36
Transitional	10	2	1.41	0.00–6.53
Psammomatous	5	–	0.93	0.00–35.94
Anaplastic	5	1	9.29	0.00–35.94
Hemangiopericytoma	6	2	2.49	0.00–13.22

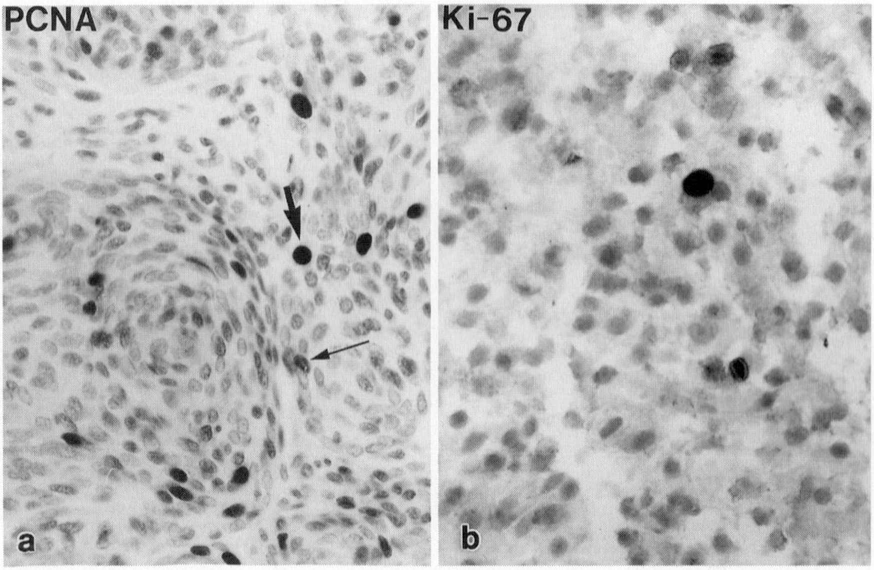

Fig. 1a. Meningothelial meningioma with PCNA immunostaining. Depending on the variability of staining pattern not only dark nuclei (*large arrow*), but also nuclei (*small arrow*) show posive reaction product. **b** Same tumor with Ki-67 labeling. The difference in cell size is caused by cryostate technique. x 500

meningiomas, Ki-67 LI has become a useful tool to define the biological malignancy more precisely. The findings above clearly show low Ki-67 LIs in benign meningiomas independently of the kind of subtype. Only the transitional type seems to reveal a tendency to slightly higher LIs. Furthermore, two transitional recurrent meningiomas had higher LIs than all the other benign recurrences. However, there is no overlapping of LIs between benign and anaplastic tumors, for the median amount of labeled cells was at least sixfold higher in malignant meningiomas. The discrepancies mentioned above either may be caused by different methods of evaluating LIs or may be based on atypical histological features, respectively. In hemangiopericytomas of the meninges, Ki-67 LIs correlate well with their different biological behavior compared to meningiomas with inconspicuous histology. Even though both tumor types are grade II according to the WHO classification, in hemangiopericytomas the frequency of recurrence is about 60%–70%, mitotic activity is often observed, and these tumors show an occasional tendency to occur in younger patients [4].

PCNA LIs were expected to be below Ki-67 LIs, in correlation with its accumulation during the S phase of the cell cycle. Bromodeoxyuridine (BrdU), another antibody identifying S-phase cells, displayed lower LIs than Ki-67 in meningiomas [6]. Thus, the over-expression of the PCNA antigen and the different gradation of immunoreactivity obviously seems not to be associated with malignancy. It might depend on the growth rate of each individual meningioma in consideration of the long biological half-life of PCNA. On the other hand, it may represent the au-

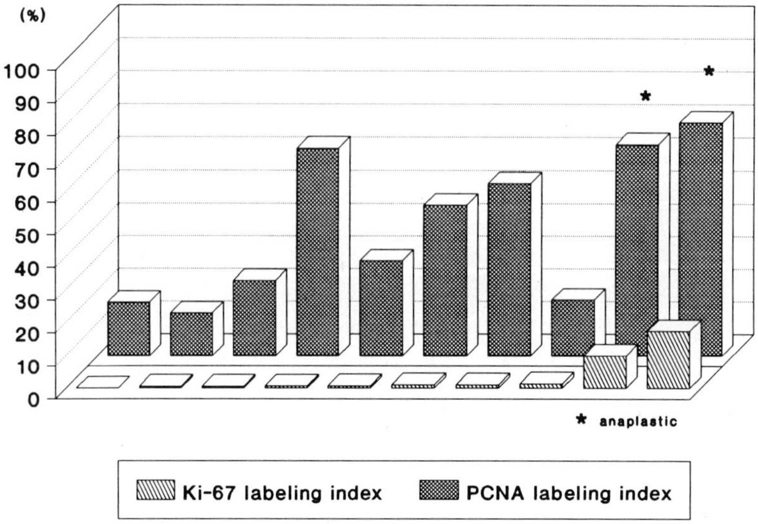

Fig. 2. Proliferation rate in meningiomas: comparison of Ki-67 and PCNA LIs

tocrine or paracrine growth factor influence on PCNA gene. In conclusion, the results seriously limit the use of anti-PCNA antibody in surgical neuropathology. Yet, as the present study implies, Ki-67 antibody still remains a confidential proliferation marker in meningiomas.

References

1. Braunsdorf WEK, Schmidt D, Mehdorn HM, Schulte HM (1991) Erste Untersuchungsergebnisse zum Proliferationsverhalten von Meningiomen mittels Ki-67 und der Geschlechtshormonrezeptorbestimmung. Neurooncological Meeting, Nov. 1–2, Kloster Banz
2. Burger PC, Shibata T, Kleihues P (1986) The use of the monoclonal antibody Ki-67 in the identification of proliferating cells: application to surgical neuropathology. Am J Surg Pathol 19:611–617
3. Gerdes J, Schwab U, Lemke H, Stein H (1983) Production of a mouse menoclonal antibody reactive with a human nuclear antigen associated with cell proliferation. Int J Cancer 31:13–20
4. Horten BC, Urich H, Rubinstein LJ, Montague SR (1977) The angioblastic meningioma: a reappraisal of a nosologic problem. Light-, electron-microscopic, tissue, and organ culture observations. J Neurol Sci 31:387–410
5. Möbius HJ, Lang C, Schlote W (1987) Zellproliferation in Meningeomen und Neurinomen: quantitative immunhistochemische Untersuchungen. Zentralbl Allg Pathol 133:5
6. Morimura T, Kitz K, Budka H (1989) In situ analysis of cell kinetics in human brain tumors. A comparative immunocytochemical study of S phase cells by a new in vitro bromodeoxyuridine-labeling technique, and of proliferating pool cell by monoclonal antibody Ki-67. Acta Neuropathol (Berl) 77:276–282
7. Ogata K, Kurki P, Celis JE, Nakamura RM, Tan EM (1987) Monoclonal antibodies to a nuclear protein (PCNA/cyclin) associated with DNA replication. Exp Cell Res 168:476–486
8. Roggendorf W, Schuster T, Peiffer J (1987) Proliferative potential of meningiomas determined with the monoclonal antibody Ki-67. Acta Neuropathol (Berl) 73:361–364

Winning Poster and Lecture Presentations

Effect of the 21-Aminosteroid U-74389F on Brain Edema Following a Cryogenic Lesion in Rats

G.-H. Schneider[1], A. Unterberg[1], and W. Lanksch[1]

Introduction

Brain edema is a major determinant of mortality and outcome after severe head injury [1, 7]. Since the clinical trials with steroids in head injury did not fulfill the hopes elicited by experimental studies, a rational treatment of posttraumatic brain swelling still remains to be found.

Acute cerebral insults, like head injury and ischemia, lead to the generation of free radicals – ionized oxygen particles that attack membranes and may cause blood-brain barrier dysfunction by peroxidation of membrane lipids [5, 11]. Lazaroids or 21-aminosteroids are a new class of steroids, amidated at the C21 position, with strong antiperoxidative characteristics [2]. Lazaroids have already been shown to attenuate neuronal damage and improve neurological outcome after experimental ischemia [6, 8].

The aim of this study was to determine whether brain edema induced by a cryogenic injury in the rat is attenuated by the aminosteroid U-74389F.

Materials and Methods

In 21 male Sprague-Dawley rats weighing 340 ± 5 g a cortical freezing lesion was applied to the right parietal region under ketamine-xylazine anesthesia [4]. Our standard lesion was made by a probe 5 mm in diameter which was cooled to –60 °C and lowered to the exposed dura for 30 s.

Ten rats were injected intraperitoneally with the aminosteroid U-74389F in three single doses 30 min before, 1 h and 12 h after trauma (total dosage: 3 mg/kg body weight, whereas the control group ($n = 11$) received the same amount of the vehicle (citric acid buffer, pH 3.0). Systemic blood pressure was monitored via a cannula in the femoral artery in the peritraumatic period.

The animals were sacrificed 24 h post trauma and the brains were quickly removed. The hemispheres were then separated and weighed for determination of brain swelling. Thereafter, they were dried for 48 h at 100 °C and weighed again. Cerebral water content was calculated as the difference between hemispheric wet and dry weight.

---

[1] Abteilung für Neurochirurgie, Universitätsklinikum Rudolf Virchow,
Freie Universität Berlin, Augustenburger Platz 1, W-1000 Berlin 65, FRG.

Advances in Neurosurgery, Vol. 21
R. Lorenz, M. Klinger, M. Brock (Eds.)

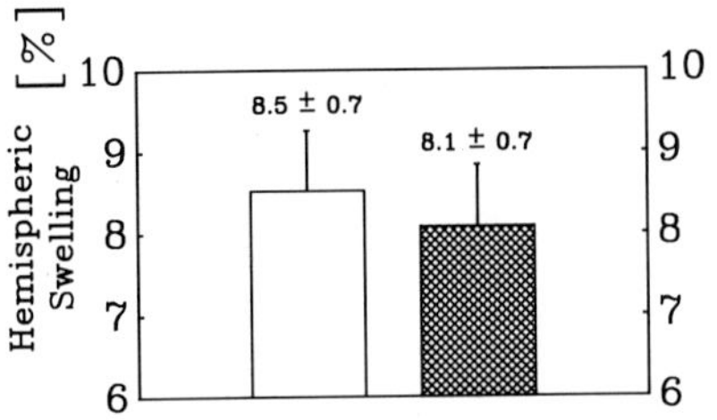

Fig. 1. Hemispheric swelling following a cryogenic lesion in rats treated with U-74389F (*shaded column*, $n = 10$), or citrate buffer (vehicle; *open column*, $n = 11$). Swelling is only slightly attenuated by the treatment with the 21-aminosteroid U-74389F

The study was conducted in blinded fashion in order to eliminate systematic errors.

Results

Treatment with the aminosteroid U-74389F attenuated brain swelling moderately (controls: 8.52% ± 0.74% vs. 8.08% ± 0.76% in treated animals, not significant; Fig. 1). Accordingly, the increase of cerebral water content due to the trauma was slightly reduced in the U-74389F-treated group (from 80.20% ± 0.13% to 79.98% ± 0.16%, not significant; Fig. 2). Water content of the nontraumatized hemispheres did not differ between vehicle and treatment group (control: 78.46% ± 0.15%, U-74389F: 78.58% ± 0.16%; Fig. 2).

Mean arterial blood pressure was comparable in both groups and did not change significantly in the peritraumatic period.

Discussion

As lipid peroxidation is one mechanism of edema generation in the cold injury model [9] and 21-aminosteroids were shown to have protective effects on the blood-brain barrier [3], lazaroids might be expected to influence brain swelling induced by a cryogenic lesion. Posttraumatic edema generation was, however, only marginally attenuated by the 21-aminosteroid U-74389F.

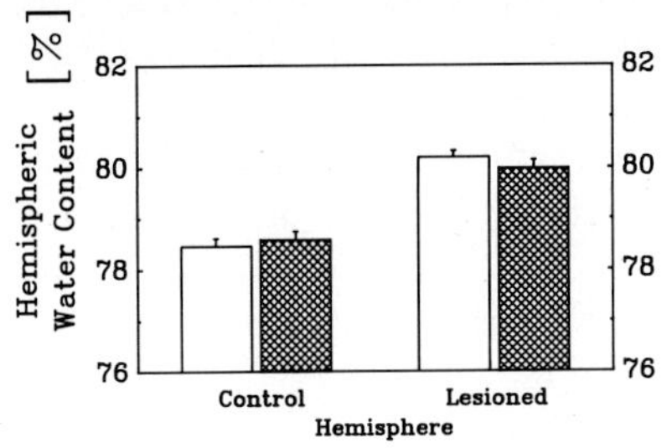

Fig. 2. Cerebral water content of treated (*shaded columns*, $n = 10$) and control (*open columns*, $n = 11$) rats in milliliters per 100 g fresh water. According to the small effect of U-74389F on posttraumatic brain swelling, there is only a marginal reduction in cerebral water content of the lesioned hemisphere, whereas the left control hemispheres of both groups do not differ in water content

The rather moderate effect of the lazaroid may be due to a minor role of free radicals in edema generation, which in fact is under debate [10], or due to insufficient free radical inhibition, i.e., insufficient lazaroid plasma concentrations. The next step is to test whether a higher dosage or intravenous administration to increase and prolong the plasma concentration of the substance will possibly enhance the beneficial effects of the lazaroid.

Acknowledgement. The excellent technical assistance of Ms. J. Kopetzki and S. Hennig is gratefully acknowledged.

References

1. Aldrich EF, Eisenberg HM, Saydjari C et al. (1992) Diffuse brain swelling in severely head-injured children. J Neurosurg 76:450–454
2. Braughler JM, Pregenzer JF, Chase RL et al. (1987) Novel 21-amino steroids as potent inhibitors of irondependent lipid peroxidation. J Biol Chem 262(22):10438–10440
3. Hall ED, Travis MA (1988) Inhibition of arachidonic acid-induced vasogenic brain edema by the nonglucocorticoid 21-aminosteroid U74006F. Brain Res 451:350–352
4. Klatzo I, Piraux A, Laskowski EJ (1958) The relationship between edema, blood-brain-barrier and tissue elements in local brain injury. J Neuropathol Exp Neurol 17:548–564
5. Kontos HA, Wei EP (1986) Superoxide production in experimental brain injury. J Neurosurg 64:803–807
6. Lesiuk H, Sutherland G, Peeling J et al. (1991) Effect of U74006F on forebrain ischemia in rats. Stroke 22:896–901
7. Marshall LF, Eisenberg HM, Jane JA et al. (1991) The outcome of severe closed head injury. J Neurosurg 75:S28–S36
8. Perkins WJ, Newberg Milde L, Milde J, Michenfelder JD (1991) Pretreatment with U74006F improves neurologic outcome following complete cerebral ischemia in dogs. Stroke 22:902–909
9. Suzuki O, Yagi K (1974) Formation of lipoperoxide in brain edema induced by cold injury. Experientia 30:248
10. Unterberg A, Wahl M, Baethmann A (1988) Effects of free radicals on permeability and vasomotor response of cerebral vessels. Acta Neuropathol (Berl) 76:238–244
11. Wahl M, Unterberg A, Baethmann A, Schilling L (1988) Mediator of blood-brain barrier dysfunction and formation of vasogenic brain edema. J Cereb Blood Flow Metab 8(5):621–634

Juxtamedullary Tumors of the Ventral, Thoracic, or Upper Lumbar Spine: A Posterolateral, Extracavital Operative Approach

S. Hussein[1], D. Woischneck[1], and H.G. Höllerhage[1]

Introduction

Juxtamedullary tumors of the ventral myelon are meningiomas or neurinomas in more than 50% of cases. Because of their benign histology, a total removal is recommended. On the other hand, owing to their slow development, extirpation may become difficult because of large tumor components in the retropleural or peritoneal space.

The ventral, transthoracic, or abdominal approach with corporectomy and final osteosynthesis has a higher operative risk. Furthermore, an optimal survey of the juxtamedullar space is difficult to achieve [2, 7]. On the other hand, costotransversectomy does not allow access to extraspinal and ventral parts of the tumor [1, 9]. We describe a modification of the costotransversectomy which allows us juxtamedullary removal of the tumor ventrally from the myelon as well as in the retropleural and peritoneal space.

Operative Procedure

The patient is positioned in the decubitus position (Fig. 1). The side of the tumor is turned upward, the patient's body is additionally rotated 45° away from the surgeon. The arm lying below is axillarily stuffed.

Skin incision is done 2 cm laterally of the midline, in a slightly curved line. For operations at the upper lumbal spine, we cut in the shape of a hockey stick. The m. erector trunci is separated from the processus spinosus subperiostally and held away by self-retaining retractors. If necessary, we cut parts of the muscle, which are readapted at the end of surgery. In the cervicothoracic area, parts of the m. trapezius, rhomboideus, or latissimus dorsi also have to be split.

We have to dissect several bony structures (Fig. 2): the vertebral arch with the lateral portion of the processus spinosus, the intervertebral joint, the processus transversus, and the rib up to its angle. The bony resection (hemilaminectomy, removal of the intervertebral joint, resection of the rib up to the angle) is done on one or more spinal levels as far as necessary. The ventral border of the access is marked by the parietal pleura or the retroperitoneum. The intercostal nerves can be

---

[1] Neurochirurgische Klinik, Medizinische Hochschule, Konstanty-Gutschow-Str. 8, W-3000 Hannover 61, FRG.

Advances in Neurosurgery, Vol. 21
R. Lorenz, M. Klinger, M. Brock (Eds.)

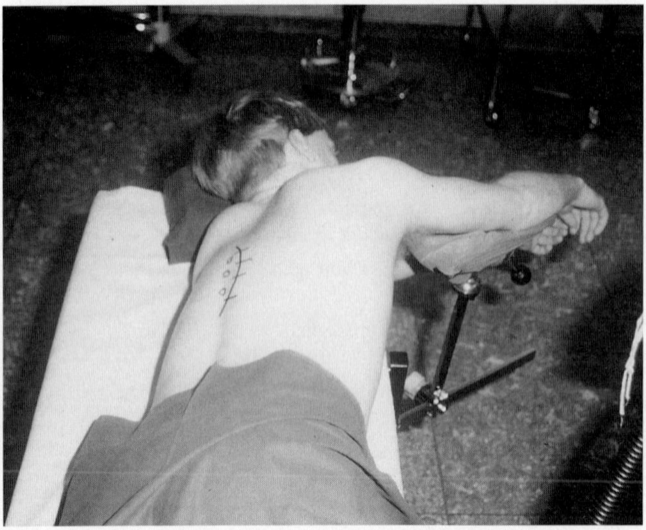

Fig. 1. Positioning of the patient: decubitus position, additional rotation 45° away from the surgeon

resected but, of course, we have to pay attention to the vascular supply of the myelon (a. radicularis magna).

If necessary, the lateral parts of the vertebral body can be removed. We can now incise the dura in a longitudinal direction between two adjacent nerve roots and remove the tumor. If necessary, the operation field can be enlarged transverse by further resection of the rib and the processus spinosus longitudinally by opening additional spinal levels. Tumor access is limited to one side; contralateral tumor components cannot be reached. After the tumor is removed, water-tight and dural closure is performed, the muscle and skin layers are closed in the usual manner.

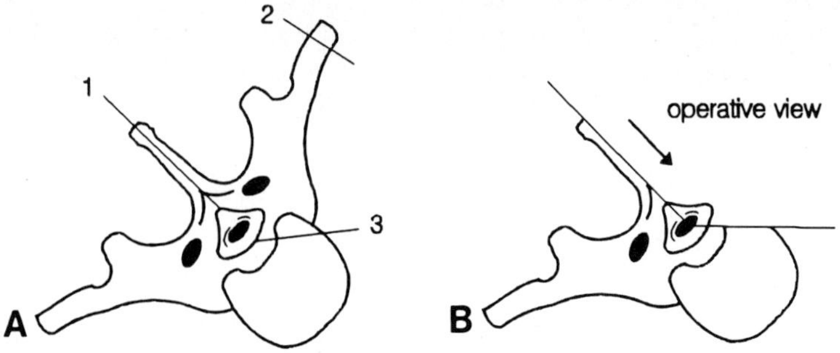

Fig. 2 A. Principles of the bony resection. *1*, Hemilaminectomy; *2*, resection of the rib (up to the angle) and the intervertebral joint; *3*, resection of the lateral parts of the vertebral body. **B** Operative view with parallel rotation of the microscope

Table 1. Summary of patients operated on

Patient no.	Sex	Age (year)	Diagnosis	Symptoms	Operative complications
1	♀	32	Meningioma Th9/10	Paraparesis, bladder dysfunction	None
2	♀	53	Meningioma Th6–8	Paraparesis bladder dysfunction	None
3	♀	48	Neurinoma Th12/L1	Radicular pain	Erosion of intercostal artery
4	♂	65	Meningioma Th1/2	Paraparesis, bladder dysfunction	None
5	♀	32	Meningioma Th11/12	Paraparesis, bladder dysfunction	None
6	♂	35	Myosarcoma Th6–8	Radicular pain	None

Operative Results

Up until now we have performed the operation on six patients (Table 1), four of them with a meningioma, one with a neurinoma. In one case, a myosarcoma could be confirmed. Four patients had a conus or cross-section syndrome which recovered after surgery. Neurological deficits due to the operation did not occur.

In one patient (no. 3 in Table 1), we noticed a wound hematoma because of an erosion of the intercostal artery 48 h after the operation. After local revision of the wound, the clinical course was without complications.

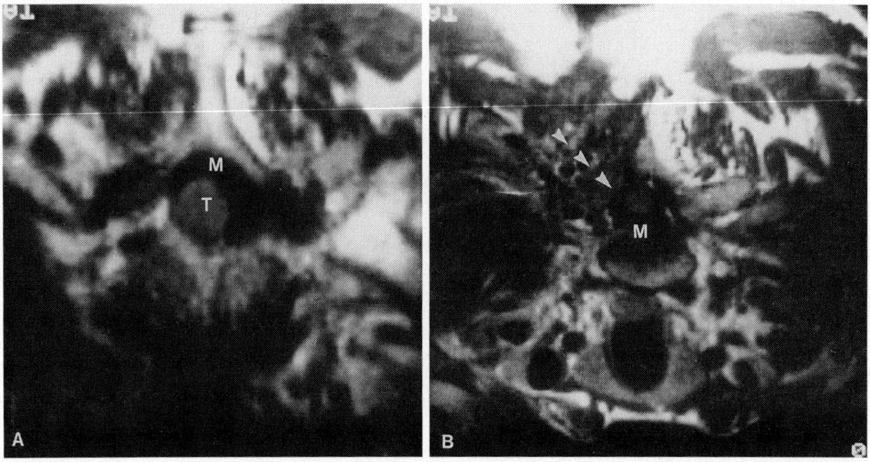

Fig. 3 A, B. Ventral-juxtamedullary meningioma Th 1 to Th 2 (patient no. 4 in Table 1) before (**A**) and after (**B**) surgery. *T*, tumor; *M*, myelon; *arrows*; operative approach

For five patients, the follow-up is now 6 months or longer: they are free of deficits; magnetic resonance gives no hints of a tumor recurrence. There are no signs of a postoperative instability of the spine. In Fig. 3 we show an example of a successful removal of a ventral juxtamedullary meningioma from Th1 to Th2 with large extraspinal components.

Discussion

The dorsal approach to ventral juxtamedullary tumors (hemilaminectomy, laminectomy) has been abandoned because of the resulting damage to the myelon. The alternative costotransversectomy, already described in 1894 [8, 9], became current again after introduction of microsurgical techniques and better preoperative radiological possibilities [6, 8, 9].

In 1954 Carpenter [3] described a modification with further bony resection pedicles, ventral parts of the vertebral body, which allowed better access laterally and ventrally from the myelon (lateral rachotomy). Brenzel [1] described an approach with resection of the intervertebral joint, the pedicle, and wider parts of the rib in order to reach dorsal parts of the vertebral body for fusion of vertebral fractures. Because of a different rotation of the patient, his modification does not allow sufficient access to the ventral juxtamedullar parts of the spinal canal. Extraspinal, retropleural, or peritoneal tumors also cannot be reached. In contrast, our modification allows a complete removal of juxtamedullar tumors of the thoracic and upper lumbar spine, especially ventral to the myelon and extraspinally. The essential points of this operation are, beside the extent of the bone resection, the correct positioning of the patient and operation microscope.

As often described [1, 6, 8], a typical complication of any kind of costotransversectomy is an erosion of the intercostal artery, which happened once in our patients. Additionally, based on the literature, we have to stress the possibility of a sealed pleura perforation. If necessary, a pleural drainage for 48 h postoperatively can easily be performed. Owing to the unilateral procedure [3, 5, 6], the costotransversectomy is believed to produce no spinal instability. Until now, 6 months after the operations, we have no signs suggesting such problems. Nevertheless, we cannot exclude such problems for the future on the basis of recent biomechanical studies [7].

References

1. Benzel EC (1989) The lateral extracavitary approach to the spine using the threequarter prone position. J Neurosurg 71:837–841
2. Benzel EC, Larson J (1986) Functional recovery after decompressive operation for thoracic and lumbal spine fractures. Neurosurgery 19:772–778
3. Capener N (1954) The evolution of lateral rachotomy. J Bone Joint Surg (Br) 36:173–179

4. Chiou SM, Laborde G, Seeger W (1989) Microsurgical unilateral approaches for spinal tumor surgery: eight years experience in 256 primary operated cases. Acta Neurochir (Wien) 100:127–133
5. Eggert HR, Scheremet R, Seeger W, Gaitzsch J (1983) Unilateral microsurgical approaches to extramedullary spinal tumors. Operative technique and results. Acta Neurochir (Wien) 67:245–253
6. Larson SJ, Holst RA, Hemmy DC (1976) Lateral extracavitary approach to traumatic lesions of the thoracic and lumbar spine. J Neurosurg 45:628–637
7. Panjabi MM, White AA (1980) Basic biomechanics of the spine. Neurosurgery 7(19):76–93
8. Rothmann RH, Simeone FA (1965) Surgical approaches to the thoracic spine. In: Rothmann RH, Simeone FA, Saunders WB (eds) The spine, vol 1. Raven, New York, pp 133–150
9. Seeger W (1982) Microsurgery of the spinal cord and surrounding structures. Anatomical and technical principles. Springer, Berlin Heidelberg New York

Activity of Ornithine Decarboxylase and Ki-67 Index in Meningiomas

R. I. Ernestus[1,2], R. Schröder[3], G. Röhn[1], N. Klug[2], K. A. Hossmann[1], and W. Paschen[1]

Introduction

Meningiomas usually are slowly growing brain tumors histologically classified as grade 1 according to the criteria of the World Health Organization (WHO) [26]. Nevertheless, some meningiomas tend to proliferate more rapidly, resulting in an increased incidence of local recurrences up to malignant meningiomatosis.

Biosynthesis of the polyamines putrescine, spermidine, and spermine is closely associated with cellular growth processes including neoplastic cell proliferation [1, 10, 12]. It has been shown that ornithine decarboxylase (ODC), the first key enzyme in polyamine metabolism, represents a biochemical marker of malignancy in brain tumors [6, 20]. Immunhistochemical labeling of a nuclear proliferation antigen by the monoclonal antibody Ki-67 is another established method for measuring the growth fraction in brain neoplasms [2–4, 9, 13–15, 18, 23–25].

We have therefore examined whether high ODC activity in combination with a high Ki-67 index in meningiomas indicates the "malignant potential" of a primarily benign brain tumor.

Material and Methods

Tissue samples of 33 meningiomas (27 primary and six recurrent tumors) were obtained during neurosurgery and, immediately after excision, frozen in liquid nitrogen. Histologically, all tumors were typical benign meningiomas WHO grade 1.

ODC activity was quantified in homogenized tissue samples by measuring the release of $^{14}CO_2$ from ^{14}C-ornithine [16]. For immunohistochemistry 11-µm thick cryostat sections were taken of each sample. Using the alkaline phosphatase anti-alkaline phosphatase method (APAAP), the percentage of Ki-67-positive cells was determined as a fraction of the total number of tumor cells [22].

---

[1] Max-Planck-Institut für Neurologische Forschung, Abteilung für Experimentelle Neurologie, Joseph-Stelzmann-Str. 9, W-5000 Köln 41, FRG.
[2] Klinik für Neurochirurgie der Universität Köln, Joseph-Stelzmann-Str. 9, W-5000 Köln 41, FRG.
[3] Institut für Pathologie, Labor für Neuropathologie, Universität Köln, Joseph-Stelzmann-Str. 9, W-5000 Köln 41, FRG.

Advances in Neurosurgery, Vol. 21
R. Lorenz, M. Klinger, M. Brock (Eds.)

Table 1. ODC activity and Ki-67 index in primary and recurrent meningiomas

	ODC activity (nmol/g per hour)		Ki-67 index (%)	
	Mean ± SD	Range	Mean ± SD	Range
Primary	4.2 ± 4.1	0.6–26.0	2.5 ± 2.5	0.3–10.4
Recurrent	7.6 ± 9.1	1.8–20.9	3.8 ± 3.6	0.8–9.9

Results

ODC Activity

Mean ODC activity was 4.2 ± 4.1 nmol/g per hour in primary and 7.6 ± 9.1 nmol/g per hour in recurrent meningiomas, respectively (Table 1). The high standard deviation of mean values reflects a wide variability of individual values. In fact, ODC activity ranged from 0.6 nmol/g per hour to 26.0 nmol/g per hour (Fig. 1). Recent investigations in gliomas suggested that values higher than 5 nmol/g per hour indicate malignancy (unpublished data). Thirteen out of the 33 meningiomas in the present series exceeded this limit, including four of the six recurrences. In three meningiomas ODC activity was even higher than 20 nmol/g per hour. We have so far observed such high values only in glioblastomas and medulloblastomas.

Ki-67 Index

Mean Ki-67 index was 2.5% ± 2.5% in primary and 3.8% ± 3.6% in recurrent meningiomas, respectively (Table 1). Similarly to ODC activity, single Ki-67 percentages widely varied in different tumors (Fig. 2). The rate of Ki-67 positive cells ranged from 0.3% to 10.4%. Previous studies of the growth fraction in meningiomas revealed mean values not exceeding 1.2% [2, 4, 11, 17, 19, 22]. Increased

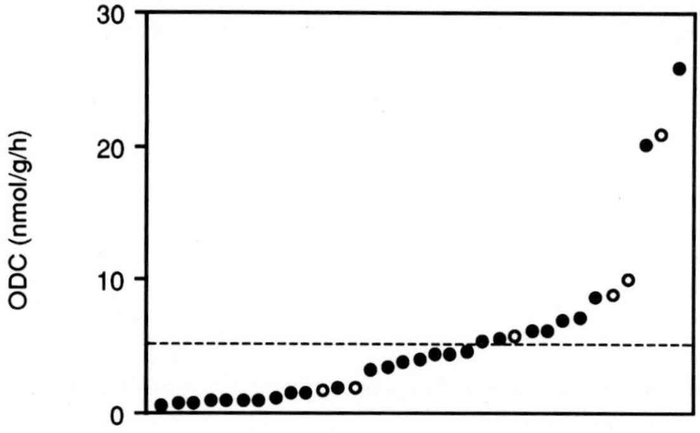

Fig. 1. ODC activity in meningiomas, single values arranged from lowest to highest activity. (*Solid circles*, primary tumors; *open circles*, recurrent tumors; *dotted line*, threshold of increased proliferation) see text

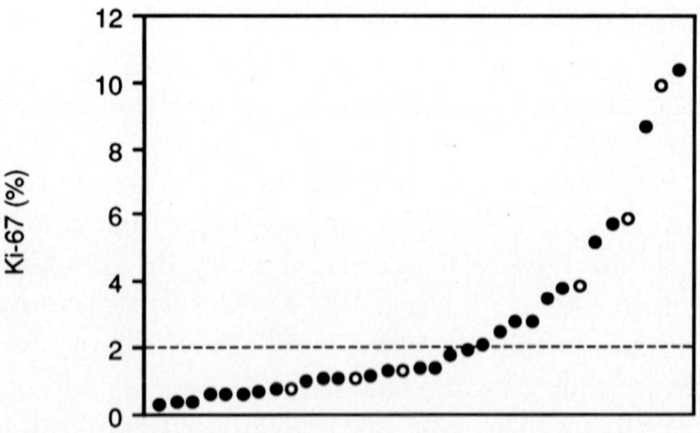

Fig. 2. Ki-67 index in meningiomas, single values arranged from lowest to highest index. (*Solid circles*, primary tumors; *open circles*, recurrent tumors; *dotted line* threshold of increased proliferation) see text

values higher than 2% were found in the present series in 13 out of all cases, including three of the six recurrent tumors. Three meningiomas had values even higher than 8%.

Correlation Between ODC Activity and Ki-67 Index

High ODC activity did not necessarily imply a high Ki-67 index, as expressed by the low correlation coefficient of $r = 0.33$ (Fig. 3). Coincidence of ODC activity higher than 5 nmol/g per hour and Ki-67 index more than 2% could be observed in seven meningiomas.

Discussion

The biochemical and immunohistochemical results of the present study underline the clinical observation of some biologically exceptional tumors within the group of benign meningiomas. None of the tumors investigated in the present series showed histological signs of anaplasia such as an increased number of mitoses, nuclear polymorphism, or others. Each tumor could be classified as a typical benign

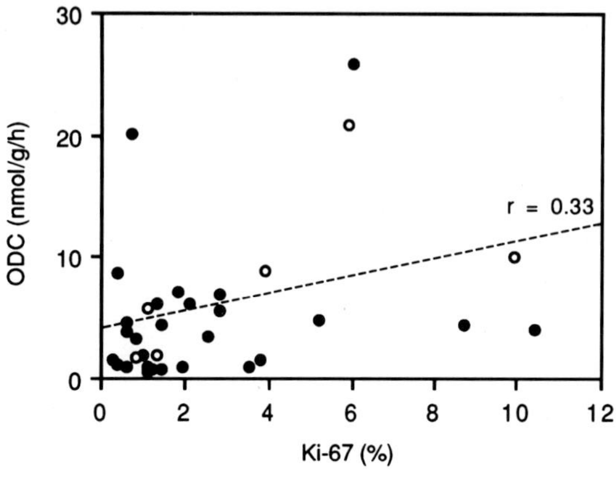

Fig. 3. Correlation between ODC activity and Ki-67 index in meningiomas. *Solid circles*, primary tumors; *open circles*, recurrent tumors

meningioma WHO grade 1. However, despite this histological homogeneity, tumors exhibited a large biochemical and immunohistochemical heterogeneity.

Both parameters investigated in the present series are assumed to reflect cellular proliferation. In experimental rat brain gliomas increased ODC activity is clearly restricted to the neoplasm and, thus, represents a marker of neoplastic growth [5]. It has been suggested that activation of ODC represents an early expression of malignancy [1]. Cell cycle studies revealed that ODC is induced during the G1 phase and is a mandatory event for cells to enter the S phase [20]. Ki-67 is a monoclonal antibody which reacts with a nuclear protein expressed in the G1, S, G2, and M phase of the cell cycle, thus indicating the growth fraction of brain tumors [7, 8].

Mean ODC activity and mean Ki-67 index were only slightly but not significantly higher in recurrent than in primary meningiomas. Thus, reports of higher Ki-67 rates in recurrent meningiomas by Roggendorf et al. [19] and Deckert et al. [4] could not be confirmed. Owing to the small number of recurrences, a correlation of Ki-67 index and the interval between primary and recurrent tumor could not be observed in the present series.

Previously determined thresholds of ODC activity and Ki-67 index were exceeded in more than one third of the meningiomas, but they did not allow a differentiation between primary and recurrent tumors. Thus, despite the substantial differences of values, no clear relationship to progressive tumor growth and consequently to malignant differentiation has been established so far. However, it cannot be excluded that the combination of both parameters might be useful for the early identification of the malignant potential of histologically benign meningiomas, but further prospective studies are required to evaluate the relationship with clinical prognosis.

Acknowledgments. This work was supported by the Deutsche Forschungsgemeinschaft, Grant Pa 266/3–2. The excellent technical assistance of Änne Pribliczki, Beate Joschko, Renate Kott, and Irmgard Meyers is gratefully acknowledged.

References

1. Bachrach U (1976) Polyamines as chemical markers of malignancy. Ital J Biochem 25:77–93
2. Böker DK, Stark HJ (1988) The proliferation rate of intracranial tumors as defined by the monoclonal antibody KI 67. Application of the method to paraffin embedded specimens. Neurosurg Rev 11:267–272
3. Burger PC, Shibata T, Kleihues P (1986) The use of the monoclonal antibody Ki-67 in the identification of proliferating cells: application to surgical neuropathology. Am J Surg Pathol 10:611–617
4. Deckert M, Reifenberger G, Wechsler W (1989) Determination of the proliferative potential of human brain tumors using the monoclonal antibody Ki-67. J Cancer Res Clin Oncol 115:179–188
5. Ernestus RI, Röhn G, Paschen W (1991) Polyamine metabolism in experimental brain tumors of rat. J Cereb Blood Flow Metab 11 Suppl 2:548
6. Ernestus RI, Röhn G, Schröder R, Klug N, Hossmann KA, Paschen W (1992) Activity of ornithine decarboxylase (ODC) and polyamine levels as biochemical markers of malignacy in brain tumors. Acta Histochem Suppl (Jena) 42:159–164

7. Gerdes J, Schwab U,. Lemke H, Stein H (1983) Production of a mouse monoclonal antibody reactive with a human nuclear antigen associated with cell proliferation. Int J Cancer 31:13–20
8. Gerdes J, Lemke H, Baisch H, Wacker H, Schwab U, Stein H (1984) Cell cycle analysis of a cell proliferation-associated human nuclear antigen defined by the monoclonal antibody Ki-67. J Immunol 31:1710–1715
9. Giangasparo F, Doglioni C, Rivano MT, Pileri S, Gerdes J, Stein H (1987) Growth fraction in human brain tumors defined by the monoclonal antibody Ki-67. Acta Neuropathol (Berl) 74:179–182
10. Horn Y, Beal SL, Walach N, Lubich WP, Spigel L, Marton LJ (1982) Further evidence for the use of polyamines as biochemical markers for malignant tumors. Cancer Res 42:3248–3251
11. Iwaki T, Takeshita I, Fukui M, Kitamaura K (1987) Cell kinetics of the malignant evolution of meningoendothelial meningioma. Acta Neuropathol (Berl) 74:243–247
12. Jänne J, Pösö H, Raina A (1978) Polyamines in rapid growth and cancer. Biochim Biophys Acta 473:241–293
13. Louis DN, Edgerton S, Thor AD, Hedley-Whyte ET (1991) Proliferating cell nuclear antigen and Ki-67 immunohistochemistry in brain tumors: a comparative study. Acta Neuropathol (Berl) 81:675–679
14. Morimura T, Kitz K, Stein H, Budka H (1991) Determination of proliferative activities in human brain tumor specimens: a comparison of three methods. J Neurooncol 10:1–11
15. Ostertag CB, Volk B, Shibata T, Burger P, Kleihues P (1987) The monoclonal antibody Ki-67 as a marker for proliferating cells in stereotactic biopsis of brain tumours. Acta Neurochir (Wien) 89:117–121
16. Paschen W, Röhn G, Meese CO, Djuricic B, Schmidt-Kastner R (1988) Polyamine metabolism in reversible cerebral ischemia. Effect of α-difluoromethylornithine. Brain Res 453:9–16
17. Patsouris E, Stocker U, Kallmeyer V, Keiditsch E, Mehraein P, Stavrou D (1988) Relationship between Ki-67 positive cells, growth rate and histological type of human intracranial tumors. Anticancer Res 8:537–544
18. Plate KH, Rüschoff J, Behnke J, Mennel HD (1990) Proliferative potential of human brain tumours as assessed by nucleolar organizer regions (AgNORs) and Ki-67-immunoreactivity. Acta Neurochir (Wien) 104:103–109
19. Roggendorf W, Schuster T, Pfeiffer J (1987) Proliferative potential of meningiomas determined with the monoclonal antibody Ki-67. Acta Neuropathol (Berl) 73:361–364
20. Russell DH, Haddox MK (1978) Cyclic AMP-mediated induction of ornithine decarboxylase in normal and neoplastic growth. Adv Enzyme Regul 17:61–79
21. Scalabrino G, Ferioli ME (1985) Degree of enhancement of polyamine biosynthetic decarboxylase activities in human tumors: a useful new index of degree of malignancy. Cancer Detect Prev 8:11–16
22. Schröder R, Bien K, Kott R, Meyers I, Vössing R (1991) The relationship between Ki-67 labelling and mitotic index in gliomas and meningiomas: demonstration of the variability of the intermitotic cycle time. Acta Neuropathol (Berl) 82:389–394
23. Shibata T, Burger PC, Kleihues P (1988) Ki-67 immunoperoxidase stain as a marker for the histological grading of nervous system tumours. Acta Neurochir Suppl (Wien) 43:103–106
24. Shibata T, Ostertag CB, Volk B (1989) Ki-67 PAP stain for histologic grading of brain tumors by squash preparations. No To Shinkei 41:55–60
25. Shiraishi T (1990) Cell kinetic analysis of brain tumors using the monoclonal antibody Ki-67: in vitro and in situ study. Acta Med Okayama 43:187–201
26. Zülch KJ (1986) Brain tumors. Their biology and pathology. 3rd edn. Springer, Berlin Heidelberg New York

Comparative Study of Monocyte-Mediated Cytotoxicity and Biological Response Modifier-Mediated Cytotoxicity Against Malignant Human Brain Tumor Cells In Vitro

G. Schackert[1], M. Kirsch[1], H. Fischer[2], H. K. Schackert[3], and S. Kunze[1]

Introduction

Monocytes/macrophages become tumoricidal subsequent to activation with biological response modifiers (BRMs), such as γ interferon (γ-IFN), β-IFN, and tumor necrosis factor α (TNF-α) [5, 7]. The killing mechanism of activated monocytes involves several factors: the secretion of TNF-α alpha and interleukin-1 (IL-1), oxygen metabolites, and lysosomal enzymes (1, 13). Activated monocytes have the property of recognizing tumor cells. They do not destroy normal cells [6, 7].

During recent years, BRMs such as β-IFN of TNF-α have been applied as soluble drugs in treatment strategies against brain tumors [9, 10, 19]. However, the results have been disappointing. Since we use the same BRMs for monocyte activation our investigation was done to compare directly the efficacy of BRM-mediated cytotoxicity with monocyte-mediated cytotoxicity against malignant brain tumor cells in vitro. Also, the central role of TNF-α in the monocyte-mediated killing mechanism is discussed.

Material and Methods

Tumor Cell Lines. Three human glioblastoma cell lines (He Ro, T739, T829) and the brain metastasis of a bronchial adenocarcinoma (T1020) were used [8]. All tumor cell lines were maintained as monolayer cultures on plastic in Eagle's basal medium (BME) supplemented with 10% fetal calf serum (FCS), sodium bicarbonate, essential amino acids, *l*-glutamine, vitamins, HEPES, and penicillin/streptomycin (Biochrom, Berlin, FRG). Cell cultures were incubated in 5% CO_2 – 95% air at 37 °C. All cultures were free of mycoplasms.

In Vitro Labeling of Human Tumor Cells. Target cells in their exponential growth phase were incubated in supplemented BME containing 0.5 μCi/ml [^{3}H] methyl thymidine (TdR, Amersham, Brunswick, FRG, specific activity 25 Ci/μmol).

[1] Neurochirurgische Klinik, Universität Heidelberg, Im Neuenheimer Feld 400, W-6900 Heidelberg, FRG.
[2] Deutsches Krebsforschungszentrum, Im Neuenheimer Feld 280, W-6900 Heidelberg, FRG.
[3] Zentrum für Chirurgie, Universität Heidelberg, Im Neuenheimer Feld 110, W-6900 Heidelberg, FRG.

Advances in Neurosurgery, Vol. 21
R. Lorenz, M. Klinger, M. Brock (Eds.)

Twenty-four hours later the cell monolayers were rinsed twice to remove non-bound [^{3}H]TdR. The cells were then incubated for another 2 h in BME, washed twice, stored on ice to extract soluble DNA precursors, and washed again. The cells were harvested by short-term trypsination (0.05% trypsin/0.2% EDTA, Biochrom, Berlin, FRG), washed three times, resuspended in endotoxin-free RPMI1640 medium (Gibco, Eggenstein, FRG) – measured by *Limulus* amebocyte assay (Pyroquant, Walldorf, FRG, sensitivity = 0.06 ng/ml) – supplemented with FCS, 15 mg gentamycin, 10 ml nonessential amino acids, and 27 ml 7.5% $NaHCO_3$, 15 ml HEPES (Gibco, Eggenstein, FRG), 20 ml vitamins, and 10 ml *l*-glutamine, and plated into 96-well plates containing the activated monocytes to obtain an initial effector-to-target cell ratio of 20:1. Triplicates of radiolabeled cells plated alone served as controls. All reagents were free of endotoxin, as measured by *Limulus* amebocyte assay (sensitivity < 0.12 ng/ml).

Isolation and Culture of Human Peripheral Blood Monocytes. Monocytes were isolated from healthy donors by Ficoll (specific gravity $d = 1.077$ g/ml) and 54% Percoll ($d = 1.068$ g/ml) gradient separation. The enriched monocyte population was suspended in RPMI1640 supplemented with 5% human AB serum and adjusted to a final concentration of 10^6 monocytes/ml, as determined by morphology, hemacolor differential blood analysis, and peroxidase staining.

Two x 10^5 monocytes were added to each 38-mm^2 well of a 96-well flat-bottomed Microtest III plate (Falcon, Becton Dickinson, Heidelberg, FRG). After allowing the monocytes to adhere for 2 h at 37 °C, the nonadherent cells were removed by washing the plates three times with warm (37 °C) RPMI1640 medium. At this point, the purity of the monocyte monolayer was > 97%.

In Vitro Activation of Human Monocytes and Monocyte-Mediated Cytoxicity Assay. Purified monocytes were incubated at 37 °C in 200 μl RPMI or RPMI with different combinations of BRMs: γ-IFN, β-IFN, and TNF. Twenty-four hours later, the monocytes were thoroughly washed three times with medium and the radiolabeled target cells were added. After 24 h the cultures were washed, refed with fresh medium, and incubated for an additional 48 h. Seventy-two hours after the addition of target cells the cultures were washed three times with phosphate-buffered saline (PBS), and the adherent viable cells were lysed with 0.2 ml 0.1 *N* NaOH. One hundred-microliter samples were added to 2 ml scintillation fluid (Aquasafe 300, Zinsser Analytic, Frankfurt, FRG) and the radioactivity of the lysate was monitored in a Wallac 1410 liquid scintillation counter. The cytotoxic activity of the monocytes was calculated as follows:

% Cytotoxicity = 100 times ([cpm with control monocytes] – [cpm with activated monocytes])/[cpm with control monocytes].

All data are based on triplicate measurements.

In Vitro Cytotoxicity Mediated by Soluble BRMs. Target cells were labeled with [^{3}H]methylthymidine (0.5 μCi/ml) and plated into a 96-well plate as described above. The cells were allowed to adhere for 2 h. Then various concentrations of

BRMs were added. Seventy-two hours later the cultures were washed three times with PBS, and the adherent viable cells were lysed with 0.2 ml 0.1 *N* NaOH. The radioactivity of the lysate was measured in a beta counter (Wallac 1410 liquid scintillation counter), and the cytotoxic activity of the BRMs was calculated as follows:

% Cytotoxicity = 100 times ([cpm target cells alone] – [cpm target cells cultured with medium containing BRM])/[cpm target cells alone].

Cytotoxicity Assay of Monocyte-Mediated Killing and Blocking with Anti-TNF-α Antibody. Using different BRMs, monocytes were activated as described above. Twenty-four hours later the radiolabeled tumor cells were added in an effector-to-target cell ratio of 20:1. At the same time, rabbit anti-recombinant human (rh)TNF-α antibody was added (dilution 1:100). The anti-TNF-α antibody was a gift from Dr. D. Männel, German Cancer Research Center, Heidelberg (final dilution to neutralize 10 ng rhTNF in L929 bioassay 1:10000). Seventy-two hours later the tumor cells were washed four times. The tumor cells were lysed by 0.1 *N* NaOH and the radioactivity measured in a beta counter.

Statistical Analysis. Experimental results from three independent assays of triplicate measurements were analyzed for their statistical significance by the two-tailed Student's *t* test.

Results

We compared the direct cytotoxic effect of BRMs on two human glioblastoma cells (T739, T829) with monocyte-mediated cytotoxicity (Fig. 1). The following BRMs were tested as single agents and in combination: γ-IFN, β-IFN, and TNF-α All BRMs were used in a concentration of 1000 U/ml. Spontaneous cytotoxicity was under 5%. The highest cytotoxicity rates mediated by soluble BRMs were achieved by use of combined treatment with γ-IFN + β-IFN for the T739 cell line (26%). TNF was cytotoxic in only 6%. The T829 glioblastoma cell line had only a very low response to TNF-α + γ-IFN (10% cytotoxicity) and was resistant to all other BRMs.

Subsequent to stimulation of monocytes with the same BRMs all cytotoxicity rates were significantly higher than those achieved with BRMs alone. Monocyte stimulation with TNF alone was very effective against T739 (51%) and T829 (73%). In addition, high cytotoxicity rates were obtained against T739 by stimulation with γ-IFN + TNF-α (58%) and γ-IFN + β-IFN (58%) and against T829 with TNF-α + γ-IFN (71%) and γ-IFN + β-IFN (63%). It was evident that monocyte-mediated cytotoxicity was two- to sixfold more effective than BRM-mediated cytotoxicity. Even the T829 cell line, which was resistant to almost all BRMs tested, responded well to monocyte-mediated cytotoxicity.

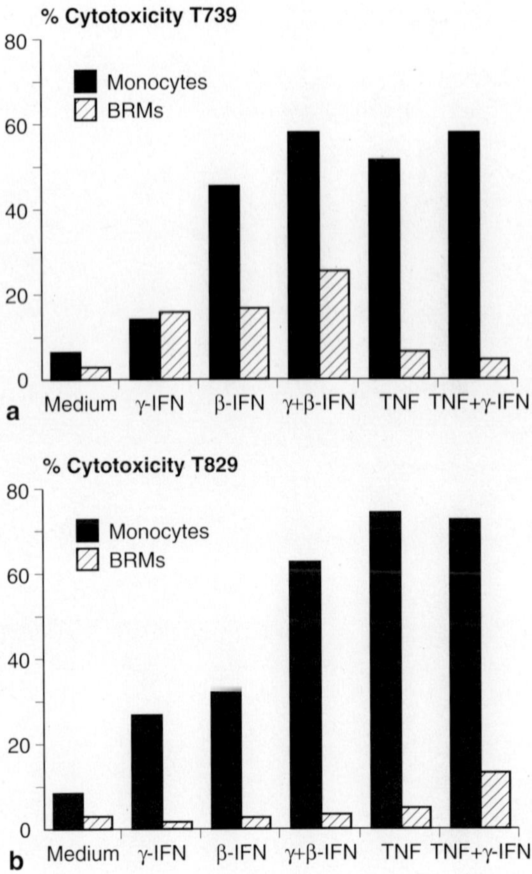

Fig. 1a,b. Cytotoxicity of glioblastoma cells T739 and T829 mediated by soluble BRMs compared to monocyte-mediated cytotoxicity (MTC) of activated monocytes. Monocytes were incubated for 24 h using the same concentrations of BRMs as for BRM-mediated cytotoxicity. The monocytes were washed three times and then incubated with target cells for 72 h. The effector to target ratio was 20:1 for MTC. Results represent means of three independent assays of triplicate measurements

Blockage of Monocyte-Mediated Cytotoxicity by Anti-TNF-α Antibody. One of the mechanisms of monocyte-mediated cytotoxicity is the secretion of TNF-α In the next set of experiments monocyte-mediated cytotoxicity was blocked by means of anti-TNF-α antibody. Three cell lines were tested: the two glioblastomas T739 and HeRo and the brain metastasis T1020 (Fig. 2). Monocytes were stimulated with different combinations of BRMs, as described above. Anti-TNF-α antibody down-regulated monocyte-mediated cytotoxicity subsequent to stimulation with TNF for T739 and HeRo glioblastoma cells. Also, after stimulation with γ-IFN + β-IFN and γ-IFN + TNF-α a partial blockage of the cytotoxic effect was noted. Both cell lines responded well to TNF-α-mediated monocyte killing (T739, 51%; HeRo, 75%), whereas even 10000 U/ml soluble TNF-α was not effective against T739 cells (13%) and lysed only 35% of HeRo glioblastoma cells (Fig. 3A,B). However, monocyte-mediated lysis of T1020 adenocarcinoma cells was generally not affected by anti-TNF-α antibody (Fig. 2C). Interestingly, this cell line did not demonstrate different susceptibility towards direct TNF or TNF-activated monocytes (Fig. 3 C). The cytotoxicity rated averaged below 30%.

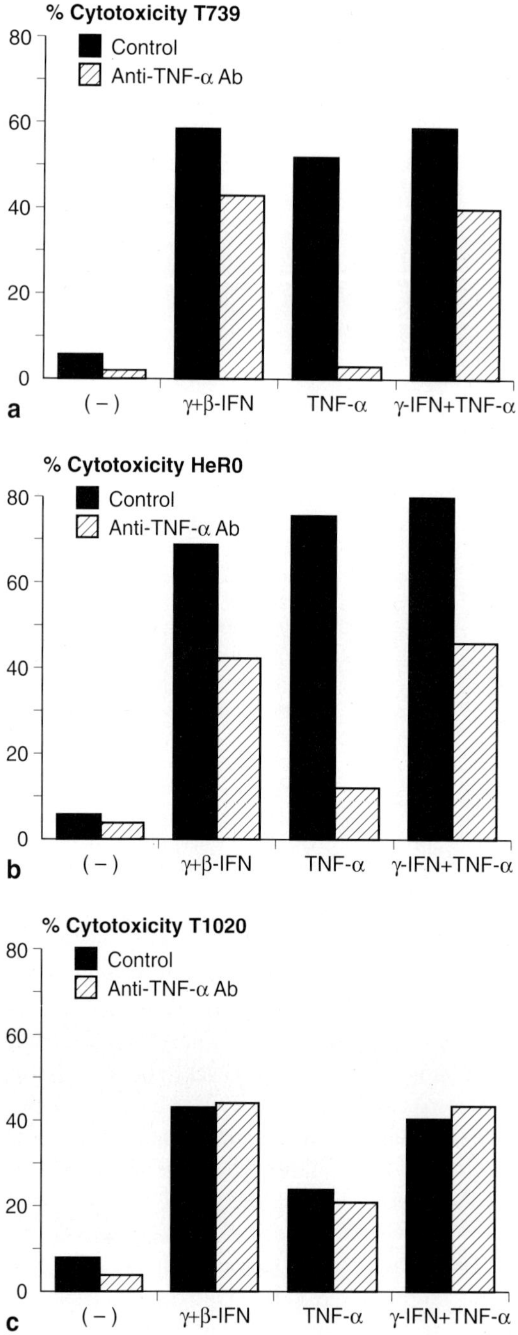

Fig. 2a–c. Influence of TNF-α antibody (dilution 1:100, final dilution to neutralize 10 ng rhTNF-α in L929 bioassay 1:1000) on monocyte-mediated cytotoxicity versus T739 and HeRo glioblastoma cells and T1020 brain metastasis cells. Prior to addition of target cells and TNF-α antibody, monocytes were activated for 24 h with different BRMs in a concentration of 1000 U/ml. Standard deviation did not exceed 10%

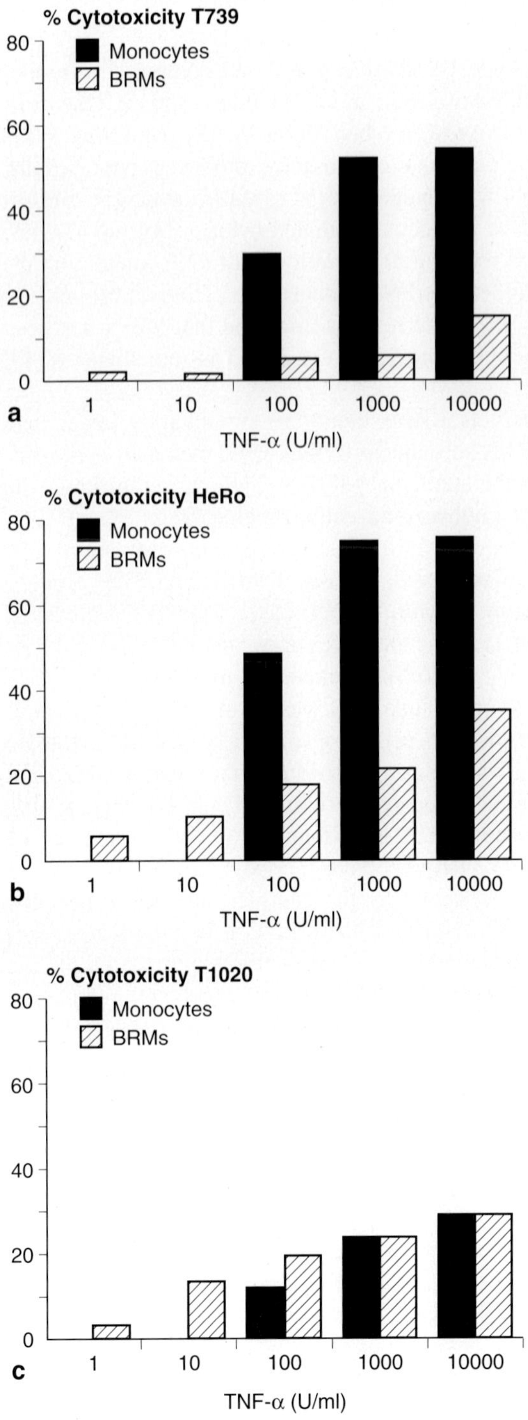

Fig. 3 a–c. TNF-α mediated cytotoxicity of 10^4 tumor cells after incubation for 72 h with various concentrations of TNF-α. These data are compared with monocyte-mediated tumor cytotoxicity (MTC). Monocytes were activated with the same concentrations of TNF-α for 24 h. Cocultivation lasted 72 h. The effector to target ratio was 20:1. Results represent mean of three independent assays of triplicate measurements

Discussion

The direct cytotoxic effect of soluble BRMs was tested and compared to monocyte-mediated lysis. γ-IFN is a central molecule in the immune response. One of its major properties involves an interaction with other BRMs [4, 12, 16]. Using γ-IFN as the only activator, monocyte-mediated cytotoxicity produces poor results, whereas the combination of γ-IFN with another BRM reveals a synergistic effect [16]. In our experiments the highest monocyte-mediated cytotoxicity (up to 73%) against glioblastoma cell lines was found after activation with TNF-α and with the combination of TNF-α + γ-IFN (71%). γ-IFN enhanced the cytotoxic property of monocytes in all combinations. One of the reasons might be that γ-IFN has been reported to stimulate the production of both TNF-α and IL-1 in macrophages [11, 12].

The cytotoxicity rates with soluble BRMs alone are significantly lower than those achieved with the same BRMs subsequent to monocyte-mediated cytotoxicity. Soluble γ-IFN β-IFN in combination, or γ-IFN + TNF-α, demonstrate the highest cytotoxicity rates against glioblastoma cells, ranging from 2% to 30%. Again, γ-IFN enhanced the cytotoxicity rate. It has been shown that tumor cells which are growth-inhibited by the synergistic action of γ-IFN and TNF produce more TNF receptors after treatment with γ-IFN [18]. The BRM-mediated cytotoxicity rates are halved and in some instances they are up to sixfold less effective than those achieved with monocyte-mediated cytotoxicity. The T829 glioblastoma cell line, for example, responded only weakly to TNF-α and was resistant to all other BRMs. Subsequent to activation of monocytes the cytotoxic response was about 60%–65%. These results demonstrate that human malignant brain tumors respond to monocyte-mediated cytotoxicity and that monocyte killing is significantly more effective in tumor cell lysis than the direct cytotoxicity of BRMs. The different susceptibility of target cells to monocyte-mediated lysis and soluble BRM cytotoxicity can be explained by the complex interaction between activated monocytes and tumor cells. Not only the secretion of monokines, e.g., TNF-α, IL-1, which are locally concentrated, but also the monocyte binding to the tumor cell play important roles; these are followed by target cell membrane destabilization, vacuolization, and lysosomal hydrolytic enzyme transfer [2].

TNF-α is an important cytokine in monocyte-mediated cytotoxicity [15]. By means of anti-TNF-α antibody we tried to evaluate the effect of the secreted cytokine by neutralizing the endogenous secretion. Our data demonstrate that the mechanism of monocyte-mediated killing is influenced by specific interactions between tumor cells and monocytes. The T1020 brain metastasis was a fair responder to TNF-mediated killing. Subsequent to activation of monocytes with TNF alone the cytotoxicity could not be enhanced. Anti-TNF-α antibody did not suppress monocyte-mediated killing. Conversely, the T739 glioblastoma cell line was almost resistant to soluble TNF. Subsequent to monocyte-mediated stimulation with TNF alone or in combination, a cytotoxicity rate of about 60% was achieved. Anti-TNF-α antibody significantly blocked the cytotoxic effect. The interaction between the tumor cell and the activated monocyte initiates a complex reaction, which is obviously different with respect to different tumor cell lines and various BRMs. TNF-α seems to play a central role in monocyte-mediated tumor cell killing [15]. Beside the secretion of endogenous TNF [15] and an exogenous carry-over phenomenon [14], the initiation of other killing mechanisms must be considered, as mentioned above [2].

Monocyte activation represents a new concept in treatment of malignant brain tumors. First investigations of monocyte function in brain tumor patients under steroid therapy demonstrate intact functional activity of the monocytes [3]. Treatment strategies in patients could involve systemic activation with BRMs encapsulated in liposomes or an adoptive immunotransfer in situ.

References

1. Adams DO, Hamilton TA (1984) The cell biology of macrophage activation. Annu Rev Immunol 2:283–318
2. Bakouche O, Ichinose Y, Heicappell R, Fidler IJ, Lackman LB (1988) Plasma membrane-associated tumor necrosis-factor. A non-integral membrane protein possibly bound to its own receptor. J Immunol 140:1142–1147
3. Barna BP, Rogers LR, Thomassen MJ, Barnett GH, Estes ML (1991) Monocuye tumoricidal activity and tumor necrosis factor production in patients with malignant brain tumors. Cancer Immunol Immunother. 33:314–318
4. Chen L, Suzuki Y, Wheelock EF (1987) Interferon-gamma synergizes with tumor necrosis factor and with interleukin 1 and requires the presence of both monokines to induce antitumor cytotoxic activity in macrophages. J Immunol 139:4096–44101
5. Cohn Z (1987) The activation of mononuclear phagocytes: fact, fancy, future. J Immunol 121:813–861
6. Fidler IJ, Kleinerman ES (1984) Lymphokine-activated human blood monocytes destroy tumor cells but not normal cells under cocultivation conditions. J Clin Oncol 2:937–943
7. Fidler IJ, Schroit AJ (1988) Recognition and destruction of neoplastic cells by activated macrophages: discrimination of altered self. Biochim Biophys Acta 948:151–173
8. Fischer H, Zeller WJ, Schwechheimer K, Hutter KJ, Wowra B, Kunze S, Sturm V (1989) Establishment and characterization of human glioblastoma cell lines in vitro and their xenografts in nude mice. Onkologie 12:169–174
9. Foon KA (1989) Biological response modifiers: the new immunotherapy. Cancer Res 49:1621–1639
10. Gillespie GY, Mahaley MS Biological response modifier therapie for patients with malignant gliomas. In: Thomas DGT (eds) Neuro-oncology – primary malignant brain tumours. Arnold, London, pp 242–282
11. Hori K, Ehrke MJ, Mace K, Mihich E (1987) Effect of recombinant tumor necrosis factor on tumoricidal activation of murine macrophages: synergism between tumor necrosis factor and gamma-interferon. Cancer Res. 47:5868–5874
12. Kildahl-Andersen O, Espevik T, Nissen-Meyer J (1985) Gamma interferon induced production of monocyte cytotoxic factor. Cell Immunol 95:392
13. Nathan CF (1987) Secretory products of macrophages. J Clin Invest 79:319–326
14. Nii A, Fidler IJ The incubation of human blood monocytes with tumor necrosis factor-alpha leads to lysis of tumor necrosis factor sensitive but not resistant tumor cells. Lymphokine Res 9:113–124
15. Philip R, Epstein LB (1986) Tumour necrosis factor as immunomodulator and mediator of monocyte cytotoxicity induced by itself, gamma-interferon and interleukin-1. Nature 323:86–89

16. Saiki I, Fidler IJ (1985) Synergistic activation by recombinant mouse interferon-gamma and muramyl-dipeptide of tumoricidal properties in mouse macrophages. J Immunol 135:684–688
17. Smith DM, Lackides GA, Epstein LB (1990) Coordinated induction of autocrine tumor necrosis factor and interleukin 1 in normal human monocytes and the implications for monocyte-mediated cytotoxicity. Cancer Res 50:3146–3153
18. Tsujimoto M, Yip YK, Vilcek J (1986) Gamma interferon enhances expression of cellular receptors for tumor necrosis factor. J Immunol 136:2441
19. Yung, WKA, Steck PA, Kelleher PJ, Moser RP, Rosenblum MG (1987) Growth inhibitory effect of recombinant alpha and beta interferon on human glioma cells. 5:323–330, 1987

Subject Index

Springer-Verlag and the Environment

We at Springer-Verlag firmly believe that an international science publisher has a special obligation to the environment, and our corporate policies consistently reflect this conviction.

We also expect our business partners – paper mills, printers, packaging manufacturers, etc. – to commit themselves to using environmentally friendly materials and production processes.

The paper in this book is made from low- or no-chlorine pulp and is acid free, in conformance with international standards for paper permanency.

Printing: Mercedesdruck, Berlin
Binding: Buchbinderei Lüderitz & Bauer, Berlin